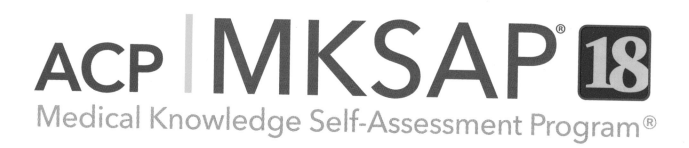

ACP | MKSAP® 18
Medical Knowledge Self-Assessment Program®

Hematology and Oncology

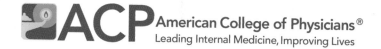

ACP American College of Physicians®
Leading Internal Medicine, Improving Lives

Welcome to the Hematology and Oncology Section of MKSAP 18!

In these pages, you will find updated information on hematopoietic stem cell disorders, multiple myeloma, bleeding disorders, hematologic issues in pregnancy, and other hematologic topics. Also addressed are issues in oncology; breast, ovarian, and cervical cancers; gastroenterologic malignancies; lung cancer; lymphoid malignancies; melanoma; the effects of cancer therapy and survivorship; and other topics in oncology. All of these topics are uniquely focused on the needs of generalists and subspecialists *outside* of hematology and oncology.

The core content of MKSAP 18 has been developed as in previous editions—all essential information that is newly researched and written in 11 topic areas of internal medicine—created by dozens of leading generalists and subspecialists and guided by certification and recertification requirements, emerging knowledge in the field, and user feedback. MKSAP 18 also contains 1200 all-new peer-reviewed, psychometrically validated, multiple-choice questions (MCQs) for self-assessment and study, including 149 in Hematology and Oncology. MKSAP 18 continues to include *High Value Care* (HVC) recommendations, based on the concept of balancing clinical benefit with costs and harms, with associated MCQs illustrating these principles and HVC Key Points called out in the text. Internists practicing in the hospital setting can easily find comprehensive *Hospitalist-*focused content and MCQs, specially designated in blue and with the 🇭 symbol.

If you purchased MKSAP 18 Complete, you also have access to MKSAP 18 Digital, with additional tools allowing you to customize your learning experience. MKSAP Digital includes regular text updates with new, practice-changing information, 200 new self-assessment questions, and enhanced custom-quiz options. MKSAP Complete also includes more than 1200 electronic, adaptive learning–enhanced flashcards for quick review of important concepts, as well as an updated and enhanced version of Virtual Dx, MKSAP's image-based self-assessment tool. As before, MKSAP 18 Digital is optimized for use on your mobile devices, with iOS- and Android-based apps allowing you to sync between your apps and online account and submit for CME credits and MOC points online.

Please visit us at the MKSAP Resource Site (mksap.acponline.org) to find out how we can help you study, earn CME credit and MOC points, and stay up to date.

On behalf of the many internists who have offered their time and expertise to create the content for MKSAP 18 and the editorial staff who work to bring this material to you in the best possible way, we are honored that you have chosen to use MKSAP 18 and appreciate any feedback about the program you may have. Please feel free to send any comments to mksap_editors@acponline.org.

Sincerely,

Patrick Alguire

Patrick C. Alguire, MD, FACP
Editor-in-Chief
Senior Vice President Emeritus
Medical Education Division
American College of Physicians

Hematology and Oncology

Acknowledgments

The American College of Physicians (ACP) gratefully acknowledges the special contributions to the development and production of the 18th edition of the Medical Knowledge Self-Assessment Program® (MKSAP® 18) made by the following people:

Graphic Design: Barry Moshinski (Director, Graphic Services), Michael Ripca (Graphics Technical Administrator), and Jennifer Gropper (Graphic Designer).

Production/Systems: Dan Hoffmann (Director, Information Technology), Scott Hurd (Manager, Content Systems), Neil Kohl (Senior Architect), and Chris Patterson (Senior Architect).

MKSAP 18 Digital: Under the direction of Steven Spadt (Senior Vice President, Technology), the digital version of MKSAP 18 was developed within the ACP's Digital Products and Services Department, led by Brian Sweigard (Director, Digital Products and Services). Other members of the team included Dan Barron (Senior Web Application Developer/Architect), Chris Forrest (Senior Software Developer/Design Lead), Kathleen Hoover (Senior Web Developer), Kara Regis (Manager, User Interface Design and Development), Brad Lord (Senior Web Application Developer), and John McKnight (Senior Web Developer).

The College also wishes to acknowledge that many other persons, too numerous to mention, have contributed to the production of this program. Without their dedicated efforts, this program would not have been possible.

MKSAP Resource Site (mksap.acponline.org)

The MKSAP Resource Site (mksap.acponline.org) is a continually updated site that provides links to MKSAP 18 online answer sheets for print subscribers; access to MKSAP 18 Digital; Board Basics® e-book access instructions; information on Continuing Medical Education (CME), Maintenance of Certification (MOC), and international Continuing Professional Development (CPD) and MOC; errata; and other new information.

International MOC/CPD

For information and instructions on submission of international MOC/CPD, please go to the MKSAP Resource Site (mksap.acponline.org).

Continuing Medical Education

The American College of Physicians is accredited by the Accreditation Council for Continuing Medical Education (ACCME) to provide continuing medical education for physicians.

The American College of Physicians designates this enduring material, MKSAP 18, for a maximum of 275 *AMA PRA Category 1 Credits*™. Physicians should claim only the credit commensurate with the extent of their participation in the activity.

Up to 33 *AMA PRA Category 1 Credits*™ are available from July 31, 2018, to July 31, 2021, for the MKSAP 18 Hematology and Oncology section.

Learning Objectives

The learning objectives of MKSAP 18 are to

- Close gaps between actual care in your practice and preferred standards of care, based on best evidence
- Diagnose disease states that are less common and sometimes overlooked and confusing
- Improve management of comorbid conditions that can complicate patient care
- Determine when to refer patients for surgery or care by subspecialists
- Pass the ABIM Certification Examination
- Pass the ABIM Maintenance of Certification Examination

Target Audience

- General internists and primary care physicians
- Subspecialists who need to remain up to date in internal medicine
- Residents preparing for the certifying examination in internal medicine
- Physicians preparing for maintenance of certification in internal medicine (recertification)

ABIM Maintenance of Certification

Check the MKSAP Resource Site (mksap.acponline.org) for the latest information on how MKSAP tests can be used to apply to the American Board of Internal Medicine (ABIM) for Maintenance of Certification (MOC) points following completion of the CME activity.

Successful completion of the CME activity, which includes participation in the evaluation component, enables the participant to earn up to 275 medical knowledge MOC points in the ABIM's MOC program. It is the CME activity provider's responsibility to submit participant completion information to ACCME for the purpose of granting MOC credit.

Earn Instantaneous CME Credits or MOC Points Online

Print subscribers can enter their answers online to earn instantaneous CME credits or MOC points. You can submit your answers using online answer sheets that are provided at mksap.acponline.org, where a record of your MKSAP 18 credits will be available. To earn CME credits or to apply for MOC points, you need to answer all of the questions in a test and earn a score of at least 50% correct (number of correct answers divided by the total number of questions). Please note that if you are applying for MOC points, you must also enter your birth date and ABIM candidate number.

Take either of the following approaches:

1. Use the printed answer sheet at the back of this book to record your answers. Go to mksap.acponline.org, access the appropriate online answer sheet, transcribe your answers, and submit your test for instantaneous CME credits or MOC points. There is no additional fee for this service.
2. Go to mksap.acponline.org, access the appropriate online answer sheet, directly enter your answers, and submit your test for instantaneous CME credits or MOC points. There is no additional fee for this service.

Earn CME Credits or MOC Points by Mail or Fax

Pay a $20 processing fee per answer sheet and submit the printed answer sheet at the back of this book by mail or fax, as instructed on the answer sheet. Make sure you calculate your score and enter your birth date and ABIM candidate number, and fax the answer sheet to 215-351-2799 or mail the answer sheet to Member and Customer Service, American College of Physicians, 190 N. Independence Mall West, Philadelphia, PA 19106-1572, using the courtesy envelope provided in your MKSAP 18 slipcase. You will need your 10-digit order number and 8-digit ACP ID number, which are printed on your packing slip. Please allow 4 to 6 weeks for your score report to be emailed back to you. Be sure to include your email address for a response.

If you do not have a 10-digit order number and 8-digit ACP ID number, or if you need help creating a username and password to access the MKSAP 18 online answer sheets, go to mksap.acponline.org or email custserv@acponline.org.

Disclosure Policy

It is the policy of the American College of Physicians (ACP) to ensure balance, independence, objectivity, and scientific rigor in all of its educational activities. To this end, and consistent with the policies of the ACP and the Accreditation Council for Continuing Medical Education (ACCME), contributors to all ACP continuing medical education activities are required to disclose all relevant financial relationships with any entity producing, marketing, re-selling, or distributing health care goods or services consumed by, or used on, patients. Contributors are required to use generic names in the discussion of therapeutic options and are required to identify any unapproved, off-label, or investigative use of commercial products or devices. Where a trade name is used, all available trade names for the same product type are also included. If trade-name products manufactured by companies with whom contributors have relationships are discussed, contributors are asked to provide evidence-based citations in support of the discussion. The information is reviewed by the committee responsible for producing this text. If necessary, adjustments to topics or contributors' roles in content development are made to balance the discussion. Further, all readers of this text are asked to evaluate the content for evidence of commercial bias and send any relevant comments to mksap_editors@acponline.org so that future decisions about content and contributors can be made in light of this information.

Resolution of Conflicts

To resolve all conflicts of interest and influences of vested interests, ACP's content planners used best evidence and updated clinical care guidelines in developing content, when such evidence and guidelines were available. All content underwent review by peer reviewers not on the committee to ensure that the material was balanced and unbiased. Contributors' disclosure information can be found with the list of contributors' names and those of ACP principal staff listed in the beginning of this book.

Hospital-Based Medicine

For the convenience of subscribers who provide care in hospital settings, content that is specific to the hospital setting has been highlighted in blue. Hospital icons (H) highlight where the hospital-only content begins, continues over more than one page, and ends.

High Value Care Key Points

Key Points in the text that relate to High Value Care concepts (that is, concepts that discuss balancing clinical benefit with costs and harms) are designated by the HVC icon [HVC].

Educational Disclaimer

The editors and publisher of MKSAP 18 recognize that the development of new material offers many opportunities for error. Despite our best efforts, some errors may persist in print. Drug dosage schedules are, we believe, accurate and in accordance with current standards. Readers are advised, however, to ensure that the recommended dosages in MKSAP 18 concur with the information provided in the product information material. This is especially important in cases of new, infrequently used, or highly toxic drugs. Application of the information in MKSAP 18 remains the professional responsibility of the practitioner.

The primary purpose of MKSAP 18 is educational. Information presented, as well as publications, technologies, products, and/or services discussed, is intended to inform subscribers about the knowledge, techniques, and experiences of the contributors. A diversity of professional opinion exists, and the views of the contributors are their own and not those of the ACP. Inclusion of any material in the program does not constitute endorsement or recommendation by the ACP. The ACP does not warrant the safety, reliability, accuracy, completeness, or usefulness of and disclaims any and all liability for damages and claims that may result from the use of information, publications, technologies, products, and/or services discussed in this program.

Publisher's Information

Disclaimer Regarding Direct Purchases from Online Retailers

CME and/or MOC for MKSAP 18 is available only if you purchase the program directly from ACP. CME credits and MOC points cannot be awarded to those purchasers who have purchased the program from non-authorized sellers such as Amazon, eBay, or any other such online retailer.

Unauthorized Use of This Book Is Against the Law

MKSAP 18 ISBN: 978-1-938245-47-3
(Hematology and Oncology) ISBN: 978-1-938245-51-0

Printed in the United States of America.

For order information in the U.S. or Canada call 800-ACP-1915. All other countries call 215-351-2600, (Monday to Friday, 9 AM – 5 PM ET). Fax inquiries to 215-351-2799 or email to custserv@acponline.org.

Errata

Errata for MKSAP 18 will be available through the MKSAP Resource Site at mksap.acponline.org as new information becomes known to the editors.

Table of Contents

Hematology and Oncology High Value Care Recommendations

The American College of Physicians, in collaboration with multiple other organizations, is engaged in a worldwide initiative to promote the practice of High Value Care (HVC). The goals of the HVC initiative are to improve health care outcomes by providing care of proven benefit and reducing costs by avoiding unnecessary and even harmful interventions. The initiative comprises several programs that integrate the important concept of health care value (balancing clinical benefit with costs and harms) for a given intervention into a broad range of educational materials to address the needs of trainees, practicing physicians, and patients.

HVC content has been integrated into MKSAP 18 in several important ways. MKSAP 18 includes HVC-identified key points in the text, HVC-focused multiple choice questions, and, for subscribers to MKSAP Digital, an HVC custom quiz. From the text and questions, we have generated the following list of HVC recommendations that meet the definition below of high value care and bring us closer to our goal of improving patient outcomes while conserving finite resources.

High Value Care Recommendation: A recommendation to choose diagnostic and management strategies for patients in specific clinical situations that balance clinical benefit with cost and harms with the goal of improving patient outcomes.

Below are the High Value Care Recommendations for the Hematology and Oncology section of MKSAP 18.

- Do not obtain a bone marrow evaluation for low-risk monoclonal gammopathy.
- Oral ferrous sulfate is the preferred treatment of iron deficiency because of its tolerability, efficacy, and cost.
- Treatment of inflammatory anemia is seldom necessary and iron replacement is ineffective.
- Avoid erythropoiesis-stimulating agents in patients with chronic kidney disease not undergoing dialysis with a hemoglobin level greater than 10 g/dL (100 g/L).
- Oral cobalamin is preferred to parenteral therapy for cobalamin deficiency.
- Avoid iron supplementation in patients with thalassemia.
- Do not test for glucose-6-phosphate dehydrogenase deficiency during an acute hemolytic episode.
- Avoid transfusions in patients with sickle cell disease and uncomplicated pain crises or chronic anemia.
- Most patients with heparin-associated thrombocytopenia and a low 4T score need no further evaluation.

- Asymptomatic patients with factor XI deficiency do not require intervention before surgery.
- Do not use prothrombin complex concentrates to manage the coagulopathy of liver disease.
- Do not evaluate for thrombophilia in most patients with acute venous thromboembolism.
- Do not perform additional testing in patients with low probability Wells criteria scores and Pulmonary Embolism Rule-Out Criteria scores of zero.
- Do not perform additional testing in patients with low probability scores for deep venous thrombosis or pulmonary embolism and normal D-dimer measurement.
- Most patients with deep venous thrombosis and those with pulmonary embolism and a good prognosis can be managed without hospitalization.
- Withholding warfarin is the preferred treatment for asymptomatic INR elevation between 4.5 and 10 (see Item 44).
- Bridging therapy during warfarin discontinuation before an invasive procedure is not necessary in most patients.
- Treatment is not required for most patients with gestational thrombocytopenia.
- Do not obtain imaging studies for localized tumors that have a low likelihood of distant metastases to certain sites, such as bone or brain.
- Do not obtain PET, CT, or bone scan for staging for newly diagnosed stage 0 to II breast cancer.
- Before administering adjuvant chemotherapy in older women with higher-risk early stage breast cancer, consider life expectancy, functional status, and medical comorbidities.
- Surveillance blood tests and other imaging tests for breast cancer should not be routinely performed and should be guided by a patient's symptoms or findings on examination that raise concern for recurrence.
- Do not offer ovarian cancer screening, even in high-risk women.
- Do not perform surveillance imaging and laboratory studies in asymptomatic cervical cancer survivors.
- Do not obtain PET scans for preoperative staging or postoperative surveillance in colorectal cancer.
- Well-differentiated neuroendocrine tumors require only observation and serial imaging.
- Routine imaging for head and neck cancer after a negative posttreatment scan is not indicated unless there are signs and symptoms suggestive of recurrent disease.

- Do not obtain nonspecific tumor markers, PET scans, and gene expression arrays in the evaluation of cancer of unknown primary.
- Outpatient treatment is reasonable for patients with febrile neutropenia expected to be of short duration, who lack significant comorbidity, and who have reliable home care and follow-up.

- Do not offer aggressive chemotherapy to patients with cancer of unknown primary and several comorbidities and poor performance status (see Item 107).
- Observation is an appropriate management strategy for men with early-stage prostate cancer who have limited life expectancy or significant medical comorbidities (see Item 117).

Hematology and Oncology

Hematopoietic Stem Cells and Their Disorders

Overview

Hematopoietic stem cells nest in the bone marrow and have the capacity to differentiate and self-renew. Hematopoietic stem cells are multipotent and can differentiate into progenitor cells; in turn, these produce leukocytes, erythrocytes, and platelets. This differentiation and proliferation to mature blood cells happens in an orderly manner called hematopoiesis. Hematopoiesis is tightly regulated by multiple factors, including the bone marrow microenvironment and hematopoietic growth factors. This includes erythropoietin, which stimulates erythrocytes; thrombopoietin, which stimulates platelet production; and granulocyte colony-stimulating factor and macrophage colony-stimulating factor, which stimulate granulocyte, monocyte, basophil, and eosinophil production. Disorders of hematopoiesis can occur at the hematopoietic stem cell or progenitor level and can lead to underproduction or overproduction of blood cells.

Bone marrow failure syndromes are characterized by the failure of hematopoiesis to keep up with physiologic demands for blood cell production, leading to peripheral cytopenias. Although rare inherited causes exist, acquired disorders are much more common and can occur secondary to intrinsic bone marrow disorders, such as myelodysplastic syndrome, or extrinsic disorders resulting from toxins or autoimmunity, as in aplastic anemia.

Myeloproliferative neoplasms are clonal myeloid neoplasms with deregulation and excess proliferation of subsets of hematopoietic stem cells. The diagnosis can be made through identification of clonal genetic abnormalities, such as *BCR-ABL* translocation and *JAK2* (*JAK2 V617F*) mutation on peripheral blood testing.

Acute leukemias, either myeloid or lymphoid in origin, are aggressive clonal neoplasms in which cells also lose the capability to differentiate into mature cells. These disorders usually require emergent evaluation and treatment.

Bone Marrow Failure Syndromes

Aplastic Anemia

Aplastic anemia (AA) is an acquired hematopoietic stem cell disorder characterized by severely decreased bone marrow cellularity and pancytopenia. Although the condition is classified as an anemia, patients usually present with a combination of anemia, neutropenia, and thrombocytopenia. Bone marrow cellularity decreases with age while the fat content of the marrow increases. These changes are amplified in AA, which is categorized as severe or very severe based on the degree of bone marrow cellularity and the severity of cytopenias.

AA is caused by a decrease in stem cells as a result of autoimmunity, toxins, and infections. Medications, such as antithyroid medications (methimazole and propylthiouracil), β-lactam antibiotics, sulfonamides, NSAIDs, anticonvulsants, and gold, have also been associated with development of AA. Discontinuing the offending medication usually improves the AA, but it can take many weeks for cell counts to recover.

Most AA is felt to be related to autoimmunity against stem cells. In patients older than 50 years and in younger patients without a suitable stem cell donor, AA is treated by immunosuppression with antithymocyte globulin, cyclosporine, and prednisone. Patients younger than 50 years with a suitable donor are usually treated with allogeneic hematopoietic stem cell transplantation. With advances in immunosuppression, bone marrow transplantation, and supportive care, the overall survival of young patients with a good risk profile has reached greater than 80%. Asymptomatic patients with mild to moderate AA can be closely monitored without immediate treatment.

Patients with AA can develop a clone of paroxysmal nocturnal hemoglobinuria cells, which lack complement-stabilizing CD55 and CD59 proteins. However, identifying the paroxysmal nocturnal hemoglobinuria clone does not routinely change treatment of AA, although it does help explain pathophysiology. AA can be differentiated from a hypoplastic variant of myelodysplastic syndrome (MDS) with decreased bone marrow cellularity by finding dysplastic cells and cytogenetic abnormalities typical for MDS. Hypoplastic MDS is also commonly treated with immunosuppressive treatment.

Pure Red Cell Aplasia

Pure red cell aplasia (PRCA) is characterized by normocytic or macrocytic anemia with decreased reticulocytes and absent or decreased erythrocyte precursors in the bone marrow. Leukocyte and platelet counts are normal. Several conditions have been implicated in the pathogenesis of PRCA, some of which are listed in **Table 1**.

Parvovirus B19 is cytotoxic to the erythrocyte precursors in the bone marrow. Parvovirus infection is usually

TABLE 1.	Causes of Acquired Pure Red Cell Aplasia
Parvovirus B19 infection	
Thymoma	
Autoimmune disease	
Lymphoid leukemias and lymphomas	
Solid tumors	
Drugs (phenytoin, isoniazid)	
Pregnancy	
Anti-EPO antibodies in patients receiving EPO	
EPO = erythropoietin.	

transient, lasting 2 to 3 weeks in immunocompetent patients, and does not usually cause clinically significant anemia in healthy patients. However, patients with chronic hemolysis (such as sickle cell anemia) who depend on increased erythrocyte production can have significant anemia with a decreased reticulocyte count. Immunocompromised patients can have sustained viremia leading to prolonged anemia requiring intravenous immune globulin treatment to hasten viral clearance.

A few patients with PRCA have an underlying occult thymoma and can improve with thymectomy. Large granular lymphocyte leukemia is a T-cell lymphoproliferative disorder that can be associated with PRCA. Flow cytometry of the peripheral blood can help identify this disorder.

A bone marrow biopsy specimen showing decreased erythrocyte precursors is required to diagnose PRCA. Idiopathic PRCA is commonly immunologically mediated and treated with immunosuppressive medications, such as prednisone, cyclosporine, and cyclophosphamide.

Neutropenia

Isolated neutropenia is a common finding in internal medicine practice. Most patients with neutropenia have a mild form (1000-1500/μL [$1-1.5 \times 10^9$/L]), but some have moderate (500-1000/μL [$0.5-1 \times 10^9$/L]) or severe (500/μL [0.5×10^9/L]) neutropenia. Clinically significant infections do not usually occur unless neutrophil counts are less than 500/μL (0.5×10^9/L). Isolated neutropenia can be secondary to congenital or acquired conditions (**Table 2**).

Benign ethnic neutropenia is a congenital neutropenia seen in black patients and those of Mediterranean descent. These patients have good neutrophil reserve and are not prone to infections. In a healthy black patient with mild neutropenia found on routine testing, no further evaluation is needed.

Cyclical neutropenia is another rare congenital condition in which neutrophil counts decrease every 2 to 5 weeks. The neutrophil count can get low enough that patients develop recurrent infections every 2 to 5 weeks.

Instead of causing leukocytosis, infections can cause neutropenia; this can happen after viral, bacterial, or rickettsial infections. Neutropenia resolves with improvement of the underlying infection. Several drugs have been implicated in causing neutropenia, including chemotherapy, NSAIDs, carbamazepine, phenytoin, propylthiouracil, cephalosporins, trimethoprim-sulfamethoxazole, and psychotropics. Drug-induced neutropenia can be dose dependent or idiosyncratic. In mild, dose-dependent neutropenia, the offending drug may be continued if clinically indicated.

Isolated neutropenia can occur with various autoimmune disorders, such as systemic lupus erythematosus. The neutropenia is usually mild, is rarely clinically significant, and improves with treatment of the underlying autoimmune disorder with immunosuppression. The triad of neutropenia, splenomegaly, and rheumatoid arthritis is called Felty syndrome; the neutropenia can be severe, and patients can have significant infections. Treatment of the underlying rheumatoid arthritis can alleviate the neutropenia, but granulocyte colony-stimulating factor is needed in some patients. Large granular lymphocyte leukemia can also be associated with clinical features of Felty syndrome.

TABLE 2.	Causes of Neutropenia
Inherited	
Cyclic neutropenia	
Benign ethnic neutropenia	
Severe congenital neutropenia	
Neutropenia associated with various congenital syndromes (such as glycogen storage disease type 1b)	
Acquired	
Autoimmune	
Associated with autoimmune conditions (systemic lupus erythematosus, rheumatoid arthritis)	
Associated with immunodeficiency	
Infection	
Viral (HIV, hepatitis, parvovirus, Epstein-Barr virus)	
Bacterial (typhoid, tuberculosis, brucellosis)	
Fungal (histoplasmosis)	
Parasitic (malaria, leishmaniasis)	
Rickettsial (ehrlichiosis, Rocky Mountain spotted fever)	
Medication (NSAIDs, antibiotics, chemotherapies, diuretics, sulfonylureas, thioamides, quinine, psychotropic drugs, anticonvulsants)	
Nutritional (folate or vitamin B_{12} deficiency)	
Idiopathic	
Sequestration and neutrophil margination (hemodialysis)	
Hematologic disorders	
Acute leukemia	
Aplastic anemia	
Myelodysplastic syndrome	
Other hematologic disorders	

Myelodysplastic Syndromes

The myelodysplastic syndromes (MDSs) are clonal stem cell disorders with ineffective hematopoiesis leading to dysplastic, hypercellular bone marrow and peripheral blood cytopenias. MDS carries a varied risk of transformation to acute myeloid leukemia (AML) that correlates with prognosis. Most MDS is idiopathic, but secondary MDS can result from chemotherapy, radiation, chemical exposure (benzene), and other factors. Other reversible causes of dysplasia that must be ruled out include vitamin B_{12}, folate, and copper deficiency; alcohol consumption; medications; and infections (such as HIV).

Macrocytic anemia is the most common cytopenia observed in MDS. The peripheral blood smear shows dysplastic cells (such as hypogranular neutrophils and platelets). These blood cells do not function well and increase the risk of infection and bleeding. MDS can have a varied presentation with numerous cell lines involved. The World Health Organization classification of MDS and its features are listed in **Table 3**. MDS is suspected in patients with otherwise unexplained cytopenias, especially with dysplastic findings on peripheral blood smear (**Figure 1**). Bone marrow biopsy is

required for diagnosis. The prognosis for patients with MDS depends on bone marrow blasts, degree of cytopenias, and cytogenetics. Patients with few blasts in the bone marrow, reasonable peripheral blood cell counts, and a favorable cytogenetic profile have a median survival of almost 9 years, whereas those with greater than 10% blasts, severe pancytopenia (hemoglobin <8 g/dL [80 g/L], platelet count <50,000/μL [50 × 10⁹/L], absolute neutrophil count <800/μL [0.8 × 10⁹/L]), and adverse cytogenetic mutations survive less than 1 year.

Older adult patients who are asymptomatic and have mild cytopenias and features of MDS can be monitored without detailed evaluation. Allogeneic hematopoietic stem cell transplantation is the only potentially curative option available. Transplantation is not an option for most patients with MDS because most are older and are usually not candidates for intensive treatment.

The two main goals of treatment of MDS are treatment of symptomatic cytopenias and reducing the risk of progression to AML. Symptomatic anemia is treated with transfusions and erythropoiesis-stimulating agents. Patients with MDS who are

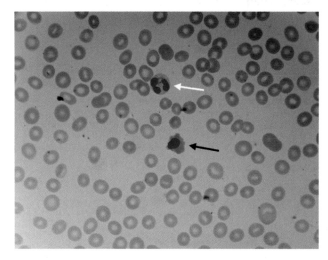

FIGURE 1. Peripheral blood smear from a patient with myelodysplastic syndrome. A dysplastic neutrophil is seen (*solid white arrow*) with hypogranular cytoplasm and a dysplastic nucleus. A nucleated erythrocyte is also seen in this field (*solid black arrow*).

Figure courtesy of Julia Choi, MD; Baylor Scott & White Health.

TABLE 3. World Health Organization Classification of Myelodysplastic Syndrome			
Category	**Frequency**	**Marrow Blasts**	**Other Features**
Refractory cytopenia with unilineage dysplasia	20%	<5%	Single cell line dysplasia (usually erythrocytes)
Refractory cytopenia with multilineage dysplasia	30%	<5%	Dysplasia in ≥2 lineages
MDS associated with isolated 5q−	Uncommon	<5%	Increased hypolobated megakaryocytes
Refractory anemia with ring sideroblasts	10%	<5%	Erythroid dysplasia, ≥15% ring sideroblasts
RAEB-1	40%	5%-9%	Unilineage or multilineage dysplasia
RAEB-2	40%	10%-19%	Unilineage or multilineage dysplasia
MDS, unclassified	Uncommon	<5%	Does not fit other categories
MDS = myelodysplastic syndrome; RAEB-1/2 = refractory anemia with excess blasts, type 1 or 2.			

at high risk have approximately a 25% risk of conversion to AML in the first year. Treatment of these patients with hypomethylating agents, such as azacytidine and decitabine, has been shown to decrease transfusion dependence and the risk of conversion to AML. A group of patients with low-risk MDS with the -5q cytogenetic abnormality could be treated with the immunomodulatory drug lenalidomide if they are transfusion dependent. Lenalidomide has been approved for this indication and is effective in decreasing transfusion requirements.

Chronic myelomonocytic leukemia has traditionally been considered a subset of MDS but is now classified as a separate entity, sharing some features of MDS with those of myeloproliferative neoplasms. Patients with chronic myelomonocytic leukemia have persistent monocytosis, often with other cytopenias; bone marrow shows dysplastic changes and less than 20% blasts. Prognosis and treatment is analogous to MDS with poor prognosis.

KEY POINTS

- Myelodysplastic syndrome is suspected in patients with cytopenias and with dysplastic findings on peripheral blood smear; bone marrow biopsy is required for diagnosis and to assess prognosis.

- The only cure for myelodysplastic syndrome is allogeneic hematopoietic stem cell transplantation, which is too toxic for most older adult patients in whom this disorder is most prevalent; however, treating patients at high risk of conversion to acute myeloid leukemia with hypomethylating agents has been shown to decrease transfusion dependence and the risk of conversion.

Myeloproliferative Neoplasms

Myeloproliferative neoplasms (MPNs) are clonal stem cell disorders characterized by proliferation of the components of the myeloid, erythroid, or megakaryocyte lineage. They are named based on the dominant cell line affected; for example, erythrocytes are increased in polycythemia, and platelets are increased in essential thrombocythemia. Overlap is considerable among these disorders, and multiple cell lines are usually elevated. A disease-defining genetic chromosomal translocation is seen in chronic myeloid leukemia (CML). Another commonly found mutation involving *JAK2 V617* is associated with polycythemia vera, essential thrombocythemia, myelofibrosis, and other myeloid disorders. Based on the type of MPN, patients are at varied risk of hepatosplenomegaly, thrombosis, and conversion to myelofibrosis or acute myeloid leukemia (AML).

Chronic Myeloid Leukemia

CML is a clonal hematopoietic stem cell disorder characterized by translocation of the long arm of chromosomes 9 and 22 [t(9;22), Philadelphia chromosome] leading to a *BCR-ABL* fusion gene. This gene codes for an abnormal activated tyrosine kinase that promotes dysregulated cell proliferation. At diagnosis,

patients with CML can be asymptomatic, with elevated neutrophil counts found on routine laboratory studies, or they can have symptoms such as fatigue, weight loss, abdominal fullness (splenomegaly), and bleeding. CML must be distinguished from a leukemoid reaction, characterized by significant elevation of the neutrophil count with left shift, increased band forms, and, at times, metamyelocytes, seen in acutely ill patients and those with infections such as *Clostridium difficile*. The clinical setting usually allows leukemoid reaction to be distinguished from CML, but in difficult presentations, chromosomal evaluation can help make the diagnosis.

CML has three phases of progression: the chronic phase, the accelerated phase, and blast crisis. The chronic phase is an indolent phase and responds well to therapy. Most patients with CML present in the chronic phase. Accelerated and blast crisis phases denote more aggressive disease that is less responsive to treatment. Blast crisis is considered to be secondary AML.

In CML, peripheral blood neutrophilia along with immature myeloid forms, such as myelocytes and metamyelocytes, are seen (**Figure 2**). In the chronic phase, fewer than 10% of blasts are present in circulation. Peripheral eosinophilia, basophilia, and thrombocytosis can also be seen. CML can be diagnosed by identifying the Philadelphia chromosome (either the fusion gene, t(9;22), or gene transcript, *BCR-ABL*) in a peripheral blood sample using fluorescence in situ hybridization or reverse transcriptase polymerase chain reaction, respectively.

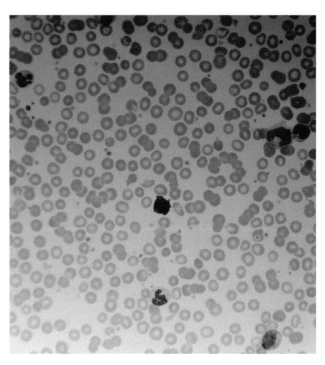

FIGURE 2. Chronic myeloid leukemia is characterized by a preponderance of mature granulocytes (*upper left*) and less mature myeloid cells such as myelocytes (*bottom right*) and metamyelocytes (*top right*). Basophils (*center*) are helpful in differentiating the myeloproliferative neoplasms from leukemoid reactions.

Figure courtesy of Deepty Bhansali, MD; Baylor Scott & White Health.

Therapy is required at diagnosis in all patients to treat symptoms and to prevent progression to blast phase and subsequent AML. Tyrosine kinase inhibitors (TKIs) are highly effective and are the treatment of choice for patients with chronic phase CML. Three TKIs, imatinib, dasatinib, and nilotinib, are FDA approved for the initial treatment of CML. TKIs bind to the BCR-ABL oncoprotein and prevent downstream signaling. Development of these TKIs has revolutionized the treatment of CML, with improved survival, and has significantly decreased the need for stem cell transplantation. Although TKIs are relatively well tolerated, they have unique adverse effects, such as fluid retention and QTc prolongation, requiring close monitoring. They also have significant drug-drug interactions that necessitate caution when starting new medications. TKIs are contraindicated during pregnancy, so either close monitoring of patients off treatment or a switch to interferon is indicated. In patients receiving TKI therapy in whom CML progresses, medication adherence or novel mutation development should be considered. Novel TKIs (bosutinib and ponatinib) are available for refractory CML. For patients with accelerated or blast phase CML, allogeneic hematopoietic stem cell transplantation is considered.

KEY POINT

- Therapy with a tyrosine kinase inhibitor is required at diagnosis in all patients with chronic myeloid leukemia to treat symptoms and to prevent progression to acute myeloid leukemia.

Polycythemia Vera

Polycythemia vera (PV) is a clonal myeloid stem cell neoplasm characterized by excess erythrocyte mass. This increase in erythrocyte mass is independent of erythropoietin level. Thrombocytosis and neutrophilia are commonly seen, justifying the term *polycythemia*, in addition to the increased erythrocyte mass. Activating mutation of the *JAK2* (*JAK2 V617F*) gene is observed in 97% of patients with PV. Most patients with PV are identified by an elevated hemoglobin level (>16.5 g/dL [165 g/L] in men or >16 g/dL [160 g/L] in women) on routine blood testing. Some patients present with symptoms such as fatigue, headache, erythromelalgia (redness and paresthesias of the extremities), pruritus, uncontrolled hypertension, and thrombosis.

Secondary erythrocytosis is much more common than PV. Refer to **Table 4** for common causes of secondary erythrocytosis

TABLE 4. Causes of Secondary Erythrocytosis			
Disorders	**Symptoms**	**Physical Examination**	**Laboratory Studies**
Polycythemia vera (primary)	Pruritus after a warm shower	Splenomegaly	Low erythropoietin
	Erythromelalgia	Plethora	Leukocytosis
	Transient ischemic attack		Basophilia
	Deep venous thrombosis/ pulmonary embolism		Thrombocytosis
			JAK2 positive
Mediated by hypoxemia	Thrombosis	Plethora	Normal leukocyte and platelet counts
COPD	Transient ischemic attack	No splenomegaly	No basophilia
Sleep apnea	Erythromelalgia uncommon	Findings consistent with underlying heart or lung disease	No leukocytosis
Congenital heart disease	Pruritus uncommon		*JAK2* negative
Intrapulmonary shunting			Decreased oxygen saturation
Elevated altitude			
Mediated by ectopic or excessive erythropoietin	Thrombosis possible	Plethora	High erythropoietin
Renal cell carcinoma	Transient ischemic attack uncommon	No splenomegaly	Microscopic hematuria (renal cell carcinoma)
Renal artery stenosis/other kidney pathology	Erythromelalgia uncommon		Abnormal finding on kidney ultrasonography
	Pruritus uncommon		No basophilia
Hepatocellular carcinoma			
Uterine fibroids			*JAK2* negative
Unusual causes	Thrombosis	Plethora	High erythropoietin
High oxygen affinity hemoglobin	Transient ischemic attack	No splenomegaly	No basophilia
	Erythromelalgia uncommon	Age <30 years	No leukocytosis
	Pruritus uncommon	Family history of erythrocytosis	*JAK2* negative
	Asymptomatic		Abnormal hemoglobin electrophoresis
			Abnormally low PaO$_2$ produces 50% hemoglobin saturation

and its clinical features. In most cases of secondary erythrocytosis, the increase in erythrocyte mass depends on the erythropoietin level. Relative polycythemia is seen in patients who have a relative decrease in plasma volume from dehydration with a normal erythrocyte mass leading to elevated hemoglobin levels.

Evaluation of a patient with PV starts with a careful history and physical examination, looking for secondary causes of polycythemia. Smoking history, occupational exposures, and use of medications should be explored. Polycythemia is a common adverse effect of testosterone supplementation, and evaluating the hematocrit level at initiation, 3 to 6 months after testosterone initiation, and annually thereafter is recommended by Endocrine Society guidelines. Guidelines also recommend interrupting the testosterone supplementation if the hematocrit value is greater than 54%. Splenomegaly is a common finding in PV. Patients with PV often have elevated leukocyte and platelet counts along with erythrocytosis. All patients suspected of having PV should undergo a complete blood count, serum erythropoietin level evaluation, and *JAK2* mutation testing. To evaluate for hypoxia, pulse oximetry should be performed. Sleep apnea can be associated with secondary polycythemia but might not be apparent, so careful assessment for signs and symptoms of sleep apnea is important; in patients at high risk, a sleep study may be necessary to evaluate for sleep apnea. Underlying causes of secondary erythrocytosis should be managed; phlebotomy decisions are more complex in these patients because the elevated hemoglobin level may be an appropriate physiologic response.

Finding a low serum erythropoietin level and *JAK2* positivity in a patient with an elevated hemoglobin level is usually diagnostic of PV.

Thrombosis is a major complication in patients with untreated PV. Whole blood viscosity is increased, with increased risk of arterial thrombosis (stroke and myocardial infarction) and venous thrombosis. *JAK2* mutation has also been implicated in thrombotic risk. Other hematologic complications in PV include progression to post-PV myelofibrosis and transformation to AML. Prognosis after transformation is poor. ▪

Treatment of PV is required at diagnosis. Phlebotomy with a goal hematocrit level of less than 45% has been shown to decrease the risk of thrombosis and is applied to all patients with PV. Phlebotomy keeps the hematocrit level under control by causing iron deficiency, so iron supplementation should not be given. Low-dose aspirin is considered in all patients with PV to decrease the risk of thrombosis. Hydroxyurea is used in patients with a high risk of thrombosis, such as those older than 60 years and those with a history of thrombosis. The *JAK1/2* inhibitor ruxolitinib is approved for treatment of patients who are intolerant of hydroxyurea or for refractory PV.

KEY POINT

- *JAK2* positivity is found in almost all patients with elevated hemoglobin levels caused by polycythemia vera.

Essential Thrombocythemia

Essential thrombocythemia (ET) is suspected in patients with sustained elevation of platelet counts greater than 450,000/μL (450 × 10⁹/L). Diagnosis of ET requires ruling out other MPNs such as CML, PV, primary myelofibrosis, and myelodysplastic syndromes. *JAK2* mutation is present in about 50% of patients with ET. Other clonal mutations in ET have been identified involving the calreticulin and *MPL* genes. In patients without these clonal mutations, diagnosis of ET requires ruling out reactive thrombocytosis. Iron deficiency anemia is a common cause for reactive thrombocytosis. Other common causes of secondary thrombocytosis are infection, inflammation, and splenectomy.

Most patients with ET are asymptomatic and present with an elevated platelet count found on routine laboratory testing. Patients can present with vasomotor symptoms such as headache, visual disturbances, dysesthesia of the palms and soles, syncope, and livedo reticularis. Other complications of ET include thrombosis and hemorrhage. Thrombosis can be venous or arterial, manifesting as a cerebrovascular accident, transient ischemic attack, digital ischemia, vision loss, or myocardial infarction. Hemorrhage in ET is commonly seen in patients with a platelet count greater than 1.5 million/μL (1500 × 10⁹/L) or use of high-dose aspirin. Extreme thrombocytosis is thought to increase bleeding risk by causing acquired von Willebrand disease. ▪

Patients with ET might not require immediate platelet-lowering therapy at diagnosis. The most important factors in defining high risk for thrombosis and the need for preventive therapy are age older than 60 years or history of thrombosis. Patients with platelet counts greater than 1,000,000/μL (1000 × 10⁹/L) are at risk for bleeding and should also be treated with hydroxyurea to lower the platelet count. Other therapies for patients who do not respond to hydroxyurea or who experience significant adverse effects include anagrelide and interferon-α. Low-dose aspirin is considered in all patients at high risk and in patients at low risk who have vasomotor symptoms. Primary care providers should be alert to the value of identifying asymptomatic thrombocytosis that may be discovered incidentally as part of a complete blood count, of ruling out a secondary cause of thrombocytosis, and, in patients with ET who are older than 60 years, of starting hydroxyurea to prevent complications. ET is less likely than other MPNs to progress to AML or myelofibrosis.

KEY POINTS

- The *JAK2* genetic mutation is seen in approximately 50% of patients with essential thrombocythemia and primary myelofibrosis.

- Most patients with essential thrombocythemia present with an elevated platelet count (>450,000/μL [450 × 10⁹/L]) found on routine laboratory testing, and they can also have vasomotor symptoms such as headache, visual disturbances, dysesthesia of the palms and soles, syncope, and livedo reticularis.

(Continued)

KEY POINTS (continued)

- Asymptomatic patients with essential thrombo-cythemia who are older than 60 years with an otherwise unexplained elevated platelet count should be treated with hydroxyurea to lower the platelet count and decrease the risk of thrombotic complications.

Primary Myelofibrosis

Primary myelofibrosis (PMF) carries the worst prognosis of the MPNs. It is a clonal myeloid stem cell disorder with characteristic marrow fibrosis and extramedullary hematopoiesis. This increased fibrosis is thought to be related to proliferation of clonal megakaryocytes, which secrete excess fibroblast growth factor. Hematopoietic progenitors are increased in the circulation, providing a leukoerythroblastic picture seen on peripheral blood smear (**Figure 3**). A leukoerythroblastic smear can also be seen in other myelophthisic disorders, such as bone involvement with carcinoma. As in ET, *JAK2* mutation test results are positive in about 50% of patients with PMF.

Most patients with PMF have significant symptoms at presentation. Cytokine-related hypercatabolic symptoms, such as fatigue, weight loss, fever, and chills, are prominent. Massive splenomegaly is common from extramedullary hematopoiesis and portal hypertension, and it is often accompanied by abdominal discomfort and early satiety. Extramedullary hematopoiesis in the gastrointestinal tract, varices from portal hypertension, and thrombocytopenia can lead to gastrointestinal bleeding. Although patients with PMF present with significant symptoms, some patients can present with more indolent disease.

Diagnosis of PMF requires bone marrow biopsy to document fibrosis in the marrow and to exclude other causes.

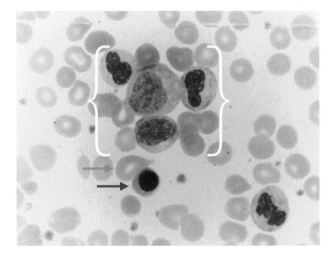

FIGURE 3. A leukoerythroblastic blood smear shows left-shifted granulopoiesis (bands on either side of a large myelocyte above a metamyelocyte in brackets) and nucleated (*blue arrow*) and teardrop-shaped erythrocytes (*green arrow*), which define a crowded myelophthisic marrow such as is seen in primary myelofibrosis or other secondary processes such as metastatic carcinoma. A mature neutrophil is seen in the bottom right.

Biopsy is usually a dry tap with no aspirate because the bone marrow is fibrotic. The Dynamic International Prognostic Scoring System has been developed using various clinical and pathological variables to stratify patients into risk categories. Patients in each risk group have significantly different prognoses; for example, patients in the low-risk group have a median survival of 185 months compared with 16 months in the high-risk group. Treatment of PMF depends on symptoms, risk of disease progression, and survival. The only treatment with potential for cure is allogeneic hematopoietic stem cell transplantation. This type of transplantation is considered in patients who have an HLA-matched donor and who are healthy enough to survive the procedure and have poor prognostic features, including older age, constitutional symptoms, more severe anemia and thrombocytopenia, and increased numbers of blasts in the marrow.

Ruxolitinib has been shown to help improve hypercatabolic symptoms and splenomegaly, with activity independent of *JAK2* mutational status. It does not alter progression to AML. Ruxolitinib is reserved for treatment in patients with debilitating symptoms who are not candidates for hematopoietic stem cell transplantation. Hydroxyurea may be used for patients with low-risk PMF. Splenectomy is only performed in patients with debilitating symptoms related to massive spleen size because it can result in significant morbidity and mortality in PMF.

KEY POINT

- The only treatment with potential for cure for primary myelofibrosis is allogeneic hematopoietic stem cell transplantation.

Eosinophilia and Hypereosinophilic Syndrome

Mild eosinophilia with an eosinophil count of 500 to 1500/µL ($0.5\text{-}1.5 \times 10^9$/L) is not commonly associated with end-organ damage. The causes for eosinophilia, recalled with the mnemonic CHINA (**Table 5**), can be varied. A common cause of eosinophilia, helminth infection should be considered in all patients. Strongyloidiasis can cause eosinophilia and is endemic in the southeastern United States. Eosinophilia may be the only manifestation of this disease, and affected patients can develop disseminated disease if glucocorticoids are mistakenly given to treat hypereosinophilic syndrome (HES).

TABLE 5.	Causes of Eosinophilia
C	Collagen vascular disease (eosinophilic granulomatosis with polyangiitis)
H	Helminthic (parasitic worm) infection (*Strongyloides*)
I	Idiopathic hypereosinophilic syndrome (cause unknown after extensive evaluation)
N	Neoplasia (lymphomas most common; myeloproliferative neoplasms)
A	Allergy, atopy, asthma (also drug induced: carbamazepine, sulfonamides)

HES is characterized by sustained eosinophil counts greater than 1500/µL (1.5×10^9/L) and associated end-organ damage attributed to eosinophilia, typically affecting the skin, lungs, heart, gastrointestinal tract, and brain, regardless of causes attributable to eosinophilia. The hypereosinophilic syndrome may be seen in patients with secondary eosinophilia or in those with a primary MPN.

Primary (neoplastic) hypereosinophilic syndrome is an MPN with eosinophilia commonly associated with activation of tyrosine kinase platelet-derived growth factor receptor α or β. Other neoplasms, such as MPNs, AML, lymphomas, and solid tumors, can also manifest with eosinophilia. Treatment of underlying conditions can alleviate eosinophilia. Glucocorticoids are used for treatment of idiopathic HES. In patients with platelet-derived growth factor receptor mutation, imatinib has been shown to be effective.

KEY POINT

- Hypereosinophilic syndrome is characterized by sustained eosinophil counts greater than 1500/µL (1.5×10^9/L) and associated end-organ damage attributable to eosinophilia; it may arise secondary to a variety of underlying causes or from a primary myeloproliferative neoplasm.

Acute Leukemias

Acute leukemia is a hematologic malignancy characterized by infiltration of the bone marrow, blood, and other tissues by uncontrolled proliferation and abnormal delayed differentiation of clonal myeloid or lymphoid precursor cells, exceeding 20% of the bone marrow or blood. In adults, acute myeloid leukemia (AML) is more common than acute lymphoblastic leukemia (ALL).

Acute Myeloid Leukemia

AML typically manifests with anemia, thrombocytopenia, or functional neutropenia secondary to bone marrow replacement with abnormal myeloblasts. Petechiae, epistaxis, and other mucosal hemorrhages occur when the platelet count dips below 20,000/µL (20×10^9/L). Symptoms of anemia vary more with patient's age and comorbidities. Although the leukocyte count is typically elevated, the absolute neutrophil count tends to be low, which confers an increased risk of infection. Myeloblasts are usually seen in the peripheral blood smear but may be absent despite unequivocal bone marrow infiltration. AML is curable in 35% to 40% of adult patients 60 years of age or younger, but the cure rate decreases to just 5% to 15% in adults older than 60 years, when comorbidities, such as cardiopulmonary disease, also preclude the use of intensive chemotherapy.

Cytogenetic and molecular classification of AML has gained increasing importance in recent years. Acute promyelocytic leukemia, characterized by poorly differentiated leukocytes with distinctive primary granules that contribute to

coagulopathy (**Figure 4**) and chromosomal translocation t(15;17), was an earlier prototype for targeted therapy in hematologic malignancies because many patients achieved, and continue to achieve, cure with all-*trans* retinoic acid, which targets the underlying defect in cell differentiation. A growing number of molecular markers are used to guide therapy. *NPM1*-mutated AML is found in about half of patients and appears overtly normal cytogenetically; it is associated with a favorable outcome. In contrast, *FLT3-ITD* identification (found in approximately one third of patients with cytogenetically normal AML) is associated with an unfavorable outcome and merits consideration for allogeneic transplantation in first remission.

The treatment of AML consists of induction therapy with an anthracycline (such as daunorubicin) and infusional cytarabine. The goal is to ablate the bone marrow, eliminating the blasts, although this transiently destroys the normal hematopoietic cells as well. Cells are expected to recover after a period of aplasia, which extends for 3 to 4 weeks, during which time the patient is supported by transfusions (erythrocytes and platelets) and prompt antibiotic treatment of neutropenic fever. A complete response is achieved in 60% to 85% of patients younger than 60 years. Consolidation therapy for responders consists of additional cycles of conventional chemotherapy in patients at low risk and allogeneic hematopoietic stem cell transplantation for patients at high risk. Treatment for older or frail patients is unsatisfactory; symptom management may include blood and platelet transfusions along with lower dose, often single-agent chemotherapy, such as oral hydroxyurea, low-dose cytarabine, and the hypomethylating agents decitabine and azacitidine. These patients are expected to survive only months. Hospice care should also be considered.

Acute Lymphoblastic Leukemia

ALL is more common in children and adolescents than in adults. Although ALL in children is often curable, survival in

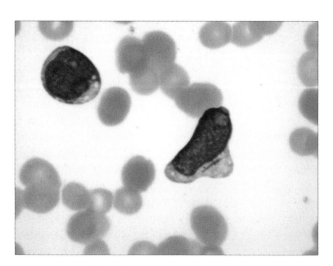

FIGURE 4. This peripheral blood smear shows an immature granulocyte with a rod-shaped inclusion body (Auer rod) characteristic of acute myeloid leukemia.

CONT.

adult patients (older than 19 years) remains inferior despite the adoption of pediatric ALL regimens. Patients with ALL present with malaise, bleeding, infections, bone pain, or a combination of these symptoms, with a small subset (<10%) having symptomatic central nervous system involvement at diagnosis. In adults, 75% of ALL is of B-cell lineage; mature B-cell ALL can present as extramedullary disease, including gastrointestinal or testicular involvement. A mediastinal mass with wheezing and stridor or skin involvement can be the presenting features of T-cell ALL. Similar to AML, ALL is classified by immunophenotype, cytogenetics, and molecular abnormalities. The most important cytogenetic abnormality in adult ALL is the Philadelphia chromosome, found in 20% to 30% of patients. Historically, Philadelphia chromosome–positive ALL had a poor prognosis. In the modern era, the use of tyrosine kinase inhibitors, such as imatinib and dasatinib, along with more traditional chemotherapy has dramatically improved remission rates. After remission induction, patients with Philadelphia chromosome–positive ALL should receive additional intensive consolidation, such as autologous or allogeneic hematopoietic stem cell transplantation.

Treatment regimens are complex. Regimen backbones include vincristine, anthracycline, corticosteroids, and L-asparaginase. Some of these agents have unique toxicities such as allergic reactions, hypofibrinogenemia and hypertriglyceridemia with L-asparaginase. Induction therapy is followed by intensification and consolidation. Unlike in AML, central nervous system prophylaxis is essential during ALL therapy, and a maintenance phase of oral mercaptopurine (daily) and methotrexate (weekly) can extend up to 2 years. Medication adherence can be problematic during the maintenance phase.

Adult survivors of childhood leukemia face higher risks of secondary cancer, cardiovascular disease, and the metabolic syndrome (high BMI, truncal obesity, dyslipidemia, insulin resistance, and hypertension) compared with age-matched controls. Primary care physicians encountering such patients should request a treatment summary from the treating facility and encourage patient participation in a local survivor clinic. Screening for lipid profile, diabetes, and hypertension is recommended. Echocardiography to screen for left ventricular dysfunction should be performed at intervals of 3 to 5 years, particularly if anthracycline exposure was high (such as doxorubicin exceeding 300 mg/m²) or if chest radiation was used. Female survivors have a higher risk of myocardial dysfunction during pregnancy. High-dose glucocorticoids, typical of ALL regimens, pose a risk for osteopenia. The cumulative incidence of secondary cancer after radiation therapy for childhood ALL reaches 11% at 30 years; tumors include skin cancer, thyroid and parotid tumors, sarcomas, and brain tumors. Cranial radiation also increases the risk for stroke and neurocognitive defects. Patients should be counseled about lifestyle risk

factors, age-based screening, and early reporting of persistent symptoms.

KEY POINTS

- Acute myeloid leukemia typically manifests with anemia, thrombocytopenia, or functional neutropenia secondary to bone marrow replacement with abnormal myeloblasts, and petechiae and other signs of mucosal bleeding are quite common when the platelet count dips below 20,000/µL (20 × 10⁹/L).

- Treatment of acute myeloid leukemia consists of induction therapy with an anthracycline and infusional cytarabine, followed by consolidation therapy for responders, consisting of additional cycles of conventional chemotherapy for patients at low risk and allogeneic hematopoietic stem cell transplantation for patients at high risk.

- After remission induction with therapy that includes a tyrosine kinase inhibitor, patients with Philadelphia chromosome–positive acute lymphoblastic leukemia should receive additional intensive consolidation such as autologous or allogeneic hematopoietic stem cell transplantation.

Hematopoietic Growth Factors

Erythropoiesis-stimulating agents (which include erythropoietin and darbepoetin) are primarily used in patients with anemia and chronic kidney disease; for patients receiving dialysis, the target hemoglobin level should be no greater than 12 g/dL (120 g/L) to avoid adverse cardiovascular outcomes. Granulocyte colony-stimulating factors (with various formulations) are used to prevent febrile neutropenia in patients receiving myelosuppressive chemotherapy who are at high risk of febrile neutropenia, such as those receiving intensive chemotherapy for high-risk breast cancer and those aged 65 or older with diffuse aggressive lymphoma being treated with curative chemotherapy. Granulocyte colony-stimulating factor is not indicated for most patients with neutropenia who are afebrile, as a routine adjunct to empiric antibiotics for patients presenting with febrile neutropenia, or for patients undergoing induction chemotherapy for acute leukemia.

Hematopoietic Stem Cell Transplantation

Autologous hematopoietic stem cell transplantation is performed in select patients who have multiple myeloma or relapsed aggressive lymphoma. Allogeneic transplantation is indicated in patients at high risk with acute leukemia and for the graft-versus-leukemia effect. Allogeneic transplantation is also used to treat patients with aplastic anemia and select patients with hemoglobinopathies such as sickle cell anemia. The allogeneic donor is typically an HLA-matched sibling or unrelated adult donor; the risk of graft-versus-host disease, which includes skin, gastrointestinal, and liver manifestations, increases with the degree of donor-recipient HLA disparity. Better supportive measures and reduced-intensity regimens have provided transplant eligibility to older adults. Although hematopoietic stem cell transplantation carries a significant risk of transplant-related mortality, survivors continue to have long-term morbidities unrelated to relapse, such as susceptibility to bacterial or viral infections and delayed pulmonary toxicity. Internists caring for patients who have undergone transplantation should evaluate patients early for symptoms suggesting infection and follow recommended immunization schedules that take into account the prolonged immunosuppressed state of these patients (see MKSAP 18 General Internal Medicine). H

Multiple Myeloma and Related Disorders

Overview

B-cell maturation to plasma cells involves early antigen-independent and antigen-dependent phases. When humoral immunity is stimulated by an infection or inflammation, multiple clones of plasma cells are expanded. These plasma cell clones can produce immunoglobulins of different classes and specificity, giving the characteristic polyclonal spike seen on protein electrophoresis. In contrast, plasma cell dyscrasias (PCDs) or monoclonal gammopathies have clonal expansion of the plasma cell or lymphoplasmacytic cells, which produce the characteristic monoclonal spike (M spike) on protein electrophoresis. This monoclonal (M) protein can be a complete immunoglobulin, with a heavy chain (IgG, IgA, IgD, or IgM) complexed with a light chain (κ or λ), or free light chains (FLCs) without a heavy chain component. Various PCDs have been described (**Table 6**). Note that M spike denotes the presence of M protein, whereas IgM is the immunoglobulin M.

Evaluation for Monoclonal Gammopathies

Monoclonal gammopathy of undetermined significance (MGUS) occurs in approximately 3% of persons older than 50 years, and most remain asymptomatic without progression. It is a clonal premalignant disorder with low risk of conversion to other PCDs. Testing is typically restricted to patients with symptoms and signs of PCD (**Table 7**).

The M protein in PCDs can be detected by serum or urine protein electrophoresis (SPEP and UPEP). Occasionally, the M protein is not a full immunoglobulin but rather isolated light chains (κ or λ) that might be missed on protein electrophoresis. SPEP and UPEP can be good initial screening tests to identify and quantify the presence of an M spike, and the serum

FLC assay is a sensitive test to identify and quantify FLCs in the serum. Neither SPEP nor UPEP can identify the subtype of immunoglobulin in the M spike, and both may miss small M proteins. Serum and urine immunofixation are more sensitive tests that can subtype the immunoglobulin and differentiate a monoclonal spike from a polyclonal spike. Polyclonal spikes are commonly found in infections, inflammatory processes, and chronic liver disease and do not usually require further hematologic evaluation. Serum FLC testing detects light chains that are not bound to heavy chains and helps quantify them. In inflammatory and infectious processes, κ and λ FLCs are increased, but the ratio remains normal because they increase proportionately. In patients with a PCD, the clonal plasma cells secrete one type of FLC, leading to an increase in the involved light chain and an abnormal FLC ratio. SPEP, serum immunofixation, and serum FLC testing are commonly used for the initial evaluation of PCDs.

Although MGUS and multiple myeloma are common causes of abnormal M proteins, other disorders can also produce an M spike (see Table 6), and patients should be evaluated for the signs and symptoms of these diseases (see Table 7). Tests considered during the evaluation of monoclonal gammopathies include complete blood count with differential; serum chemistries, including creatinine, calcium, and albumin levels; β_2-microglobulin; SPEP; UPEP; serum and urine immunofixation; serum FLC tests; and quantitative immunoglobulins. Plain radiographs of the bones (skeletal surveys) are used to assess for the presence of lytic lesions. Skeletal surveys

TABLE 6. Disorders Associated with Monoclonal Gammopathies
Plasma Cell Disorders
Monoclonal gammopathy of undetermined significance[a]
Multiple myeloma
Immunoglobulin light-chain (AL) amyloidosis
Monoclonal immunoglobulin deposition disease
Proximal tubulopathy (with or without Fanconi syndrome)
Solitary plasmacytoma
Solitary plasmacytoma of bone
Solitary extramedullary plasmacytoma
POEMS syndrome[b]/osteosclerotic myeloma
B-cell Disorders
Waldenström macroglobulinemia/lymphoplasmacytic lymphoma
Marginal zone lymphoma
Chronic lymphocytic leukemia/small lymphocytic lymphoma
Heavy chain disease

[a]Many diseases may be associated with monoclonocal gammopathy of undetermined significance, including but not limited to connective tissue diseases, hepatitis C, HIV, cryoglobulinemia, and cold agglutinin disease.

[b]Polyneuropathy, Organomegaly, Endocrinopathy, presence of M protein, and Skin changes.

TABLE 7.	Common Clinical Scenarios for Consideration of Plasma Cell Dyscrasia Testing[a]		
Clinical Scenario	**Disease Considerations**	**Disease Characteristics**	**Additional Investigative Evaluation[b]**
Lytic bone lesions or hypercalcemia	MM	Osteolytic bone lesions, PTH-independent hypercalcemia	Standard investigative evaluation
Age-inappropriate bone loss[c]	MGUS, MM	Osteopenia or osteoporosis with or without associated fractures	Standard investigative evaluation
Peripheral neuropathy	AL amyloidosis; MM, WM (rare), MGUS	Sensorimotor axonal polyneuropathy	Tissue aspirate/biopsy for amyloid
	POEMS syndrome; MGUS, MM, solitary plasmacytoma of bone	Sensorimotor inflammatory demyelinating polyneuropathy, hepatosplenomegaly, endocrinopathies (hypogonadism, adrenal insufficiency), hyperpigmentation, hypertrichosis, multicentric Castleman disease, osteosclerotic bone lesions	VEGF, endocrine evaluation (e.g., testosterone level)
	Cryoglobulinemic vasculitis; MGUS, MM, B-cell non-Hodgkin lymphoma (e.g., WM)	Sensory or sensorimotor polyneuropathy, mononeuropathy multiplex	Cryoglobulins, complement levels, hepatitis evaluation
Kidney disease	Cast nephropathy; MM	Acute kidney injury, nonalbumin proteinuria (monoclonal FLCs), bland urine sediment	Kidney biopsy
	AL amyloidosis; MGUS, MM	Nephrotic syndrome	Tissue aspirate/biopsy for amyloid
	Monoclonal gammopathy of renal significance	Varied kidney manifestations in patients who otherwise meet criteria for MGUS with a small plasma clone	Kidney biopsy
	Proximal tubulopathy +/− Fanconi syndrome	Normal anion gap, hyperchloremic metabolic acidosis, hypophosphatemia, hypouricemia, renal glucosuria, amino aciduria	Kidney biopsy, serum phosphorus and uric acid, urinalysis
	Cryoglobulinemic vasculitis	Membranoproliferative glomerulonephritis with proteinuria and active urinary sediment	Cryoglobulins, complement levels, hepatitis evaluation
Anemia	MM	Normocytic (occasionally macrocytic) anemia	Standard investigative evaluation

AL amyloidosis = immunoglobulin light-chain amyloidosis; FLC = free light chain; MGUS = monoclonal gammopathy of undetermined significance; MM = multiple myeloma; POEMS = Polyneuropathy, Organomegaly, Endocrinopathy, M protein, and Skin changes; PTH = parathyroid hormone; VEGF = vascular endothelial growth factor; WM = Waldenström macroglobulinemia.

[a]This is not an all-inclusive list; other less common conditions can be associated with plasma cell dyscrasias.

[b]Evaluation beyond the standard evaluation for a monoclonal gammopathy.

[c]Premenopausal women or men <65 years of age with no additional risk factors for bone loss.

CONT.

are used to assess for lytic lesions in multiple myeloma. Bone scans, which detect increased osteoblast activity in most bone metastases, may not detect the more purely lytic lesions in multiple myeloma and should not be used. In select patients, PET scans and MRI are required to accurately evaluate bone lesions.

Bone marrow aspirate and biopsy quantifies the percentage of plasma cells in the marrow and help classify the PCD. Cytogenetic evaluation of the bone marrow aspirate helps establish an accurate prognosis. Bone marrow testing can be deferred in patients with low-risk features, such as an IgG gammopathy measuring less than 1.5 g/dL, a normal serum FLC ratio, and no evidence of end-organ damage. **H**

KEY POINTS

- Tests useful in the evaluation of monoclonal gammopathies include complete blood count with differential, serum chemistries, β_2-microglobulin, serum and urine protein electrophoresis, serum and urine immunofixation, serum free light chain testing, and quantitative immunoglobulins.

- Bone marrow evaluation need not be undertaken in patients with a monoclonal gammopathy and low-risk features, such as an IgG gammopathy less than 1.5 g/dL, normal serum free light chain ratio, and no end-organ damage.

HVC

Monoclonal Gammopathy of Undetermined Significance

MGUS is characterized by an M protein level less than 3 g/dL (or less than 500 mg/24 h of urinary monoclonal FLCs), clonal plasma cells comprising less than 10% of the bone marrow cellularity, and the absence of related signs and symptoms of end-organ damage (**Table 8**). MGUS is diagnosed incidentally during evaluation for various signs and symptoms such as neuropathy, vasculitis, elevated protein, or end-organ damage.

The prevalence of MGUS increases with age and is noted in approximately 5% of persons older than 70 years. When an asymptomatic condition has a high prevalence rate and low risk of progression to symptomatic disease, it is important to provide an accurate prognosis and appropriate counseling and management. Non-IgM, IgM, and light-chain MGUS are the three types, based on type of M protein. Non-IgM MGUS can progress to multiple myeloma and, although less likely, to other PCDs at a rate of 1% per year. IgM MGUS has the potential to progress to Waldenström macroglobulinemia at a rate of 1.5% per year. Light-chain MGUS can progress to other PCDs at a rate of 0.3%. In addition to the type of M protein, factors that predict the risk of progression include the quantity of M protein and an abnormal serum FLC ratio (**Table 9**).

TABLE 8. Diagnostic Criteria for the Plasma and Lymphoplasmacytic Cell Dyscrasias

Diagnosis	M Protein	Bone Marrow Clonal Plasma Cells or Lymphoid Cells	Disease-Specific Signs/Symptoms
MGUS			
Non-IgM (IgG, IgA)	<3 g/dL	<10%	No
IgM	<3 g/dL	<10%	No
Light chain[a]	Affected serum FLC increased and serum FLC ratio increased	<10%	No
	Urinary M protein <500 mg/24 h		
Smoldering myeloma[b]	IgG or IgA ≥3 g/dL or κ or λ urinary FLC M protein ≥500 mg/24 hr	10%-59%	No
Smoldering WM[b]	IgM ≥3 g/dL	≥10%	No
Multiple myeloma requiring therapy	Present (absent in nonsecretory disease)	≥10% or biopsy evidence of a bony or extramedullary plasmacytoma	Yes
WM requiring therapy	Present	≥10%	Yes

CRAB Criteria for Myeloma-Related Signs and Symptoms

HyperCalcemia: Serum calcium >11 mg/dL (2.8 mmol/L) or >1 mg/dL (0.3 mmol/L) higher than the upper limit of normal

Renal failure: Serum creatinine >2 mg/dL (177 μmol/L) or creatinine clearance <40 mL/min

Anemia: Hemoglobin <10 g/dL (100 g/L) or 2 g/dL (20 g/L) below the lower limit of normal

Bone disease: ≥1 lytic bone lesions on imaging studies

Myeloma-Defining Biomarkers for Myeloma-Related Signs and Symptoms

≥60% clonal plasma cells on bone marrow examination

Involved: uninvolved serum FLC ratio ≥10[c]

≥1 focal lesion on MRI

WM-Related Signs and Symptoms

Systemic symptoms: Fatigue, B symptoms (fevers, night sweats, weight loss), neuropathy, hyperviscosity

Physical examination findings: Symptomatic lymphadenopathy or hepatosplenomegaly

Laboratory findings: Cytopenias (anemia, thrombocytopenia)

FLC = free light chain; MGUS = monoclonal gammopathy of undetermined significance; WM = Waldenström macroglobulinemia.

[a]Light-chain MGUS does not have a heavy-chain component.

[b]Smoldering myeloma or WM may have the diagnostic M protein level with or without the percentage of bone marrow clonal plasma or lymphoid cells.

[c]Involved light chain must be greater than 100 mg/dL.

Data from Rajkumar SV, Dimopoulos MA, Palumbo A, Blade J, Merlini G, Mateos MV, et al. International Myeloma Working Group updated criteria for the diagnosis of multiple myeloma. Lancet Oncol. 2014;15:e538-48. [PMID: 25439696] doi:10.1016/S1470-2045(14)70442-5

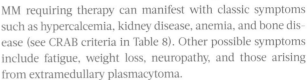

TABLE 9.	Risk of MGUS Progression to a Clinically Symptomatic Plasma Cell Dyscrasia	
Diagnosis	**Risk Factors**	**Progression**
Non-light chain MGUS (IgG, IgA, IgM)	M protein ≥1.5 g/dL	At 20 years:
	Non-IgG M protein	3 RFs: 58%
	Abnormal serum FLC ratio	2 RFs: 37%
		1 RF: 21%
		0 RFs: 5%
Smoldering myeloma	M protein ≥3 g/dL	At 5 years:
	Bone marrow plasma cells ≥10%	3 RFs: 76%
		2 RFs: 51%
	Serum FLC ratio <0.125 or >8 mg/dL	1 RF: 25%

FLC = free light chain; MGUS = monoclonal gammopathy of undetermined significance; RF = risk factor.

Data adapted from Rajkumar SV, Kyle RA, Therneau TM, Melton LJ 3rd, Bradwell AR, Clark RJ, et al. Serum free light chain ratio is an independent risk factor for progression in monoclonal gammopathy of undetermined significance. Blood. 2005;106:812-7. [PMID: 15855274]; and Dispenzieri A, Kyle RA, Katzmann JA, Therneau TM, Larson D, Benson J, et al. Immunoglobulin free light chain ratio is an independent risk factor for progression of smoldering (asymptomatic) multiple myeloma. Blood. 2008;111:785-9. [PMID: 17942755]

In addition to the risk of progression, patients with MGUS are at higher risk of osteoporosis and fracture of the axial skeleton, and bone mineral density testing should be considered. Treatment is not required at diagnosis. Patients commonly undergo follow-up for signs and symptoms of progression, initially at 6 months and then yearly, if stable.

Kidney disease in patients with monoclonal gammopathy has traditionally been linked to light-chain nephrotoxicity in those with multiple myeloma or amyloid infiltration in those with amyloidosis. More recent data suggest that some patients with features otherwise quite consistent with MGUS may, nonetheless, have significant kidney disease related to the abnormal immunoglobulin. If other, more likely causes of kidney injury are excluded (for example, diabetes or hypertension), these patients should be diagnosed with monoclonal gammopathy of renal significance and require aggressive myeloma-like therapy to prevent progressive and irreversible kidney injury.

KEY POINT

- Monoclonal gammopathy of undetermined significance is characterized by an M protein level less than 3 g/dL, clonal plasma cells comprising less than 10% of the bone marrow cellularity, and the absence of related signs and symptoms of end-organ damage.

Multiple Myeloma

Multiple myeloma (MM) is a clonal plasma cell neoplasm. MM can present as smoldering (asymptomatic) disease with risk of progression or as symptomatic disease, which requires immediate treatment to prevent complications. Smoldering MM has a higher clonal plasma cell burden than MGUS and a higher risk of transformation to MM requiring therapy.

Clinical Manifestations and Findings

MM requiring therapy can manifest with classic symptoms such as hypercalcemia, kidney disease, anemia, and bone disease (see CRAB criteria in Table 8). Other possible symptoms include fatigue, weight loss, neuropathy, and those arising from extramedullary plasmacytoma.

Normocytic anemia is a common finding in MM requiring therapy. Anemia is caused by bone marrow plasma cell infiltration and kidney disease. The peripheral blood smear may show rouleaux formation (**Figure 5**). Patients can also be immunosuppressed from leukopenia, impaired lymphocyte function, and hypogammaglobulinemia. Although patients with MM can have increased total immunoglobulin, normal immunoglobulins are usually reduced. Patients are at increased risk of respiratory infections, and chemotherapy for MM can further increase this risk.

Bone pain is a common symptom of MM. Osteoclast activation and osteoblast inactivation occur, leading to development of lytic lesions (**Figure 6**) and vertebral body compression fracture. This increased bone resorption leads to hypercalcemia. Patients with MM are prone to developing pathologic fractures with minimal or no trauma.

Kidney dysfunction with an elevated creatinine level or occult injury is seen in a significant proportion of patients. The two main causes of kidney disease are elevated FLCs causing cast nephropathy and hypercalcemia. Cast nephropathy, commonly termed myeloma kidney, is caused by deposition of FLCs in the distal tubules, leading to tubulointerstitial damage. Underlying cast nephropathy makes these patients especially vulnerable to additional kidney injury through dehydration, NSAID use, or exposure to radioiodine contrast. Other causes of kidney dysfunction in MM include

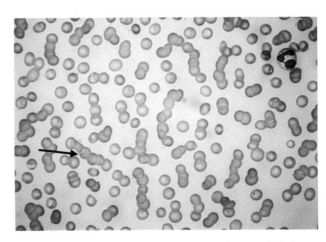

FIGURE 5. Peripheral blood smear showing rouleaux formation. This finding can be seen in patients with multiple myeloma. Rouleaux refers to the appearance of erythrocytes stacked on each other (*arrow*). Various conditions can cause rouleaux formation, including poor preparation of the blood smear.

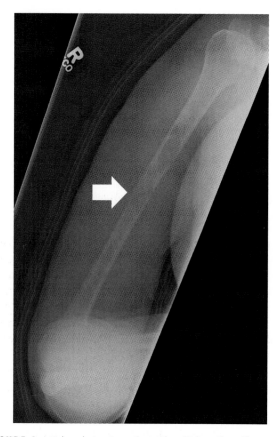

FIGURE 6. Lytic bone lesions in a patient with multiple myeloma. The arrow denotes an oblique pathologic fracture through a mid-humerus lytic lesion. Other lytic lesions can be seen both proximal and distal to the fracture.

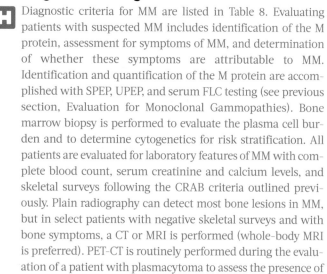

CONT. immunoglobulin light-chain amyloidosis, cryoglobulinemic glomerulonephritis, and proximal tubulopathy.

Diagnosis and Prognosis

Diagnostic criteria for MM are listed in Table 8. Evaluating patients with suspected MM includes identification of the M protein, assessment for symptoms of MM, and determination of whether these symptoms are attributable to MM. Identification and quantification of the M protein are accomplished with SPEP, UPEP, and serum FLC testing (see previous section, Evaluation for Monoclonal Gammopathies). Bone marrow biopsy is performed to evaluate the plasma cell burden and to determine cytogenetics for risk stratification. All patients are evaluated for laboratory features of MM with complete blood count, serum creatinine and calcium levels, and skeletal surveys following the CRAB criteria outlined previously. Plain radiography can detect most bone lesions in MM, but in select patients with negative skeletal surveys and with bone symptoms, a CT or MRI is performed (whole-body MRI is preferred). PET-CT is routinely performed during the evaluation of a patient with plasmacytoma to assess the presence of additional occult extramedullary tumors.

Symptoms of organ dysfunction should not necessarily be attributed to the underlying PCD. Kidney biopsy is performed to document myeloma kidney when it is clinically difficult to differentiate kidney injury from another diagnosis, such as diabetic nephropathy. Evaluation for alternative causes of hypercalcemia and anemia should be completed, especially when the patient has low-risk disease.

Smoldering MM has a risk of conversion to MM requiring therapy of about 10% per year for the first 5 years. The risk of progression decreases after the first 5 years. This risk is not uniform; risk factors for progression include a high M protein level, a large burden of clonal plasma cells, and an abnormal serum FLC ratio (see Table 9). Patients with smoldering MM at imminent risk of progression in the next 2 years and therefore requiring immediate therapy include those with 60% or more plasma cells in the bone marrow, more than one focal bone lesion on MRI, or a serum FLC ratio of 0.01 or less or 100 or greater.

MM is staged based on serum markers such as β2-microglobulin and albumin. However, cytogenetics of the bone marrow more accurately predict prognosis and sometimes guide better treatment decisions.

Treatment

Patients with smoldering MM are usually monitored for progression to MM requiring therapy every 3 to 6 months without beginning treatment. Recent studies have shown improved survival with treatment of high-risk smoldering MM; however, defining these patients at high risk is somewhat controversial, and it is not routine practice to treat them. Bisphosphonates do not decrease the risk of progression in smoldering MM.

Treatment of MM requiring therapy has been revolutionized over the last few years with the advent of new treatment options, which have significantly improved survival (averaging almost 10 years from diagnosis). Patients are initially evaluated for autologous hematopoietic stem cell transplantation (HSCT) eligibility. Autologous HSCT with high-dose melphalan is not curative in MM but does improve progression-free and overall survival. Patients eligible for transplant typically undergo induction therapy with multiagent chemotherapy followed by autologous HSCT and close observation or maintenance therapy. Induction chemotherapy involves various combinations of immunomodulatory drugs (lenalidomide or thalidomide), proteasome inhibitors (bortezomib), glucocorticoids (dexamethasone), and alkylating agents (melphalan or cyclophosphamide).

Treatment for MM is not curative, so all patients eventually present with relapsed or refractory disease. Several new drugs have been approved in this setting, including proteasome inhibitors (carfilzomib and ixazomib), the immunomodulatory drug pomalidomide, histone deacetylase inhibitors (panobinostat), and monoclonal antibodies (daratumumab and elotuzumab). These new agents are effective, and studies are under way evaluating them in the first-line setting.

Agents used to treat MM have unique side effects. Lenalidomide and pomalidomide carry a risk of venous thromboembolism (VTE), and patients are considered for thromboprophylaxis. Bortezomib and thalidomide cause peripheral neuropathy. Bortezomib is associated with a high risk of herpes zoster reactivation; prophylactic therapy with acyclovir is recommended.

Pain is a dominant symptom in patients with MM requiring therapy, and many patients require treatment with opioids; NSAIDs can worsen kidney disease in these patients. Surgical stabilization of impending fracture is undertaken to prevent morbidity. Bisphosphonates (zoledronic acid and pamidronate) are used to prevent skeletal events. Zoledronic acid has also been shown to improve survival in MM requiring therapy. Patients taking bisphosphonates should be closely monitored for hypocalcemia and osteonecrosis of the jaw.

Nephrotoxic agents and contrast studies should be used judiciously in patients with MM and a risk of worsening kidney disease. Hypercalcemia is treated with hydration and bisphosphonates. Annual influenza vaccination (inactivated) should be administered to all patients with MM. Because of the immunocompromised state of MM, pneumococcal vaccination with the 13-valent pneumococcal conjugate vaccine and 23-valent pneumococcal polysaccharide vaccine should be administered in accordance with Advisory Committee on Immunization Practices guidelines (see MKSAP 18 General Internal Medicine). Select patients with recurrent infections and hypogammaglobulinemia benefit from intravenous immune globulin infusions. **H**

KEY POINTS

- Hypercalcemia, kidney disease, anemia, and bone disease are classic symptoms of multiple myeloma requiring therapy, which is defined by the presence of an M protein and 10% or more clonal plasma or lymphoid cells in the bone marrow.

- Smoldering multiple myeloma is defined by immunoglobulin levels and the percentage of plasma cells exceeding limits for monoclonal gammopathy of undetermined significance in patients with no disease-specific symptoms; most of these patients do not require immediate chemotherapy but should be closely monitored to assess disease progression.

(Continued)

KEY POINTS *(continued)*

- Bisphosphonates should be routinely prescribed in patients with myeloma requiring therapy because they prevent skeletal events and improve survival.

- Patients with multiple myeloma eligible for transplant typically receive induction therapy with multiagent chemotherapy followed by autologous hematopoietic stem cell transplantation and close observation or maintenance therapy.

Immunoglobulin Light-Chain Amyloidosis

Amyloidosis refers to a varied group of disorders associated with extracellular deposition of low-molecular-weight proteins in a β-pleated sheet configuration. These are usually abnormal proteins that circulate in the blood and deposit in various organs. Various proteins have been implicated in amyloidosis (**Table 10**). All amyloid deposits have a characteristic apple-green birefringence under polarized light microscopy of the tissue with Congo red staining.

Light-chain amyloidosis (AL) is the most common type. It is a clonal plasma cell dyscrasia characterized by production of amyloidogenic λ or κ free light chains. These light chains can deposit in various organs, resulting in varying clinical presentations of the disease (**Table 11**, **Figure 7**). Diagnosis requires biopsy of the affected tissue that shows the characteristic pathological findings. To avoid invasive biopsy, fat pad or bone marrow biopsy is sometimes performed initially. After confirmation of the amyloid in the tissue, immunohistochemical staining can confirm the light-chain composition of the amyloid deposit or identify alternative components, such as transthyretin or amyloid A protein. Patients with AL amyloidosis should undergo analysis for clonal plasma cell dyscrasias with serum and urine protein electrophoresis, serum FLC testing, and bone marrow biopsy.

All patients are evaluated for extent of organ involvement. Cardiac involvement is common with AL amyloidosis,

TABLE 10.	The Amyloidoses	
Type	**Disease Association**	**Amyloid Protein**
AL amyloidosis	Plasma cell dyscrasias (MGUS, multiple myeloma), Waldenström macroglobulinemia (rare)	Monoclonal free λ or κ light chains
Hereditary amyloidosis	Inherited	Mutated transthyretin (TTR), fibrinogen α chain[a]
AA amyloidosis	Rheumatoid arthritis, inflammatory bowel disease, familial Mediterranean fever, chronic infection	Serum amyloid A protein
Age-related (senile) amyloidosis	Age	Wild-type TTR
Dialysis-related amyloidosis	Dialysis for any reason	β_2-microglobulin

AA = amyloid A (secondary) amyloidosis; AL = immunoglobulin light-chain amyloidosis; MGUS = monoclonal gammopathy of undetermined significance.

[a]Not an all-inclusive list.

Multiple Myeloma and Related Disorders

TABLE 11. Clinical Manifestations of AL Amyloidosis by Organ System

Organ System	Clinical Manifestations	Findings
Kidney	Anasarca, lower extremity edema, foamy urine	Nephrotic range proteinuria with bland urine sediment, hypoalbuminemia, elevated creatinine, nephromegaly on kidney ultrasonography
Gastrointestinal	Gastrointestinal bleeding, dysphagia, early satiety, abdominal distention, steatorrhea	Anemia, iron deficiency, submucosal hematomas on endoscopy, hypoalbuminemia, delayed gastric emptying, intestinal pseudo-obstruction, malabsorption, small bowel bacterial overgrowth
Liver	Weight loss, abdominal pain, features of chronic liver disease and portal hypertension	Cholestatic liver test abnormalities, hepatosplenomegaly, ascites, varices, evidence of portal hypertension
Neurologic	Distal numbness, paresthesias, neuropathic pain, weakness, autonomic nerve dysfunction	Distal sensorimotor polyneuropathy on electromyography/nerve conduction studies, autonomic neuropathy
Cardiac	Chest pain, symptoms from chronic heart failure or arrhythmia	Echocardiographic changes (ventricular hypertrophy with granular appearance, restrictive cardiomyopathy with diastolic heart failure greater than systolic heart failure), electrocardiographic changes (low voltages, pseudoinfarct pattern, conduction system changes, arrhythmias), abnormal cardiac MRI (late gadolinium enhancement)
Coagulation	Bleeding diathesis, periorbital purpura	Factor X deficiency with prolonged PT and aPTT, prolonged PT and aPTT from advanced liver impairment, blood vessel fragility from vascular amyloid deposition
Musculoskeletal	Macroglossia (see Figure 7), muscle pseudohypertrophy, symmetric arthropathy, submandibular gland enlargement, carpal tunnel syndrome	Carpal tunnel syndrome on electromyography/nerve conduction studies, joint space widening on plain radiographs, periarticular soft tissue and muscle infiltration on MRI

aPTT = activated partial thromboplastin time; PT = prothrombin time.

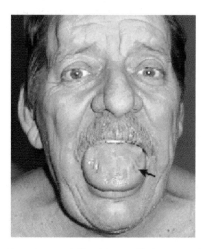

FIGURE 7. Macroglossia is a hallmark feature of light-chain amyloidosis. Heavy infiltration of amyloid restricts mobility of tongue. The tongue cannot be extended, and obstruction of the pharynx causes problems with deglutition and breathing. Note the indentations from teeth pressing on the enlarged tongue (*arrow*).

CONT.

and evaluation with echocardiography, electrocardiography, B-type natriuretic peptide, and serum troponin T is commonly performed. Cardiac MRI is more sensitive than echocardiography and has a distinctive pattern. Kidney involvement usually manifests as nephrotic range proteinuria; 24-hour urine assessment of the protein assists diagnosis. Other organs that can be involved and their clinical features are listed in Table 11. **H**

Prognosis of AL amyloidosis depends on the presence and extent of cardiac involvement; survival ranges from almost 8 years to only 6 months.

Treatment of AL amyloidosis starts with evaluating the patient for autologous HSCT. Eligibility for transplantation is based on age (younger than 70 years), performance status (independence completing activities of daily living), and the extent of organ involvement. Patients with advanced cardiac disease, stage 4 chronic kidney disease, or large effusions are generally not eligible for transplantation. Autologous HSCT has been shown to improve organ function and survival. Patients ineligible for transplant should receive treatment with melphalan- or bortezomib-based chemotherapy regimens. Supportive care to treat symptoms is necessary.

KEY POINTS

- Diagnosis of immunoglobulin light-chain amyloidosis requires biopsy of the affected tissue showing characteristic pathological findings of apple-green birefringence under polarized light microscopy of the tissue with Congo red staining; immunohistochemical staining then determines the light-chain nature of the amyloid.

- Patients with immunoglobulin light-chain amyloidosis who are ineligible for autologous hematopoietic stem cell transplantation should receive treatment with melphalan- or bortezomib-based chemotherapy regimens.

Waldenström Macroglobulinemia

Waldenström macroglobulinemia (WM) is an indolent B-cell lymphoma with clonal lymphoplasmacytic cells in the bone or lymph nodes that secrete clonal IgM in the blood. WM is differentiated from MGUS by the presence of more than 10% clonal lymphoplasmacytic cells in the bone marrow, greater than 3 g/dL of M protein, symptoms from the disease, or a combination of the three. As in multiple myeloma, patients with smoldering, asymptomatic WM can be observed without therapy.

Patients can present with classic "B symptoms" of drenching night sweats, fever, and weight loss and may have anemia and fatigue. Tissue infiltration leads to hepatosplenomegaly, lymphadenopathy, gastrointestinal dysfunction, and kidney disease. Peripheral sensorimotor neuropathy is seen in 20% of patients and can be associated with antimyelin-associated glycoprotein. Increased serum viscosity from the circulating IgM can lead to hyperviscosity syndrome. Hyperviscosity syndrome can include diverse central nervous system symptoms, including headache, altered mental status, change in vision and hearing, nystagmus, and ataxia. Funduscopic evaluation may reveal dilated retinal veins, papilledema, and flame hemorrhages. Mucosal bleeding is related to platelet dysfunction and dysfibrinogenemia (prolonged thrombin time).

 Symptomatic hyperviscosity requires emergent treatment with plasmapheresis to remove excess IgM. Therapy to decrease IgM production is instituted simultaneously in patients with hyperviscosity symptoms and should be initiated in other patients with symptomatic WM. Rituximab, either as a single agent or in combination with chemotherapy such as cyclophosphamide, bendamustine, and bortezomib, along with glucocorticoids, is commonly used. Recently, ibrutinib (a Bruton's tyrosine kinase inhibitor) has been approved for treatment of WM.

KEY POINT

- Patients with Waldenström macroglobulinemia can develop a hyperviscosity syndrome, with symptoms including altered mental status and diverse central nervous system symptoms, dilated retinal veins on funduscopic examination, and mucosal bleeding from impaired platelet function and dysfibrinogenemia.

Cryoglobulinemia

Cryoglobulinemia denotes the presence of clonal or polyclonal immunoglobulins that precipitate in the serum at temperatures less than 37 °C (98.6 °F) and dissolve with rewarming. Cold agglutinins, which are often confused with cryoglobulins, are antibodies against erythrocyte antigens that agglutinate erythrocytes in blood at temperatures less than 37 °C (98.6 °F) and can sometimes cause cold agglutinin autoimmune hemolytic anemia.

Cryoglobulinemias are classified as types I, II, and III based on the composition of the cryoglobulins. Type I cryoglobulinemia involves a monoclonal immunoglobulin, usually IgM, and is associated with plasma cell dyscrasias. Types II and III are called mixed cryoglobulinemias; they are composed of a mixture of polyclonal IgG and monoclonal or polyclonal IgM. Mixed cryoglobulinemias are usually seen in association with infections such as hepatitis C, with connective disorders, and rarely with lymphoproliferative disorders.

Type I cryoglobulinemia is usually asymptomatic but can rarely cause symptoms of hyperviscosity and thrombosis. Patients can present with digital cyanosis, ulcers, Raynaud phenomenon, or gangrene. Patients with neurologic symptoms from the hyperviscosity are treated with emergent plasmapheresis, along with treatment of the underlying plasma cell dyscrasia to prevent production of cryoglobulins. Vasculitic symptoms, such as palpable purpura, glomerulonephritis, and neuropathy, are less common in type I (see MKSAP 18 Rheumatology for further information on mixed cryoglobulinemias).

KEY POINTS

- Type I cryoglobulinemia involves a monoclonal immunoglobulin, usually IgM, is associated with plasma cell dyscrasias, and is typically asymptomatic.
- Types II and III mixed cryoglobulinemias are composed of a mixture of polyclonal IgG and monoclonal or polyclonal IgM and are usually seen in association with hepatitis C, connective disorders, or lymphoproliferative disorders.

Erythrocyte Disorders

Approach to Anemia

Anemia is a pathologic state resulting in an insufficient number of erythrocytes to deliver oxygen to organs and tissues. Anemia can arise from blood loss, underproduction of erythrocytes, destruction of erythrocytes (hemolysis), or a combination of these factors. Patients with chronic anemia may be entirely asymptomatic or may experience symptoms of dyspnea, decreased exercise tolerance, palpitations, lightheadedness, or fatigue. Symptoms generally reflect the degree of anemia and the rapidity with which anemia develops. Symptoms are also determined by end-organ function and vascular disease. Anemia developing over the same period in a young, otherwise healthy person may be asymptomatic, whereas in someone with critical coronary artery atherosclerosis, it may manifest with severe chest pain.

From a laboratory perspective, the automated complete blood count (CBC) identifies the severity of the anemia. The CBC includes the erythrocyte count, hematocrit level (percentage of total blood volume composed of erythrocytes), hemoglobin concentration in the blood, and erythrocyte indices such as mean corpuscular volume (MCV) and the red cell distribution width (indication of the range of erythrocyte size). Physiologically, men have a higher hemoglobin concentration than women because of the erythropoietic effects of androgens.

Normal pregnancy is associated with a dilutional anemia resulting from an increase in plasma volume that exceeds the increase in erythrocyte mass to deliver oxygen to the developing fetus at low viscosity. Other pathophysiologic states can affect hemoglobin levels. Because erythrocyte production is controlled by erythropoietin synthesized in the kidney in response to hypoxia, kidney disease can lead to anemia. Similarly, patients deficient in iron, cobalamin, or folate can develop anemia because these vitamins and minerals are required for hemoglobin production. Whether anemia is a normal result of the aging process is a subject of debate, although it is clear that associated pathophysiologic states and, likely, nutritional deficiencies contributing to anemia are more common in older adults.

In assessing patients with anemia, reviewing the CBC along with the peripheral blood smear can lead to valuable diagnostic clues. Defining the anemia as microcytic, macrocytic, or normocytic can narrow the differential diagnosis. Furthermore, reviewing erythrocyte morphology microscopically can provide a diagnosis. **Table 12** lists common erythrocyte morphologic features and their interpretations. Anemia in adults is commonly caused by iron deficiency, absolute or relative erythropoietin deficiency (kidney disease or the anemia of inflammation, respectively), or acute blood loss. Acquired hemolytic anemia is much less common. Anemia in hospitalized patients most often results from acute blood loss, the anemia of inflammation, or the anemia of kidney disease.

In addition to the CBC, a reticulocyte count provides information on the marrow response to anemia. A normal marrow will produce reticulocytes in response to anemia or hypoxia. In contrast, patients with vitamin B_{12}, folate, or iron deficiency or those with marrow diseases such as myelodysplasia or aplastic anemia cannot make adequate erythrocytes and therefore have a low reticulocyte count for their degree of anemia. The reticulocyte count may be reported as a percentage of the total erythrocyte count or as the absolute number of reticulocytes as determined by flow cytometry.

An algorithm for the evaluation of anemia can be found in **Figure 8**. In addition to the CBC and review of the peripheral blood smear, a bone marrow aspirate and biopsy can be helpful in the diagnosis of anemia, especially in assessing stem cell disorders such as aplastic anemia, dysmyelopoietic syndrome, and acute leukemia. Anemia combined with other cytopenias increases the likelihood of a primary marrow cause. Prussian blue staining can identify marrow iron stores, although interpretation of serum ferritin levels is often sufficient for that purpose. Anemia should never be considered a final diagnosis;

TABLE 12. Common Erythrocyte Findings on Peripheral Blood Smear	
Peripheral Blood Smear Finding	**Interpretation**
Bite cells (erythrocytes with a nonstaining, clear zone)	Glucose-6-phosphate dehydrogenase deficiency
Burr cells (echinocytes; erythrocytes with a small number of spicules of uniform size and distribution on the cell surface)	Uremia
Elliptocytes (erythrocytes that are elongated, oval, or elliptically shaped)	Hereditary elliptocytosis
Macrocytes or macro-ovalocytes	Cobalamin or folate deficiency, myelodysplasia, use of antimetabolites
Microcytosis, anisopoikilocytosis	Iron deficiency
Nucleated erythrocytes	Marrow stress (hemolysis, hypoxia)
Rouleaux formation ("stacked-coin" appearance of erythrocytes)	Paraproteinemia (myeloma)
Schistocytes (irregularly shaped, jagged fragments of erythrocytes)	Microangiopathy (TTP, HUS, DIC)
Sickle cells (drepanocytes; erythrocytes with spiculated shape)	Sickle cell anemia
Spherocytes (small hyperchromic erythrocytes without central pallor)	Hereditary spherocytosis, warm autoimmune hemolytic anemia
Spur cells (acanthocytes; erythrocytes with a small number of spicules of variable size and distribution on the cell surface)	Severe liver disease
Stomatocytes (erythrocytes with a mouth-shaped area of central pallor)	Artifact, hereditary stomatocytosis
Target cells (codocytes; erythrocytes with an area of central density surrounded by pallor and then a rim of density)	Hemoglobinopathy, liver disease, splenectomy, iron deficiency
Teardrop cells (dacryocytes; cells with round main body part and an elongated end)	Fibrosis, marrow granuloma, marrow infiltration

DIC = disseminated intravascular coagulation; HUS = hemolytic uremic syndrome; TTP = thrombotic thrombocytopenic purpura.

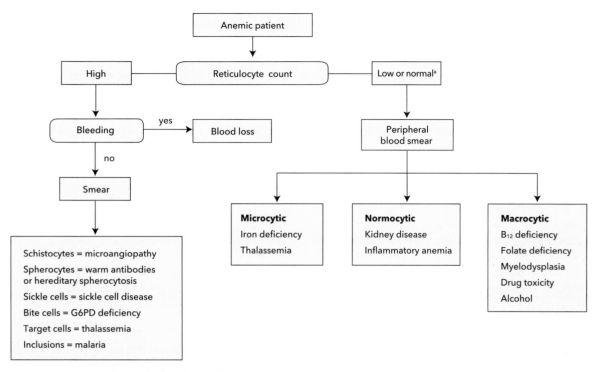

FIGURE 8. Diagnostic algorithm for the evaluation of a patient with anemia.

ᵃReticulocyte count may be low or normal in some patients with bleeding or hemolysis.

the cause must be identified. Recognizing the underlying cause leads to more focused treatment beyond transfusion to correct the anemia, as well as other prevention or therapeutic opportunities linked to the specific cause.

KEY POINTS

- Symptoms from anemia are related to its severity and how rapidly it occurs, as well as to the presence or absence of underlying organ or vascular disease.

- Anemia in hospitalized patients is most likely related to acute blood loss, the anemia of inflammation, or the anemia of kidney disease.

Anemia Due to Erythrocyte Underproduction or Maturation Defects

Iron Deficiency

Iron is an essential component of the hemoglobin molecule. In addition to its critical role in oxygen delivery, iron is also necessary for DNA synthesis and cellular transport. Most of the iron in the body is contained in the erythron; each milliliter of packed red blood cells contains about 1 mg of elemental iron. Hepcidin, the key peptide involved in iron regulation, is produced in the liver and is a negative regulator of iron absorption. Hepcidin production increases with inflammation and decreases in response to hypoxia, anemia, and iron deficiency. Hepcidin production is regulated by several proteins, including human hemochromatosis, hemojuvelin, matriptase-2, and transferrin receptor 1 and 2. These proteins are important in hereditary iron overload states discussed later in this chapter. Hepcidin causes internalization and proteolysis of ferroportin in the enterocyte and macrophage leading to decreased iron absorption from the gut and decreased iron release from macrophages.

Iron is derived from the diet as heme-based iron from red meat, poultry, and fish and non–heme-based iron from green leafy vegetables, lentils, beans, and peas. Vegetable iron has a more limited uptake because of phytates and oxalates that form complexes with iron and limit bioavailability. The typical adult diet contains 5 mg of iron for every 1000 calories. Only 10% to 20% of oral iron is absorbed. Because iron loss cannot efficiently be increased, in a normal physiologic state, iron absorption is about equal to iron loss. The typical adult man loses approximately 1 mg of iron daily from gastrointestinal mucosal turnover, whereas the typical adult woman loses approximately 1.5 mg of iron daily through mucosal turnover and menstrual blood loss.

Iron intake, use, and loss require a fine balance. Iron deficiency is a significant problem because of increased iron requirements during pregnancy and lactation and endemic helminthic infections that increase iron loss. Iron requirements are increased during normal growth and development, making iron deficiency in infants and children a widespread occurrence. Iron deficiency in adults rarely occurs secondary to decreased oral intake but is more commonly secondary to blood loss. For premenopausal women, this is typically secondary to menstrual blood loss, but for men or postmenopausal women, occult gastrointestinal blood loss should be suspected. Numerous lesions in the upper and lower gastrointestinal tracts may cause such bleeding, but identifying an occult colonic neoplasm may be especially important. Iron is absorbed in the proximal small bowel, and patients with celiac disease, inflammatory bowel disease, or surgical resection can experience iron malabsorption. Importantly, iron malabsorption may occur in the absence of diarrhea, steatorrhea, and weight loss, which are common symptoms of malabsorption. *Helicobacter pylori* infection is associated with iron deficiency because of impaired iron uptake (this mechanism is not well established) and increased iron loss from gastritis or peptic ulcer disease. Common causes of iron deficiency anemia are listed in **Table 13**.

Patients with iron deficiency may be asymptomatic or may experience fatigue, lack of a sense of well-being, irritability, headache, and decreased exercise tolerance. Pica, the tendency to eat or crave starch, clay, paper, ice, or other crunchy foodstuffs, is sometimes seen in severe iron deficiency. The pathophysiology of pica remains poorly understood.

Physical examination findings may be normal in patients with early anemia from iron deficiency. Symptomatic patients can experience tachycardia, conjunctival rim pallor (inferior conjunctival rim same color as palpebral conjunctiva), glossitis, and stomatitis. Severe iron deficiency can cause spooning of the nails (koilonychia).

A low MCV, elevated red-cell distribution width, and peripheral blood smear showing microcytosis and anisopoikilocytosis (**Figure 9**) are virtually diagnostic of iron deficiency, especially in premenopausal women; these findings may obviate the need for additional laboratory testing, provided that a follow-up CBC is performed to assess response to iron therapy.

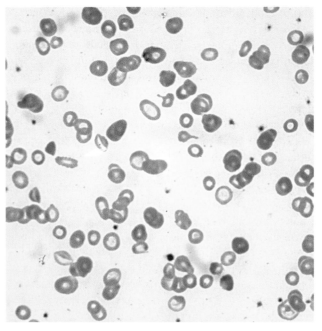

FIGURE 9. Hypochromia and microcytosis with anisopoikilocytosis in a patient with iron deficiency. Note the relatively small erythrocytes compared with the lymphocytes on the smear. Note also the abnormalities in shape and size of the erythrocytes (anisopoikilocytosis).

A low serum iron level, elevated total iron-binding capacity, low transferrin saturation (iron/total iron-binding capacity × 100), and serum ferritin level less than 14 ng/mL (14 µg/L) confirm the diagnosis of iron deficiency. Although ferritin is an acute phase reactant that increases with inflammation, a ferritin level greater than 100 ng/mL (100 µg/L) virtually excludes iron deficiency. Measuring serum levels of zinc protoporphyrin and soluble transferrin receptor was previously suggested in the evaluation of iron deficiency, but because of considerable overlap in patients with and without iron deficiency, these measurements are no longer recommended. Thrombocytosis occurs frequently with iron deficiency caused by blood loss. Although a bone marrow stained with Prussian blue can detect iron stores, this test is seldom necessary in the diagnosis of iron deficiency.

Iron deficiency is typically treated with oral iron salts. Oral ferrous sulfate is the least expensive preparation, with each 325-mg tablet containing 65 mg of elemental iron. Oral absorption can be increased with supplemental vitamin C; conversely, medications such as antacids and fiber can reduce absorption. It has become increasingly recognized that frequent dosing (two or three times daily) of oral iron can lead to increased hepcidin production, which actually reduces iron absorption. For this reason, a single daily or every-other-day dose of oral iron sulfate may be the best replacement dose. Although oral ferrous fumarate, ferrous gluconate, and other oral iron salts are available, none have proven superior to ferrous sulfate in tolerability, efficacy, or cost. Delayed-release and slow-release preparations may be better tolerated but are also associated with reduced

TABLE 13.	Causes of Iron Deficiency Anemia
Loss of iron	
Bleeding	
Menstruation	
Gastrointestinal bleeding (can be microscopic)	
Other overt or occult blood loss	
Decreased intake	
Nutritional deficiency	
Decreased absorption	
After gastric/duodenal surgery	
Celiac disease	
Helicobacter pylori infection	
Autoimmune atrophic gastritis	
Increased iron requirements	
Pregnancy	
Lactation	

iron absorption because these products can bypass the intestinal sites where iron absorption occurs. Although oral iron is typically well tolerated, symptoms can include gastrointestinal upset, constipation, and abdominal pain. Iron replacement typically results in a reticulocytosis within days. Hemoglobin levels typically increase by approximately 1 g per week. Oral iron replacement typically lasts 3 to 6 months after normalization of hemoglobin to replace iron stores.

 For patients undergoing dialysis who have large iron requirements or for patients with celiac disease, inflammatory bowel disease, or those who have undergone resection of the stomach or small bowel, oral iron may not be adequate treatment. These patients typically require parenteral iron. Iron dextran was the principal intravenous iron product used in the past, but with the risk of anaphylaxis and relatively poor bioavailability, newer parenteral iron preparations with a better safety profile and better ferrokinetics are more often used. These include iron sucrose, ferric gluconate, ferumoxytol, and ferric carboxymaltose. Data are inadequate to recommend one newer parenteral agent over another for patients requiring parenteral iron. **H**

KEY POINTS

HVC • A low mean corpuscular volume, elevated red-cell distribution width, and peripheral blood smear showing microcytosis and anisopoikilocytosis are virtually diagnostic of iron deficiency, especially in premenopausal women; these findings may render additional testing unnecessary, provided the response to iron therapy is monitored.

HVC • Iron deficiency is typically treated with oral iron salts, optimally dosed once daily, with oral ferrous sulfate being the preferred preparation because of its tolerability, efficacy, and cost.

Inflammatory Anemia

For decades, anemia has been recognized in conjunction with either chronic infections such as tuberculosis or osteomyelitis or in conjunction with malignancy. Because these types of infection and malignancy are "chronic diseases," these anemic states were often referred to as "anemia of chronic disease." From a pathophysiologic standpoint, "inflammatory anemia" is a more appropriate term, because these anemias are related to increased hepcidin production in response to inflammatory mediators such as interleukin-6. Hepcidin causes decreased iron absorption from the enterocyte through internalization and proteolysis of ferroportin. No FDA-approved assays for hepcidin evaluation are available, although several enzyme-linked immunosorbent assays and spectrometry-based assays are in development. Inflammatory cytokines also blunt the erythropoietin response to anemia.

In patients with inflammatory anemia, the peripheral blood smear typically shows a normochromic, normocytic anemia. Over time, as iron absorption decreases, microcytosis can be seen. Typically, patients with inflammatory anemia have a hemoglobin level of 8 to 10 g/dL (80-100 g/L). Because of impaired erythropoiesis, caused by a blunted response to erythropoietin, the reticulocyte count is typically low for the degree of anemia. The characteristic iron study pattern seen in inflammatory anemia is increased serum ferritin level, low serum iron level, and a reduced total iron-binding capacity. **Table 14** lists characteristic laboratory features useful in distinguishing iron deficiency from inflammatory anemia. Although seldom necessary, a bone marrow biopsy specimen would show adequate stainable iron stores.

Patients with diabetes or heart failure can also have an increase in inflammatory cytokines and related inflammatory anemia. In some patients with findings consistent with inflammatory anemia, the inflammatory state is not obvious. Such patients do not require extensive evaluation for the source of inflammation.

Inflammatory anemia seldom requires treatment. Iron replacement is ineffective. Although supplemental erythropoietin can correct anemia in inflammatory states, it can also lead to hypertension and thrombosis and should be used with extreme caution. Patients with cancer who experienced anemia with chemotherapy and who received erythropoietin felt better and had better blood counts, but cancer mortality was increased. **H**

TABLE 14.	Laboratory Characteristics of Inflammatory Anemia, Iron Deficiency Anemia (IDA), and IDA with Inflammation		
Finding	**Type of Anemia**		
	Inflammatory Anemia	**Iron Deficiency Anemia**	**IDA with Inflammation**
MCV	72-100 fL	<80 fL	<100 fL
Serum iron	<60 µg/dL (11 µmol/L)	<60 µg/dL (11 µmol/L)	<60 µg/dL (11 µmol/L)
TIBC	<250 µg/dL (45 µmol/L)	>400 µg/dL (72 µmol/L)	<400 µg/dL (72 µmol/L)
TIBC saturation	2%-20%	<15% (usually <10%)	<15%
Ferritin	>35 ng/mL (35 µg/L)	<15 ng/mL (15 µg/L)	<100 ng/mL (100 µg/L)
Serum soluble transferrin receptor concentration	Normal	Increased	Increased
Stainable iron in bone marrow	Present	Absent	Absent

MCV = mean corpuscular volume; TIBC = total iron-binding capacity.

KEY POINTS

- Patients with inflammatory anemia have a hemoglobin level of 8 to 10 g/dL (80-100 g/L) and a peripheral blood smear showing a normochromic, normocytic anemia associated with an elevated serum ferritin level, low serum iron level, and a reduced total iron-binding capacity.

HVC
- Treatment is seldom necessary in inflammatory anemia, and iron replacement is ineffective; although supplemental erythropoietin improves anemia, it is associated with worsening hypertension, thrombotic complications, and, in patients with cancer, increased mortality.

Anemia of Kidney Disease

Because erythropoietin is made in the renal cortex in response to anemia and hypoxia, patients with kidney disease can have anemia that is typically normochromic and normocytic. In kidney disease, the reticulocyte count is typically low because of a relative deficiency of erythropoietin. The peripheral blood smear may show burr cells (echinocytes) in patients with features of uremia.

Because kidney disease is also associated with platelet defects and gastrointestinal bleeding from ulcer disease or angiodysplasia, microcytosis in the setting of kidney disease should raise the suspicion for iron deficiency. In some patients, minor elevations in serum creatinine level can be associated with low erythropoietin levels and anemia. Although it is important to first rule out other causes of anemia, measuring the erythropoietin level can be helpful in evaluating anemia in patients with mild kidney disease.

Anemia of kidney disease can be associated with fatigue, depression, dyspnea, and decreased exercise tolerance. Anemia is also associated with increased morbidity and mortality from heart disease and stroke in patients undergoing dialysis. Supplemental use of erythropoiesis-stimulating agents (ESAs) can improve anemia in patients with kidney disease. Guidelines recommend that ESAs be withheld in patients with chronic kidney disease (CKD) not requiring dialysis who have a hemoglobin level greater than 10 g/dL (100 g/L). For patients with CKD with a hemoglobin level less than 10 g/dL (100 g/L), ESA treatment should be individualized based on symptoms, rapidity of hemoglobin decline, and transfusion needs. For patients undergoing dialysis, ESAs should be initiated for hemoglobin levels less than 10 g/dL (100 g/L), but hemoglobin concentrations should not exceed 11.5 g/dL (115 g/L) to avoid adverse effects, including worsening hypertension, volume overload, and thrombotic complications. Patients with CKD require iron replacement because of gastrointestinal blood loss and the need for freely available iron to maintain adequate response to ESAs. Because of high iron requirements in patients taking ESAs, parenteral iron is typically used to maintain a serum ferritin level greater than 100 ng/mL (100 µg/L) with a transferrin saturation of at least 20%. Although more than 95% of patients respond to ESAs, insufficient response can result from iron deficiency, folate deficiency, aluminum toxicity, blood loss, or inflammation.

KEY POINT

- Patients with anemia of kidney disease who are not yet **HVC** undergoing dialysis and have a hemoglobin level greater than 10 g/dL (100 g/L) should not receive erythropoiesis-stimulating agents (ESAs); patients with chronic kidney disease who are not yet undergoing dialysis and have a hemoglobin level less than 10 g/dL (100 g/L) should receive individualized ESA therapy based on symptoms, rapidity of hemoglobin decline, and transfusion needs.

Cobalamin (Vitamin B$_{12}$) Deficiency

Cobalamin is necessary for DNA synthesis. Humans cannot synthesize cobalamin but must consume it in their diet; it is found in animal meats, liver, shellfish, and dairy products. Dietary deficiency is an uncommon cause of cobalamin deficiency because body stores are typically available for many years. Instead, cobalamin deficiency is nearly always a result of malabsorption. Dietary cobalamin is more available for absorption in an acid environment and requires binding with intrinsic factor to enhance absorption in the terminal ileum.

Cobalamin deficiency may be the result of decreased bioavailability, which may be the result of age-related gastric achlorhydria or the use of proton pump inhibitors, or both. Cobalamin malabsorption can also occur in more generalized malabsorptive states such as inflammatory bowel disease, pancreatic insufficiency, and bacterial overgrowth.

Pernicious anemia, characterized by autoimmune gastritis and intrinsic factor deficiency, is another cause of cobalamin deficiency. Antibodies to parietal cells are found in 90% of patients with pernicious anemia, whereas antibodies to intrinsic factor are detected in about 70% of patients. Although antibody testing is sometimes used in the diagnosis of pernicious anemia, the varied sensitivity and specificity of these tests limits the utility of such testing. The Schilling test is no longer used in the evaluation of cobalamin deficiency because of the limited availability of radioactive intrinsic factor.

Patients with cobalamin deficiency can present with weight loss, glossitis, and "lemon yellow" skin because of pallor and jaundice resulting from ineffective erythropoiesis. Severe cobalamin deficiency can cause neurologic symptoms, including loss of vibratory sense, loss of proprioception, spastic ataxia, and other dorsal column symptoms. Psychiatric symptoms (megaloblastic mania) can manifest as dementia, hallucinations, and frank psychosis.

In patients with cobalamin deficiency, the peripheral blood smear shows oval macrocytes and hypersegmented neutrophils (**Figure 10**). Pancytopenia resulting from ineffective hematopoiesis can also be seen. Other laboratory findings are consistent with intramedullary hemolysis caused by ineffective erythropoiesis, including decreased haptoglobin, elevated lactate dehydrogenase, and elevated indirect bilirubin levels. The reticulocyte count is low in patients with cobalamin deficiency.

Although serum cobalamin levels may be low, serum cobalamin, especially in the low-normal range, may not

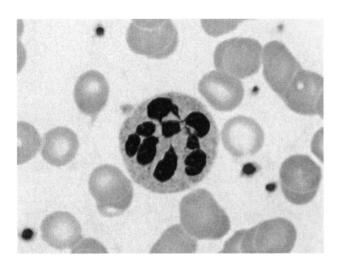

FIGURE 10. Hypersegmented polymorphonuclear (PMN) cell in a patient with pernicious anemia. The presence of hypersegmented PMNs becomes significant when they constitute greater than 5% of PMNs with five or more lobes or 1% with six or more lobes.

adequately represent tissue cobalamin levels. As such, an elevated concentration of methylmalonic acid is a more sensitive indicator of cobalamin deficiency.

Although supplemental folate can improve the anemia found in cobalamin deficiency, folate does not correct or prevent the associated neuropsychiatric complications. An important distinction to make is that folate deficiency leads to an elevation in homocysteine levels with normal levels of methylmalonic acid, whereas cobalamin deficiency has increases in both metabolites.

Patients with cobalamin deficiency can be treated with oral cobalamin, 1000 to 2000 μg daily, regardless of cause; an adequate amount of this dose will be absorbed, even if intrinsic factor is lacking or malabsorption is ongoing. Parenteral cobalamin is more expensive and more cumbersome to administer. Intranasal and oral gel preparations are also available but are not clearly superior to tablet preparations. When cobalamin is replaced, megaloblastic changes in the marrow improve within hours. Reticulocytosis appears in several days, and hemoglobin level increases by approximately 1 g per week. If the response to cobalamin is inadequate, an alternative diagnosis, such as myelodysplasia, should be considered. Neurologic changes may not be reversible with replacement.

KEY POINTS

- An elevated serum methylmalonic acid level accurately reflects tissue cobalamin stores and confirms cobalamin deficiency in patients with borderline or low-normal serum cobalamin levels.

- **HVC** Treatment for cobalamin deficiency should be instituted with 1000 to 2000 μg/d of oral cobalamin, which is absorbed well even in patients with malabsorption, eliminating the need for parenteral therapy.

Folate Deficiency

Folate is a common component of most diets in the United States; it is found in green leafy vegetables, bananas, lemons, melons, and most other fruits. Supplemental folate has been added to grains in the United States for many years to prevent birth defects. As such, dietary folate deficiency is uncommon except in patients with malnutrition. Persons who consume excess alcohol are apt to ingest inadequate amounts of folate as well as having impaired absorption. Folate is poorly stored and deficiency can develop in weeks to months in patients with insufficient folate ingestion. Patients with disease states characterized by rapid cell turnover, such as pregnancy, hemolysis, or desquamating skin disorders (psoriasis), have increased folate requirements.

Drugs such as triamterene, phenytoin, or methotrexate can lead to folate deficiency by either inhibiting folate absorption or conversion to its active form. Because folate is absorbed in the jejunum, small bowel diseases such as amyloidosis, celiac disease, or inflammatory bowel disease can also inhibit folate absorption.

The peripheral blood smear in folate deficiency is identical to that seen with cobalamin deficiency. Serum folate measurement, if very low, helps establish the diagnosis; however, a normal level may be unreliable because a single meal can normalize levels. Although folate levels in erythrocytes may better reflect chronic folate balance, an elevated serum homocysteine level has a sensitivity and specificity of greater than 90% in diagnosing folate deficiency and is the preferred test when deficiency is suspected despite a normal serum folate level.

After cobalamin deficiency is excluded, patients with folate deficiency should receive oral folate, 1 to 5 mg/d.

KEY POINTS

- A very low serum folate level confirms the diagnosis of folate deficiency; however, a normal level may be seen in patients with clearly reduced tissue stores, so an elevated homocysteine level supports folate deficiency in these patients.

- Cobalamin deficiency should be excluded before patients receive folate therapy; although blood abnormalities may improve with folate supplementation, the neurologic complications of cobalamin deficiency would continue to progress.

Thalassemia

Thalassemia is associated with erythrocyte underproduction and ineffective erythropoiesis and can be considered a disorder of erythrocyte production. Hemoglobin is a tetramer containing two α chains, two β chains ($\alpha_2\beta_2$), and the iron-containing tetrapyrrole heme moiety. Production of α and β chains normally occurs in a balanced fashion from genes located on chromosomes 16 and 11, respectively. Mismatched production of either α or β chains results in impaired production of hemoglobin and ineffective erythropoiesis. The worldwide incidence of impaired β-chain synthesis is 1% to 5%, with impaired α-chain synthesis being even higher. Thalassemia is common in African and Mediterranean countries, the Middle East, and Southeast Asia. Homozygous α-thalassemia leads to intrauterine demise, and homozygous β-thalassemia causes severe symptomatic anemia invariably diagnosed at an early age. Internists are likely to manage patients with heterozygous forms of thalassemia.

The peripheral blood smear typically shows microcytosis, nucleated erythrocytes, and target cells in patients with thalassemia (**Figure 11**). Unlike other underproduction anemias, patients with heterozygous thalassemia typically have a preserved or even an increased erythrocyte count associated with a decreased MCV. Although patients with iron deficiency typically have considerable variation in cell shape and size (anisopoikilocytosis), leading to elevation in red cell distribution width, the microcytic cells in thalassemia are more uniform, and the red cell distribution width is normal. Because of ineffective erythropoiesis, thalassemia is associated with increased lactate dehydrogenase, increased unconjugated bilirubin, and decreased haptoglobin levels.

α-Thalassemia

The α-globin gene is duplicated on chromosome 16 leading to several genotypes. Patients with a single α gene mutation are silent carriers and are clinically healthy. A two-gene mutation results in α-thalassemia trait characterized by a hemoglobin level of approximately 10 g/dL (100 g/L) with microcytosis. Unlike patients with iron deficiency, patients with α-thalassemia trait have normal or elevated iron stores. Diagnosis is usually achieved by excluding other causes of hypochromic microcytic anemia. Select reference laboratories can establish the diagnosis through direct sequencing of the globin genes. Patients with a three-gene mutation have more severe anemia and make a tetramer of β globin called hemoglobin H that can be identified on electrophoresis. In contrast, hemoglobin electrophoresis is normal for α-thalassemia trait.

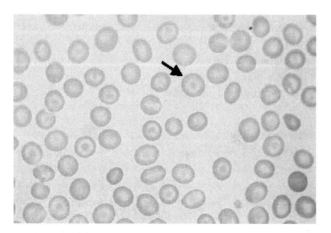

FIGURE 11. This peripheral blood smear in a patient with β-thalassemia major shows target cells (erythrocytes with an area of central density surrounded by pallor and then a rim of density) and a prominent nucleated erythrocyte.

Patients with α-thalassemia trait should receive supplemental folate and genetic counseling before starting a family. Patients with hemoglobin H disease typically have hemoglobin concentrations of approximately 7 to 8 g/dL (70-80 g/L) and are seldom transfusion dependent. Care should be taken to avoid supplemental iron in patients with thalassemia because these patients absorb iron well; transfusion should also be avoided. In such circumstances, these patients may develop iron overload with resultant heart and liver failure requiring iron chelation therapy with parenteral desferrioxamine or oral iron chelators (deferasirox or deferiprone).

β-Thalassemia

More than 250 mutations have been described in the β-globin gene resulting in a spectrum of diseases from mild reduction in β-chain synthesis (β$^+$-thalassemia) to complete absence of β-chain synthesis (β^0-thalassemia). As such, the clinical spectrum of disease in β-thalassemia includes β-thalassemia minor, β-thalassemia intermedia, and β-thalassemia major. β-Thalassemia minor (trait) is characterized by a microcytic anemia (MCV, 60-70 fL) with a hemoglobin level of 10 to 12 g/dL (100-120 g/L). Unlike α-thalassemia trait, β-thalassemia minor produces an abnormal hemoglobin electrophoresis with an increase in hemoglobin A$_2$ ($\alpha_2\delta_2$) because of a substitution of δ globin for β globin. Hemoglobin F may also be increased depending on the specific mutation. Patients with β-thalassemia intermedia have hemoglobin levels of 7 g/dL (70 g/L) without need for transfusion.

Patients with β-thalassemia should be treated with folate; as with α-thalassemia, supplemental iron should be avoided.

> **KEY POINT**
>
> - Patients with thalassemia should receive supplemental folate and avoid iron supplementation because they may develop iron overload requiring chelation therapy.

HVC

Hemolytic Anemias

Hemolysis occurs when excessive erythrocyte destruction occurs, either through ineffective erythropoiesis; clearance in the reticuloendothelial system of the spleen or liver; immune injury mediated by immunoglobulins or complement; or physical destruction by fibrin, valves, or other intracirculatory devices.

Hemolysis may be accompanied by a bone marrow response (reticulocytosis) and is invariably accompanied by findings consistent with erythrocyte destruction, such as an increase in unconjugated bilirubin, increased lactate dehydrogenase, increased serum free hemoglobin, and hemoglobinuria. Symptoms of hemolysis depend on the degree of anemia and its chronicity. Pigmented gallstones from insoluble calcium bilirubinate are common in chronic hemolytic disorders.

Hemolysis can be broken down into congenital and acquired causes. Congenital disorders segregate into hemoglobinopathies (sickle cell), disorders of the erythrocyte

CONT.

membrane (hereditary spherocytosis), enzyme defects (glucose-6-phosphate dehydrogenase deficiency), and the thalassemia syndromes.

Acquired hemolysis can occur secondary to medications (fludarabine, bendamustine, quinine, penicillins, α-methyldopa); can be immune in nature; or can occur secondary to micro- or macroangiopathic processes, infections, or physical agents.

Congenital Hemolytic Anemia
Hereditary Spherocytosis
Hereditary spherocytosis (HS) is typically an autosomal dominant disorder more common in people of Northern European descent. HS is not confined to a single mutation; rather, mutations in α spectrin, β spectrin, ankyrin, band 3, and protein 4.2 have been described in patients with HS. Mutations in these scaffolding proteins adversely affect the interaction between the lipid bilayer and cytoskeleton in the erythrocyte cell wall resulting in a spherocyte (**Figure 12**) characterized by reduced surface-to-volume ratio, osmotic fragility, and splenic sequestration.

Symptoms of HS can be quite variable, and even though HS is a congenital disorder, patients may adapt to mild anemia without symptoms until well into adulthood. An acute episode of bone marrow suppression, typically associated with infection, can lead to new anemia symptoms in patients who were previously able to compensate for hemolysis. In addition to anemia, symptomatic patients typically present with splenomegaly or, more rarely, splenic infarction or rupture, and calcium bilirubinate (pigmented) gallstones are common.

Laboratory findings in HS include spherocytosis on the peripheral blood smear and varying degrees of anemia, reticulocytosis, and hyperbilirubinemia. The mean corpuscular hemoglobin concentration is elevated in patients with HS. Erythrocytes in these patients have increased osmotic fragility when exposed to fluids with high osmolarity. This is the basis of the osmotic fragility test sometimes used to diagnose HS. Flow cytometry can identify characteristic cell surface abnormalities that establish the diagnosis.

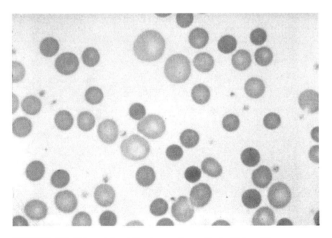

FIGURE 12. This peripheral blood smear in a patient with hereditary spherocytosis shows round cells of uniform density (without central pallor) characteristic of spherocytes.

Patients with HS, as with other hemolytic states, have increased folate requirements and should receive supplemental folate. For severe hemolysis, splenectomy is effective, and partial splenectomy has proven effective in young children whose immune function is improved with a functioning spleen. As with other conditions requiring splenectomy, vaccination for *Streptococcus pneumoniae, Haemophilus influenzae,* and *Neisseria meningitides* is important before the procedure.

Other congenital disorders of the erythrocyte membrane that can lead to hemolysis include hereditary elliptocytosis and hereditary pyropoikilocytosis. Hereditary elliptocytosis is less commonly associated with anemia.

Glucose-6-Phosphate Dehydrogenase Deficiency
The gene for glucose-6-phosphate dehydrogenase (G6PD) is located on the X chromosome, and as such G6PD deficiency primarily affects men. It can affect women who are homozygous for G6PD disease, through the process of lyonization (inactivation of one of the two X chromosomes) with preference of expression for the defective gene, or who have Turner syndrome (XO karyotype). G6PD deficiency is the most common enzyme deficiency in humans and has been associated with more than 160 gene mutations. G6PD is important in the pentose phosphate pathway, allowing for reduction of nicotinamide adenine dinucleotide phosphate (NADP to NADPH). NADPH is necessary to reduce oxidative stress in response to drugs (chloroquine), infection, or toxins. Two G6PD variants, G6PD A, which produces mild disease that is often asymptomatic, and G6PD Mediterranean are most commonly seen. G6PD Mediterranean is associated with favism, or hemolysis in people who consume fava beans. G6PD variants are thought to provide partial protection for malarial infections. G6PD deficiency occurs most commonly in people of African, Asian, Mediterranean, and Middle Eastern descent and among Kurdish Jews.

G6PD deficiency has a varied presentation. It can be associated with neonatal jaundice and, in later life, with acute hemolysis typically occurring within 1 to 3 days after exposure to oxidative stress. Typical triggers include drugs such as chloroquine, sulfonamides, rasburicase, dapsone, and phenazopyridine, and environmental toxins such as naphthalene from mothballs. The peripheral blood smear may show bite cells (**Figure 13**) and Heinz bodies (denatured hemoglobin) visible on supravital stain. Although very uncommon, severe hemolysis can lead to kidney injury and dialysis.

G6PD evaluation involves a fluorescent spot test used to detect NADPH. A positive result shows lack of fluorescence. Evaluation should not be performed during an acute hemolytic episode because, with hemolysis, the older, more enzyme-deficient erythrocytes are preferentially destroyed leaving younger erythrocytes with higher G6PD levels in the circulation; this often leads to a false-negative result. Qualitative G6PD enzyme activity and subtyping can provide a more specific diagnosis.

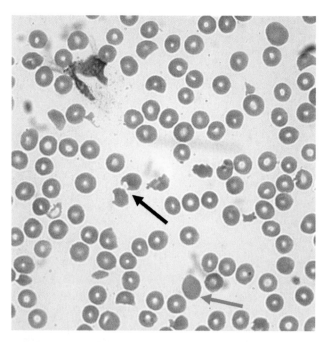

FIGURE 13. Bite cells seen at the center of this slide are typical findings in glucose-6-phosphate dehydrogenase deficiency and are characterized by a membrane defect that appears as though a semicircular bite has been taken out of the erythrocyte. The defect is caused by removal of denatured hemoglobin by macrophages in the spleen. A polychromatophilic macro-ovalocyte can also be seen (bottom), indicating a reticulocyte response.

CONT.

Typical management of G6PD deficiency includes recognition and diagnosis of the disorder and avoidance of offending agents. During hemolytic episodes, treatment is supportive, with transfusion reserved only for severely symptomatic patients. **H**

Other less common enzyme defects leading to congenital hemolysis include enzyme deficiencies in the glycolytic pathway, pyruvate kinase deficiency, and aldolase A deficiency.

Sickle Cell Syndromes

There is perhaps no hemolytic anemia as clinically dramatic as sickle cell anemia. Affecting nearly every organ system and characterized by extraordinarily painful vaso-occlusive crises, sickle cell disease (SCD) is prevalent among black patients. SCD is characterized by homozygosity for a single point mutation in the sixth position of the β-globin gene resulting in abnormal hemoglobin S (Hb S) that polymerizes under hypoxic conditions, leading to deformed erythrocytes that can adhere to the endothelium of capillaries throughout the circulation. Because of hemolysis, free hemoglobin scavenges nitric oxide, and hemolyzed erythrocytes release arginase, depleting the body of arginine, a necessary precursor to nitric oxide. As a result, patients with SCD experience vasoconstriction and platelet activation, complicating their clinical course.

Hb S is more common in patients of African origin, and most patients homozygous for Hb S (Hb SS) are black, with about 8% of black persons in the United States having sickle cell trait (Hb S). Hb S can be coinherited with hemoglobin C (Hb SC), β-thalassemia (Sβ⁺-thalassemia), or other hemoglobins, which tends to lead to milder disease than Hb SS. Characteristic electrophoretic patterns for sickling disorders are shown in **Table 15**.

Sickle Cell Disease Complications and Their Management

Chronic hemolysis, vaso-occlusive disease with acute and chronic end-organ damage, nitric oxide depletion, and immune compromise from functional asplenia lead to the myriad of problems faced by patients with SCD. The only potential "cure" for SCD is allogeneic bone marrow transplantation, but the timing and appropriate population for transplantation have not been adequately determined. Hydroxyurea modulates many of the complications of SCD and even prolongs life expectancy because of its ability to increase fetal

TABLE 15. Characteristics of Adult Sickle Cell Syndromes							
Disease Type	Hb (g/dL [g/L])	MCV (fL)	Hb S (%)	Hb A (%)	Hb A₂ (%)	Peripheral Blood Smear Findings	Clinical Severity[a] 0 to +++
Sickle trait (AS)	NL	NL	40	60	<3.5	NL	0
Hb SS	6-8 (60-80)	NL	>90	0	<3.5	Sickle cells	+++
Sβ⁺-thalassemia	9-12 (90-120)	70-75	>60	10-30	>3.5	Rare sickle cells Target cells	+ to ++
Sβ⁰-thalassemia	7-9 (70-90)	65-70	>80	0	>3.5	Sickle cells Target cells	+++
SCD	10-15 (100-150)	75-NL	50	0	Hb A₂ = 0 Hb C = 50[b]	Sickle cells Target cells	+ to ++

Hb = hemoglobin; Hb SS = homozygous sickle cell anemia; MCV = mean corpuscular volume; NL = normal; Sβ⁺ = sickle β⁺; Sβ⁰ = sickle β⁰; SCD = hemoglobin SC disease.

[a]Clinical severity is variable within each genotype.

[b]Note that Hb C comigrates with Hb A₂ on standard alkaline cellulose acetate electrophoresis but will separate on citrate agar electrophoresis.

NOTE: Hb percentages may not total 100% because Hb F is not included in this table.

CONT.

hemoglobin levels and generate nitric oxide. Hydroxyurea is not used often enough and is not always used at the appropriate dose. It should be prescribed for all patients with frequent pain crises, severe symptomatic anemia, or previous acute chest syndrome or stroke. Managing SCD requires a team of providers and must include preventive, acute, and chronic treatment goals (**Table 16**).

Painful vaso-occlusive events are the hallmark of SCD. The frequency and severity of acute painful events varies considerably among patients with SCD, the reasons for which remain poorly understood. In most communities, a few patients with recurrent acute painful events account for most hospitalizations. Research has shown that many practitioners do not properly assess and manage pain in this population, often leaving pain undertreated. Painful events are associated with morbidity and mortality in patients with SCD, and the number of painful crises is inversely related to life expectancy.

For these reasons, recognition and treatment of painful events should be immediate. Opiates are the preferred analgesic, with the exception of meperidine, which can cause seizures. Chronic pain is more difficult to treat in SCD, and the pathophysiology is poorly understood. Chronic pain is exacerbated by emotional stress, anxiety, insomnia, and depression and is perhaps best treated with a holistic approach emphasizing nonopioid options such as NSAIDs, relaxation techniques, massage, and biofeedback. A few patients with SCD develop opioid dependence, although the prevalence is no greater than in a comparable age- and illness-matched population.

Two new treatments to prevent painful crisis have recently been approved. Oral L-glutamine, a precursor of nicotinamide adenine dinucleotide (NAD), is necessary to form the antioxidant NADH. It is believed that sickle cell crises are partially related to oxidant stress. A randomized trial in patients receiving L-glutamine showed benefit with reduction in the number

TABLE 16. Common Complications and Treatments in Adults with Sickle Cell Disease

Complications	Treatment
Vaso-occlusive pain episode	**Acute:** rest, relaxation, warmth, NSAIDs, oral and IV hydration, narcotic analgesia
	Recurring: HU for more than 3 episodes/year, pain that interferes with daily activities; avoidance of triggers; nonnarcotic or narcotic analgesia
Acute chest syndrome	**Acute:** oxygen, incentive spirometry, analgesics, empiric antibiotics, IV fluids, simple or erythrocyte exchange transfusions
	Preventive: HU for recurrent acute chest syndrome, incentive spirometry in hospitalized patients
Aplastic crisis	**Acute:** supportive care, blood transfusions as needed
Infection	**Acute:** appropriate and immediate antibiotic management (particular concern for encapsulated bacteria)
	Prevention: influenza, pneumococcal, and meningococcal vaccines
Hyperhemolytic crisis	**Acute:** supportive care, avoid further blood transfusions, immunosuppression might be helpful
	Preventive: avoid blood transfusions if possible, extended antibody screen can lessen but not eliminate recurrence
Multiorgan failure	**Acute:** erythrocyte exchange transfusions
Ischemic stroke	**Acute:** erythrocyte exchange transfusions, aspirin
	Preventive: chronic simple transfusions or erythrocyte exchange transfusions (target Hb S <30%-50%)
Hepatic crisis	**Acute:** supportive, transfusion or exchange transfusion if anemia is symptomatic
Cholelithiasis	**Acute:** if symptomatic, cholecystectomy with preoperative transfusions to hemoglobin of 10 g/dL (100 g/L)
Chronic kidney disease/ proteinuria	**Preventive:** blood pressure control to <130/80 mm Hg
	Secondary preventive: ACE inhibitor or ARB in patients with microalbuminuria
Priapism	**Acute:** relaxation, hydration, narcotic analgesics, aspiration of blood from corpora cavernosa and irrigation with dilute epinephrine, transfusions, shunt procedure
	Preventive: oral α-adrenergic agonists, HU. The role of leuprolide and sildenafil is not clear.
Pulmonary hypertension	No proven therapy established for prevention or treatment
Retinopathy	Annual ophthalmologic examination, laser phototherapy for retinopathy
Osteopenia/osteoporosis	Supplementation with calcium and vitamin D, bone mineral density measurements
Avascular necrosis	Analgesics and physical therapy, arthroplasty
Foot and leg ulcers	**Acute:** early aggressive treatment, debridement, bandage impregnated with zinc oxide
	Preventive: proper footwear to prevent pressure points

ARB = angiotensin receptor blocker; Hb S = hemoglobin S; HU = hydroxyurea; IV = intravenous.

CONT.

of sickle cell crises. Similarly, the recently approved P-selectin inhibitor, crizanlizumab, has been shown to reduce painful crises by preventing cellular adhesion.

Pulmonary complications are a common source of morbidity and mortality in patients with SCD. Acute chest syndrome (ACS) is a clinical diagnosis based on the constellation of fever (>38.6 °C [101.5 °F]), tachypnea, hypoxia, cough, shortness of breath, and a new pulmonary infiltrate. ACS can be the result of infection, in situ thrombosis, thromboembolism, fat embolism, or a combination of these factors. In addition to supportive measures, including oxygen to treat hypoxia and the use of empiric antibiotics to treat infection, patients with ACS require erythrocyte transfusion, either with packed red blood cells (PRBCs) or as exchange transfusion. In addition to ACS, pulmonary hypertension is a recognized complication of SCD found in up to 30% of patients, typically presenting as worsening right heart failure. Although associated with increased mortality, the appropriate management of pulmonary hypertension in patients with SCD has not been determined. Phosphodiesterase inhibitors, such as sildenafil, have been associated with increased painful crises.

Stroke and other central nervous system disease remain major complications of SCD. Approximately 30% of patients with Hb SS, Hb SC, or Sβ⁺-thalassemia can have silent or symptomatic strokes. Monthly transfusion begun after a stroke can reduce the incidence of subsequent stroke by 50% but carries the risk of iron overload necessitating iron chelation. Hydroxyurea may also help in stroke prevention. In addition to thrombotic stroke, patients with SCD can have moyamoya disease (irregular perforating vascular networks near occluded or stenotic vessels in the region corresponding to lenticulostriate and thalamoperforate arteries) predisposing to cerebral bleeding in the third and fourth decade of life. Adults with SCD have lower cognitive function than healthy adults, perhaps secondary to silent ischemia or chronic anemia. It is unclear whether such cognitive decline can be prevented.

Recently, the National Institutes of Health and the U.S. Department of Health and Human Services published evidence-based guidelines for the treatment of SCD. Strong recommendations from this report are listed in **Table 17**.

Erythrocyte Transfusions in Sickle Cell Disease

Transfusion management in SCD is complicated. Inappropriate transfusion can lead to alloimmunization, iron overload, and infectious complications. Antibody formation can lead to hyperhemolysis, a presumed immune response leading to hemolysis of nearly all transfused blood in addition to native blood. Simple transfusions with PRBCs are used to increase oxygen delivery and should not be used for uncomplicated pain crises or to treat chronic anemia. Patients undergoing surgical procedures requiring general anesthesia should receive PRBC transfusion for a target hemoglobin level of 10 g/dL (100 g/L) to avoid surgical complications. Monthly transfusions (hypertransfusion) in patients with an initial stroke can reduce the incidence of subsequent stroke and reduce stroke

TABLE 17. Strong Recommendations from the National Institutes of Health/U.S. Department of Health and Human Services Guidelines for the Management of Sickle Cell Disease
Rapid initiation of opioids for vaso-occlusive crisis
Use of incentive spirometry in hospitalized patients
Use of analgesics and physical therapy for treatment of avascular necrosis
Use of ACE inhibitors in patients with microalbuminuria
Regular ophthalmologic examinations and referral for laser photocoagulation for retinopathy
Use of echocardiography to evaluate signs of pulmonary hypertension
Hydroxyurea for patients with more than 3 vaso-occlusive crises per year, for those with pain or chronic anemia interfering with daily activities, or those with recurrent acute chest syndrome
Preoperative transfusion to serum hemoglobin level of 10 g/dL (100 g/L) for surgeries requiring general anesthesia
Assess for iron overload and begin oral iron chelation if necessary

occurrence in patients at risk for stroke based on cranial Doppler arterial velocity. Exchange transfusion is often used in the treatment of acute stroke, complicated acute chest syndrome, and acute retinal artery occlusion. With any transfusion, care should be taken to keep hemoglobin concentrations less than 10 g/dL (100 g/L) to avoid problems with blood hyperviscosity.

Other Hemoglobinopathies

More than 1000 mutations have been identified in the α- or β-globin gene, including hemoglobin C, hemoglobin D, and hemoglobin E. Most of these are only clinically relevant if coinherited with Hb S.

KEY POINTS

- Patients with hereditary spherocytosis may remain asymptomatic well into adulthood but may develop acute anemia symptoms when an acute infection suppresses the bone marrow, leading to decompensated hemolysis.

- Evaluation for glucose-6-phosphate dehydrogenase deficiency should not be performed during an acute hemolytic episode, because the older enzyme-deficient erythrocytes are preferentially destroyed during these episodes, which would lead to a false-negative result on testing.

- Painful events are associated with morbidity and mortality in patients with sickle cell disease, and the number of painful crises is inversely related to life expectancy; recognition and treatment of pain should be immediate.

- In patients with frequent acute vaso-occlusive events or other serious complications of sickle cell anemia, hydroxyurea decreases subsequent acute pain events, reduces the risk of acute chest syndrome or stroke, and prolongs survival.

(Continued)

HVC

- In patients with sickle cell disease, simple transfusions with packed red blood cells (PRBCs) should not be used for uncomplicated pain crises or to treat chronic anemia; however, patients undergoing surgical procedures requiring general anesthesia should receive PRBC transfusion for a target hemoglobin level of 10 g/dL (100 g/L) to avoid perioperative complications.

Acquired Hemolytic Anemia

Immune-Mediated Hemolysis

Immune-mediated hemolysis is characterized by antibody binding to erythrocytes causing complement-mediated and phagocyte-mediated destruction. Antibodies responsible for immune-mediated hemolysis are divided into warm antibodies, typically IgG, that react at normal body temperature and cold agglutinins, usually IgM, that bind at cooler temperatures. The laboratory hallmark of immune-mediated hemolysis is a positive direct antiglobulin (Coombs) test that detects either IgG or complement (C3) on the erythrocyte surface. Characteristics of immune-mediated hemolysis are shown in **Table 18**.

Warm Autoimmune Hemolytic Anemia

In warm autoimmune hemolytic anemia (WAIHA), pathogenic IgG antibodies are directed against Rh-type antigens on the erythrocyte surface. IgG-coated erythrocytes can be completely phagocytized by splenic macrophages via the Fc receptor and are cleared from the circulation. Warm IgG antibodies can bind and activate complement in a portion of these patients. Partial phagocytosis of the erythrocyte surface area results in spherocytes, which can be viewed on the peripheral blood smear. The direct antiglobulin test result is positive for

IgG and is also sometimes positive for C3. Although WAIHA can be a primary disorder, it can also occur secondary to drugs (penicillins or α-methyldopa); lymphoproliferative disorders, such as chronic lymphocytic leukemia; or diseases with disordered immune regulation, such as systemic lupus erythematosus.

Treatment of symptomatic WAIHA involves alleviating immune destruction of erythrocytes using glucocorticoids, intravenous immune globulin, or rituximab. Splenectomy is also effective in nearly 70% of patients. Patients with hemolysis and life-threatening anemia may require blood transfusion (see Transfusion). Although donor blood will also be destroyed at an accelerated rate, improved hemoglobin levels may be sustained while waiting for therapy directed at eliminating the autoantibody to take effect.

Cold Agglutinin Disease

In cold agglutinin disease, pathogenic IgM antibodies are directed against erythrocyte glycoprotein antigens (I or i antigen). Cold agglutinins bind at temperatures lower than normal body temperature (for example, the temperature of distal extremities during cold exposure). Cold agglutinins cause complement fixation, and C3-coated cells are both cleared by hepatic Kupffer cells and destroyed in circulation. The peripheral blood smear shows erythrocyte agglutination leading to a markedly elevated MCV on laboratory testing (**Figure 14**). In cold agglutinin disease, the direct antiglobulin test result is positive for C3. Cold agglutinin disease should always raise suspicion for an underlying lymphoproliferative abnormality, and it can also be seen in *Mycoplasma* and Epstein-Barr virus infections.

Treatment of cold agglutinin disease is primarily directed at avoidance of cold exposure, including warming of all infusates in hospitalized patients. Treatment with glucocorticoids,

TABLE 18.	Characteristics of Warm Autoimmune Hemolytic Anemia (WAIHA) and Cold Agglutinin Disease	
Characteristic	**WAIHA**	**Cold Agglutinin Disease**
Temperature for optimal antibody binding to erythrocytes	37.0 °C (98.6 °F)	<37.0 °C (98.6 °F)
Immunoglobulin class	IgG	IgM
Typical AGT pattern	IgG positive, C3 positive or negative	IgG negative, C3 positive
Peripheral blood smear findings	Spherocytes	Erythrocyte agglutination
Clinical manifestations[a]	Anemia, fatigue, dyspnea, jaundice, splenomegaly	Anemia, fatigue, dyspnea, jaundice, acrocyanosis, splenomegaly
Associated conditions	Autoimmune, lymphoproliferative (chronic lymphocytic leukemia, B-cell non-Hodgkin lymphomas), drug-induced[b]	Infectious (*Mycoplasma* and Epstein-Barr virus), lymphoproliferative (IgM MGUS, Waldenström macroglobulinemia, other B-cell non-Hodgkin lymphomas)
Treatment	Glucocorticoids, splenectomy, immunosuppression, treatment of underlying condition	Cold avoidance, rituximab, plasmapheresis, treatment of underlying condition

AGT = antiglobulin (Coombs) test; MGUS = monoclonal gammopathy of undetermined significance.

[a]Manifestations in cold agglutinin disease are worse upon exposure to the cold. Lymphadenopathy in either entity should raise suspicion of a lymphoproliferative disorder.

[b]Cephalosporins, penicillins, NSAIDs, isoniazid, procainamide, methyldopa, levodopa.

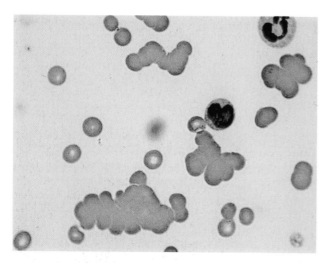

FIGURE 14. Cold agglutinin disease. Notice the erythrocyte agglutination on the slide, which can lead to a spuriously high mean corpuscular volume on automated counters.

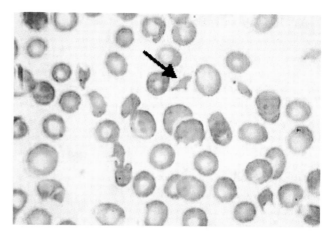

FIGURE 15. Peripheral blood smear showing schistocytes, or fragmented erythrocytes.

CONT.

intravenous immune globulin, or splenectomy is seldom effective. Rituximab, fludarabine, or a combination of both has demonstrated activity in case series. **H**

KEY POINTS

- Treatment of symptomatic warm autoimmune hemolytic anemia involves alleviating immune destruction of erythrocytes using glucocorticoids, intravenous immune globulin, or rituximab; splenectomy is also effective in nearly 70% of patients.

- Treatment of cold agglutinin disease is primarily directed at avoidance of cold exposure, including warming of all infusates in hospitalized patients; the use of glucocorticoids, intravenous immune globulin, or splenectomy is seldom effective.

Nonimmune Hemolytic Anemia

Microangiopathic Hemolytic Anemia

Microangiopathic hemolytic anemia is characterized by the presence of fragmented erythrocytes (schistocytes) on the peripheral blood smear (**Figure 15**) and is typically caused by erythrocyte destruction resulting from shearing as erythrocytes circulate through fibrin strands. Microangiopathy can be caused by thrombotic thrombocytopenic purpura or the hemolytic uremic syndrome (see Platelet Disorders); malignancy; disseminated intravascular coagulation; hypertensive crisis; drugs such as cyclosporine, mitomycin, or gemcitabine; or eclampsia. Microangiopathy is often accompanied by thrombocytopenia, kidney injury, and central nervous system disturbance. Treatment is directed toward the underlying disease process.

Macroangiopathic Hemolytic Anemia

Patients with artificial valves or those with left ventricular assist devices can develop anemia resulting from erythrocyte fragmentation known as macroangiopathic hemolysis.

Similarly, patients with giant hemangiomas, such as those with Kasabach-Merritt syndrome, can develop erythrocyte fragmentation from localized intravascular coagulation.

Paroxysmal Nocturnal Hemoglobinuria (PNH) [FATIGUE AB PAIN]

Patients with PNH lack proteins on the erythrocyte surface that are anchored by glycophosphatidylinositol due to acquired mutations in the *PIGA* gene that persist in bone marrow stem cells. Two of these proteins, CD55 and CD59, protect the erythrocyte from complement-mediated destruction. Patients lacking these proteins develop episodic hemolysis, marrow aplasia, and thrombosis. The cause of thrombosis is unclear. Patients with PNH are at higher risk for leukemia or myelodysplasia. Diagnosis involves demonstrating absence of glycophosphatidylinositol-linked proteins such as CD55 and CD59 on leukocytes by flow cytometry. PNH therapy includes folate supplementation, glucocorticoids, and a novel monoclonal antibody to C5, eculizumab, which inhibits activation of the terminal complement cascade, decreases hemolysis, reduces thrombotic complications, and improves quality of life. Eculizumab is associated with *Neisseria* infections, so patients should receive meningococcal vaccination before use. **H**

KEY POINTS

- Treatment of patients with microangiopathic hemolytic anemia is directed toward the underlying disease process, which can include hemolytic uremic syndrome, malignancy, drugs, and thrombotic thrombocytopenic purpura.

- Patients with paroxysmal nocturnal hemoglobinuria develop episodic hemolysis, marrow aplasia, and thrombosis; therapy with eculizumab, a monoclonal antibody to C5 that inhibits terminal complement activation, decreases complications and improves quality of life.

Other Causes of Hemolysis

March Hemoglobinuria

March hemoglobinuria develops after physical erythrocyte destruction in the soles of the feet in response to long-distance running or marching. March hemoglobinuria has also been described in hand drummers and karate enthusiasts.

Hemolysis Associated with Chemical and Physical Agents

Arsenic or arsine gas exposure, elevated serum copper levels, the bite of the brown recluse spider, and severe burns are rare causes of hemolysis.

Hemolysis from Infections

Malaria, babesiosis, clostridia, and *Bartonella* (Oroya fever) are all associated with hemolysis.

Iron Overload Syndromes

Primary/Hereditary Hemochromatosis

Hereditary hemochromatosis (HH) is the most common inherited genetic disorder in whites, with a prevalence of 1 in 250 persons of northern European descent. Approximately 85% to 90% of patients with HH are homozygous for the C282Y mutation in the *HFE* gene; the remaining patients are typically compound heterozygotes for C282Y and the H63D or S65C mutations. *HFE* mutations result in hepcidin deficiency and increased ferroportin expression on duodenal enterocytes, which results in increased iron absorption and eventual organ injury because no physiologic mechanism allows for excreting excess iron. Cirrhosis and cardiomyopathy are major causes of morbidity, small joint arthritis is common, and diabetes mellitus and other endocrinopathies may be seen.

Patients may be diagnosed late in the disease course through evaluation of decompensated liver disease or symptomatic cardiomyopathy, although liver and heart damage are largely irreversible at this late stage even if iron stores are actively reduced. The diagnosis may also be made earlier in the disease course through evaluation of abnormal aminotransferase levels that precede cirrhosis, characteristic arthropathy involving the second and third metacarpophalangeal joints (**Figure 16**), or endocrinopathy such as androgen insufficiency arising from pituitary or endocrine organ injury. Skin hyperpigmentation, accounting for the "bronze diabetes" terminology for HH, is likely caused by pituitary infiltration and excess melatonin secretion. The diagnosis is also made through screening family members of patients with known hemochromatosis.

The diagnosis is suspected by finding an elevated transferrin saturation greater than 45% and an elevated serum ferritin level; diagnosis is confirmed through genetic testing.

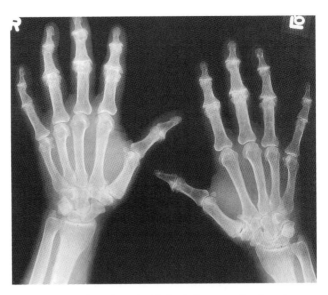

FIGURE 16. A plain radiograph of the hands shows osteophyte formation involving the distal interphalangeal and proximal interphalangeal joints and the metacarpophalangeal (MCP) joints. These "hook" osteophytes, particularly of the second and third MCP joints, are a characteristic finding in patients with hereditary hemochromatosis.

MRI is used to noninvasively assess the extent of cardiac and liver iron overload and generally obviates the need to perform organ biopsy to quantitate iron deposits. Liver biopsy may still be useful in patients who have hepatitis C infection or alcohol dependence as alternate options for causing liver disease.

First-degree relatives of patients with HH should be counseled about their risks and advised to undergo medical evaluation and screening. Asymptomatic family members of patients with hemochromatosis and a serum ferritin level less than 500 ng/mL (500 μg/L) can be safely observed. Symptomatic patients or those with signs of end-organ injury should undergo therapeutic phlebotomy, the goal of which is to reduce total body iron stores; each unit (450-500 mL) of blood removed contains 200 to 250 mg iron, which unloads parenchymal deposition over time. Phlebotomy should be performed once or twice per week depending on the patient's hematocrit level. Iron stores in patients with HH may exceed 30 g, requiring phlebotomy over 2 to 3 years. The serum ferritin level should be evaluated every 3 months, with a target goal of 50 to 100 ng/mL (50-100 μg/L). When this goal is reached, maintenance phlebotomy should be instituted; schedules vary from 2 to 6 units of blood per year. Patients with HH without hepatic fibrosis or cardiomyopathy can expect a normal life expectancy with phlebotomy and judicious alcohol intake. Although advanced liver disease is not reversible with phlebotomy, patients benefit from screening for hepatocellular carcinoma and other secondary prevention as indicated for patients with cirrhosis. Similarly, phlebotomy is much less effective in patients who already manifest cardiac toxicity from iron overload.

Secondary Iron Overload

Secondary iron overload occurs in patients who require chronic transfusion (most commonly in hereditary hemoglobinopathies such as thalassemia major); in subsets of patients with sickle cell anemia; or in acquired bone marrow failure conditions, such as myelodysplastic syndrome. End-organ involvement in secondary iron overload overlaps with that seen in HH, particularly regarding hepatic deposition, although endocrinopathy and cardiac effects are more common and arthropathy is less common. Therapeutic phlebotomy should not be performed, because these patients are anemic. The iron chelator deferoxamine has traditionally been the mainstay of therapy, but it requires continuous infusion, either intravenously or subcutaneously. Several oral iron chelators, including deferasirox and deferiprone, are available and may be more convenient. Monitoring is accomplished by serial serum ferritin measurements.

Porphyria cutanea tarda is a less common cause of secondary iron overload unrelated to chronic transfusion, but it is typically associated with acquired abnormalities in porphyrin metabolism and underlying liver disease, especially hepatitis C infection. Porphyria cutanea tarda is characterized by cutaneous blisters, often on the hands, and hypertrichosis; it responds well to phlebotomy.

Platelet Disorders
Normal Platelet Physiology

Platelets are cell fragments released from megakaryocytes that circulate in an inactive state in the blood for 8 to 10 days. One third of the platelets are sequestered in the spleen and released back into the circulation in response to epinephrine.

Platelet activation, the first step in hemostasis, occurs in a three-stage process. Platelets adhere to exposed subendothelial surfaces of injured vessel walls (mediated by von Willebrand factor [vWF]). Platelets then change shape and release adenosine diphosphate and triphosphate, serotonin, fibrinogen, vWF, and factor V. Clopidogrel irreversibly binds to the P2Y12 adenosine diphosphate receptor, blocking platelet activation and aggregation. During shape change, glycoprotein IIb/IIIa receptors are exposed, bind fibrinogen, and initiate reversible platelet-platelet aggregation. The intravenous antiplatelet agents abciximab, eptifibatide, and tirofiban inhibit fibrinogen binding during this stage. In the final stage, arachidonic acid is released and converted to thromboxane A_2, promoting irreversible platelet aggregation and resulting in a platelet plug (aspirin acts by irreversibly acetylating thromboxane A_2). Finally, platelets provide the phospholipid membrane necessary to complete the coagulation cascade (see Bleeding Disorders).

Approach to the Patient with Thrombocytopenia

Thrombocytopenia must be evaluated according to the platelet count and the clinical setting. Platelet counts greater than 100,000/µL (100×10^9/L) do not increase bleeding risk. Counts between 50,000 and 100,000/µL ($50\text{-}100 \times 10^9$/L) do not require treatment and are adequate for surgical procedures, although 100,000/µL (100×10^9/L) is desirable for neurosurgery. Platelet counts between 30,000 and 50,000/µL ($30\text{-}50 \times 10^9$/L) must be corrected before surgical intervention, and counts less than 10,000/µL (10×10^9/L) are associated with risk of spontaneous bleeding.

The first step of the evaluation is to review the peripheral blood smear and confirm the count. Pseudothrombocytopenia occurs when a patient has antibodies to ethylenediaminetetraacetic acid (EDTA), causing platelets to clump together in vitro. An accurate count can be obtained from blood drawn in citrate or heparin instead of EDTA. Inaccurate platelet counts may also occur if the platelets are exceptionally large (complete blood count machine may count them as erythrocytes) or if erythrocyte fragments (schistocytes) are counted by the machine as if they were platelets (leading to a higher than actual platelet count).

When thrombocytopenia is confirmed, symptoms are assessed, with attention paid to mucocutaneous bleeding (epistaxis, gum bleeding, menorrhagia, hematuria, melena, or hematochezia) and easy bruising. A thorough review of medications and supplements is required, especially in relation to the timing of onset of the thrombocytopenia. Drug and alcohol exposure must be documented and quantified, and dietary restrictions noted (for example, vegans may be deficient in vitamin B_{12}). The patient's medical history may show related disorders, such as HIV infection, hepatitis C infection, or thyroid diseases (hyperthyroidism and hypothyroidism may be associated with thrombocytopenia).

The physical examination may reveal blood blisters in the mouth ("wet purpura"), petechiae or ecchymoses on the skin, or splenomegaly. ▣

Thrombocytopenic Disorders

Decreased Production
Disorders associated with bone marrow infiltration (myelofibrosis, metastatic tumors, granulomatous diseases) can decrease platelet production, as can nutritional deficiencies (vitamin B_{12} or folate) or abnormalities in stem cell maturation (aplastic anemia and myelodysplasia). Other cytopenias often accompany the low platelet count.

Increased Destruction
Non–Immune-Mediated Thrombocytopenia
Splenomegaly is a common medical problem that causes thrombocytopenia without platelet destruction through increased sequestration. The thrombocytopenia is usually associated with anemia and leukopenia.

Unlike sequestration, non-immune platelet destruction is caused by abnormal platelet aggregation occurring in the setting of disseminated intravascular coagulation or a microangiopathic hemolytic anemia (MAHA) such as thrombotic thrombocytopenic purpura (TTP) or hemolytic uremic syndrome (HUS) (see following sections).

Thrombotic Thrombocytopenic Purpura
Patients with TTP present with MAHA and thrombocytopenia. Acquired TTP is caused by a deficiency in the metalloprotease ADAMTS13, which is responsible for cleaving high-molecular-weight vWF multimers. These multimers accumulate, generating platelet-rich thrombi in small vessels. These thrombi consume platelets and shear erythrocytes, fragmenting them into schistocytes (see Erythrocyte Disorders for figure) and may cause end-organ injury. Autoantibodies to ADAMTS13 are responsible for the deficiency in most patients, but hereditary TTP has been reported in some. Drugs such as ticlopidine, quinine, cyclosporine, gemcitabine, and vascular endothelial growth factor inhibitors (such as bevacizumab) can cause TTP. Drug abuse with oxymorphone, 3,4-methylenedioxymethamphetamine ("ecstasy"), and cocaine has also been reported to cause TTP.

Acquired TTP presents with MAHA (evidenced by elevated lactate dehydrogenase and decreased haptoglobin levels, schistocytes on peripheral blood smear, and a negative direct antiglobulin [Coombs] test result) and thrombocytopenia

(with normal coagulation study results). An ADAMTS13 level less than 10% supports the diagnosis; an ADAMTS13 level greater than 50% should suggest an alternate diagnosis. The clinical picture is described in **Table 19**. All patients have MAHA and thrombocytopenia, but only 5% of patients present with all the aforementioned signs. The mortality rate associated with TTP is high, so treatment must begin immediately without waiting for ADAMTS13 test results. Treatment is successful in 85% of patients.

Initial treatment involves therapeutic plasma exchange to remove the high-molecular-weight vWF multimers and replace the deficient ADAMTS13 (plasma infusion, although not a definitive treatment, can be started if therapeutic plasma exchange is delayed). Glucocorticoids are added to decrease autoantibody production. Remission is defined by a normalization of the platelet count and is usually seen after 7 to 10 plasma exchange treatments. Rituximab may be added for patients with refractory disease.

Hemolytic Uremic Syndrome
HUS is characterized by thrombocytopenia, MAHA, and acute kidney injury. Classic HUS presents after an acute diarrheal illness caused by enterotoxin-producing *Escherichia coli* O157:H7 (although other strains have also been implicated). Diagnosis is confirmed by stool culture and polymerase chain reaction for Shiga toxin, free Shiga toxin, or O157:H7 antigen testing. Management is supportive (fluids and transfusions as needed). Antibiotics do not alter the course of the disease. Classic HUS has a 4% associated mortality rate, and long-term sequelae include hypertension and mild kidney disease. Atypical HUS presents without diarrhea and may be caused by complement

TABLE 19. Clinical Characteristics of Thrombotic Thrombocytopenic Purpura	
Clinical Features	**Laboratory Findings/ Pathologic Explanation**
Pallor and fever	Microangiopathic hemolytic anemia in 100% of patients (schistocytes); fever likely from microinfarcts
Bruising, petechiae	Thrombocytopenia in 100% of patients; normal prothrombin time, activated partial thromboplastin time, and fibrinogen level
Kidney injury	Mild kidney disease, proteinuria, hematuria from microthrombi
Fluctuating neurologic findings (confusion, headache, transient numbness, coma)	CT scan may demonstrate cerebrovascular accident; transient microthrombi lead to reversible findings
Nausea, vomiting, diarrhea	Bowel ischemia
Chest pain, arrhythmia	Myocardial injury; abnormal findings on electrocardiogram, troponin elevation

CONT.

dysregulation or may occur secondary to drugs (see drugs listed in the TTP section previously), systemic lupus erythematosus, or other infection (HIV, *Streptococcus pneumoniae*). In severe cases of HUS or when the distinction from TTP is unclear, treatment with plasma exchange should begin immediately, with eculizumab (a monoclonal antibody that binds to complement C5 and prevents generation of the membrane attack unit, C5b-9) added if atypical HUS is suspected. Drug-induced HUS is managed supportively with drug avoidance.

KEY POINTS

- All patients with acquired thrombotic thrombocytopenic purpura have microangiopathic hemolytic anemia and thrombocytopenia; other clinical features may include fever, kidney disease, and fluctuating neurologic abnormalities.

- The mortality rate associated with thrombotic thrombocytopenic purpura is high, so treatment with therapeutic plasma exchange should be started as soon as a diagnosis is suspected, without awaiting laboratory results confirming ADAMTS13 deficiency.

- Hemolytic uremic syndrome is usually caused by enterotoxin-producing *Escherichia coli*, and management is supportive for most patients; antibiotics do not alter the natural course of disease.

Immune-Mediated Thrombocytopenia

Immune Thrombocytopenic Purpura

Peripheral destruction of platelets with decreased production is a feature of immune thrombocytopenic purpura (ITP) and is caused by autoantibodies directed against glycoproteins on the platelet surface membrane. Because only 6% of patients with platelet counts between 100,000 and 150,000/μL (100-150 × 10⁹/L) develop persistent thrombocytopenia, many guidelines suggest the diagnosis of ITP be limited to patients with platelet counts less than 100,000/μL (100 × 10⁹/L). ITP can occur alone, can be triggered by medications, or can be associated with other disorders, such as systemic lupus erythematosus, chronic lymphocytic leukemia, HIV, hepatitis C, or *Helicobacter pylori* infection.

ITP is characterized by the duration of the thrombocytopenia. Acute ITP lasts fewer than 3 months, persistent ITP lasts 3 to 12 months, and chronic ITP lasts longer than 12 months. Many patients are asymptomatic until the platelet count decreases to less than 10,000/μL (10 × 10⁹/L). Petechiae and ecchymoses without lymphadenopathy or splenomegaly are notable physical signs. Laboratory findings are limited to a low platelet count. Antiplatelet antibody testing is not sensitive or specific. Testing for HIV and hepatitis C should be performed. Bone marrow evaluation is not necessary unless clinical findings suggest an alternate diagnosis.

Treatment of acute ITP is instituted when patients become symptomatic or if the platelet count decreases to less than 30,000/μL (30 × 10⁹/L). Asymptomatic patients can be managed with careful observation. Initial therapy involves either glucocorticoids or intravenous immune globulin (IVIG). Glucocorticoids are less expensive and easier to administer, but the response to IVIG is faster. Complications from glucocorticoids may include mood disorders, insomnia, fluid retention, hyperglycemia, and hypertension; complications from IVIG may include infusion reactions (headache, chills, anaphylaxis), kidney disease, and thrombosis. Those patients who relapse or have ITP refractory to these treatments require second-line treatments, which include splenectomy or rituximab.

If ITP remains refractory to second-line treatment, thrombopoietin receptor agonists, such as eltrombopag (given orally daily) and romiplostim (given subcutaneously weekly), may be beneficial (with a target platelet count of 50,000/μL [50 × 10⁹/L]), but they must be taken continuously to prevent relapse.

Because patients with chronic ITP may be asymptomatic, treatment decisions must balance the risk of bleeding against treatment-related toxicities.

Heparin-Induced Thrombocytopenia

Type I heparin-induced thrombocytopenia (HIT) refers to a non-immune-mediated decrease in platelets occurring within the first few days of exposure to heparin. No intervention is needed because type I is clinically benign. Type II HIT is an immune-mediated thrombocytopenia occurring 5 to 10 days after exposure. It is caused by antibodies against platelet factor 4 (complexed to heparin). Associated thrombosis, which includes typical deep venous thrombosis, pulmonary embolism, or more unusual acute arterial occlusions, can be life threatening. The risk is highest with unfractionated heparin compared with low-molecular-weight heparin. Most patients with HIT develop platelet counts less than 150,000/μL (150 × 10⁹/L), but severe thrombocytopenia is unusual. In patients with high baseline platelet counts, a decrease of greater than 50%, even if still within the "normal" range, warrants concern. Skin necrosis at the site of heparin injection or progressive thromboembolic events in patients receiving heparin are signs of possible HIT, even if the platelet count remains normal. The 4T scoring system (**Table 20**) is useful for diagnosis. A low probability score reliably excludes the diagnosis; a high score should prompt empiric therapy pending confirmatory tests.

Testing for heparin-associated antibodies is necessary to confirm the diagnosis. Testing for HIT involves a screening test and a confirmatory test. The enzyme-linked immunosorbent assay for platelet factor 4 antibodies is a very sensitive screening test (a negative test result rules out the diagnosis) but is not specific. The diagnosis must be confirmed with a functional test such as the serotonin release assay or the heparin-induced platelet aggregation assay. Classic platelet aggregation assays provide a more detailed evaluation of platelet function, but they are labor intensive and not used in initial screening.

Heparin must be discontinued immediately. An alternate anticoagulant should then be started (unless the patient is actively bleeding). Argatroban is an intravenous alternative,

TABLE 20. The 4T Scoring System for Predicting Heparin-Induced Thrombocytopenia and Thrombosis			
4 Ts	**2 Points**	**1 Point**	**0 Points**
Thrombocytopenia	Platelet count decrease >50% and platelet nadir ≥20,000/µL (20 × 10⁹/L)	Platelet count decrease 30%-50% or platelet nadir 10,000-19,000/µL (10-19 × 10⁹/L)	Platelet count decrease <30% or platelet nadir <10,000/µL (10 × 10⁹/L)
Timing of platelet count decrease	Clear onset between days 5-10 or platelet count decrease ≤1 day (with heparin exposure within 30 days)	Consistent with platelet count decrease between days 5-10, but unclear (e.g., missing platelet counts); onset after day 10; or decrease ≤1 day (heparin exposure 30-100 days ago)	Platelet count decrease <4 days without recent exposure
Thrombosis or other sequelae	New thrombosis (confirmed); skin necrosis; acute systemic reaction after intravenous unfractionated heparin bolus	Progressive or recurrent clot; nonnecrotizing (e.g., erythematous) skin lesions; suspected thrombosis (not proved)	None
Other causes for thrombocytopenia	None apparent	Possible	Definite

High probability: 6-8 points.

Intermediate probability: 4-5 points.

Low probability: 0-3 points.

but recent reports support the use of non–vitamin K antagonist oral anticoagulants (such as rivaroxaban). Warfarin should not be the initial alternate anticoagulant because antithrombotic efficacy requires 3 to 5 days of therapy, during which time declining levels of protein C increase the thrombotic risk. Transitioning to warfarin is safe after thrombocytopenia resolves. Anticoagulation should be continued for 2 to 3 months in patients with HIT without documented thromboembolic events or 3 to 6 months for patients with HIT with associated thrombosis. Patients should be instructed to avoid heparin for life. **H**

KEY POINTS

- Antiplatelet antibody testing is not sensitive or specific for immune thrombocytopenic purpura and should not be done.

- Treatment for immune thrombocytopenic purpura is instituted with glucocorticoids or intravenous immune globulin when patients become symptomatic or if the platelet count decreases to less than 30,000/µL (30 × 10⁹/L); asymptomatic patients can be managed with careful observation.

- Heparin-induced thrombocytopenia should be suspected in any patient treated with heparin whose platelet count decreases by greater than 50% from baseline or is less than 150,000/µL (150 × 10⁹/L).

- The 4T scoring algorithm should be used to stratify the likelihood of heparin-induced thrombocytopenia, and heparin should be discontinued and an alternate anticoagulant started for patients with intermediate or high risk for disease while awaiting confirmatory results of heparin-associated antibodies.

(Continued)

KEY POINTS *(continued)*

- Most patients taking heparin who develop thrombocytopenia but have a low 4T score need no further evaluation. **HVC**

- Diagnosis of heparin-induced thrombocytopenia requires a screening test (enzyme-linked immunosorbent assay for platelet factor 4 antibodies) followed by a confirmatory test (serotonin release assay or heparin-induced platelet aggregation assay).

Qualitative Platelet Disorders

Acquired Platelet Dysfunction

Patients presenting with mucocutaneous bleeding and normal complete blood count, prothrombin time, and activated partial thromboplastin time should be evaluated for platelet dysfunction, which can result from rare hereditary disorders or acquired disorders (**Table 21**). Von Willebrand disease is a much more common inherited cause of coagulation factor deficiency leading to platelet dysfunction (see Bleeding Disorders). After platelet dysfunction is identified, treatment depends on the clinical situation. Acute bleeding can be managed with platelet transfusions, but complete reversal of antiplatelet agent effects may be detrimental if the therapy is lifesaving (for example, patients with recent cardiac stents). Minor dental procedures or menorrhagia can be managed with antifibrinolytic agents (tranexamic acid or ε-aminocaproic acid).

Platelet Function Testing

Platelet function can be assessed by a variety of laboratory tests. The Platelet Function Analyzer-100 is useful as a screening device, replacing the traditional bleeding time. The test is run on a citrated blood sample exposed to collagen and either epinephrine or adenosine diphosphate. It is a sensitive screen

TABLE 21.	Causes of Platelet Dysfunction		
	Comments	**Severity**	**Treatment**
Congenital Platelet Defects			
Glanzmann thrombasthenia	Defect in glycoprotein IIb-IIIa	Severe	Platelets or recombinant factor VIIa, ε-aminocaproic acid
Bernard-Soulier syndrome	Defect in glycoprotein Ib-IX	Severe	Platelets, ε-aminocaproic acid
Wiskott-Aldrich syndrome	Triad of eczema, thrombocytopenia, immunodeficiency	Moderate	Platelets, ε-aminocaproic acid
Gray platelet syndrome	Patients may develop myelofibrosis	Moderate	Platelets, ε-aminocaproic acid
Storage pool disease	Collection of diseases characterized by defect in platelet granules	Moderate to mild	Platelets, ε-aminocaproic acid; some may respond to desmopressin
Acquired Platelet Defects			
Uremia	Does not correlate with severity of kidney disease	Mild	Dialysis, desmopressin, ε-aminocaproic acid
Liver disease	Also associated with hyperfibrinolysis and coagulopathy	Mild to severe	Platelets, ε-aminocaproic acid
Myeloproliferative neoplasms	If platelet count is >1-1.5 million/μL (1000-1500 × 10⁹/L), may be associated with acquired von Willebrand disease	Mild to severe	Before surgical procedures, normalize the platelet count Platelet transfusion may be necessary if bleeding occurs
Post-cardiac bypass	Multifactorial, including interaction with bypass machine	Mild	Platelets, if necessary
Antiplatelet drugs			
IIb-IIIa inhibitors	Antiplatelet effects range from irreversible (abciximab) to reversible (eptifibatide and tirofiban)	Severe	Platelets
Aspirin	Irreversible	Mild	Platelets, if necessary
Clopidogrel	Irreversible	Mild	Platelets, if necessary
NSAIDs	Temporary	Mild	None usually needed
Other drugs and herbs (β-lactams, vitamin E, ginkgo, turmeric, garlic, Chinese tree fungus)		Mild	None usually needed

for von Willebrand disease and will detect abnormalities caused by antiplatelet medications. The Verifynow® test assesses for continued antiplatelet activity of aspirin or clopidogrel, but guidelines do not recommend using it to guide therapy. Thromboelastography and rotational thromboelastometry are bedside devices that analyze platelet function, coagulation, and clot stability and may be useful as screening tests in patients with unexplained bleeding. ⊞

KEY POINTS

- Patients presenting with mucocutaneous bleeding and normal complete blood count, prothrombin time, and activated partial thromboplastin time should be evaluated for von Willebrand disease or acquired platelet dysfunction.

- The Platelet Function Analyzer-100 is a useful screening test for assessing qualitative platelet disorders.

Bleeding Disorders
Normal Hemostasis

Hemostasis is the process by which bleeding is controlled through a complex network of prothrombotic and fibrinolytic activity. Clot generation occurs on phospholipid membranes through the activation of procoagulant factors (**Figure 17**). Traditionally, the process was described as a waterfall coagulation cascade (**Figure 18**), which is still used to understand screening tests and the factors that influence them.

Primary hemostasis describes the interaction between platelets, von Willebrand factor (vWF), and the vessel wall (see Platelet Disorders for platelet activation and vWF activity). Secondary hemostasis refers to the activation of coagulation factors that eventually lead to fibrin clot formation. Clots are then degraded through fibrinolysis.

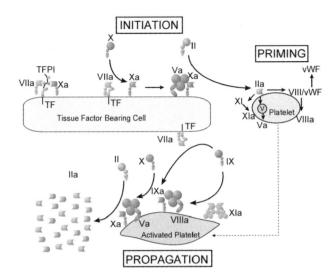

FIGURE 17. The cell-based model of hemostasis is useful for understanding coagulation as it occurs in vivo. The initiation of coagulation takes place on the surface of a tissue factor–bearing cell, such as a macrophage, a tumor cell, or an activated endothelial cell. Tissue factor (TF) and a small amount of factor VIIa generate factor Xa, which joins with factor Va to form a small amount of thrombin (factor II). In the priming step, this small amount of thrombin proceeds to activate platelets and factor VIII, which joins with factor IX to generate factor Xa. On the platelet surface, the prothrombinase complex can generate a large thrombin burst in the propagation step, allowing for cleavage of fibrinogen into fibrin.

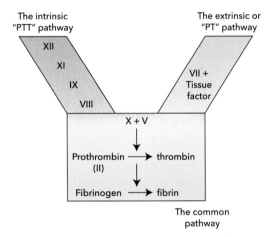

FIGURE 18. The "waterfall" model of hemostasis is useful for teasing out coagulation disorders affecting the prothrombin time (PT) and the activated partial thromboplastin time (aPTT). In this model, factors common to the PT and the aPTT are X, V, II, and fibrinogen. Factor VII is unique to the PT, and factors XII, XI, VIII, and IX are unique to the aPTT.

Evaluation of Patients with Suspected Bleeding Disorders

Patients with bleeding disorders present with symptoms of easy bruising, bleeding gums, menorrhagia, gastrointestinal bleeding, or postoperative bleeding. The clinical history provides guidance regarding how to proceed in the evaluation, with attention paid to history of tooth extraction, menstrual bleeding, minor and major surgical procedures, and family history of bleeding. Medication use and exposure to alcohol or

recreational drugs must be documented. The physical examination focuses on finding evidence of petechiae, ecchymoses, deep tissue hematomas, or joint effusions.

Laboratory tests used to measure hemostasis are the prothrombin time (PT) and the activated partial thromboplastin time (aPTT). The PT, expressed as the INR, is more sensitive to the effects of the vitamin K–dependent factors (II, VII, and X), whereas the aPTT is a more sensitive measurement of factors VIII, IX, XI, and XII. The thrombin time measures fibrinogen convergence to fibrin clot, and the Platelet Function Analyzer-100 (PFA-100®) measures platelet function. Specialized tests include mixing studies to evaluate inhibitors, specific factor level assays, and tests for fibrin degradation products and D-dimers.

Differential diagnoses for patients experiencing bleeding and who have abnormal findings on specific clotting assays are outlined in **Table 22**.

KEY POINT

• Basic laboratory tests used to evaluate hemostasis are the prothrombin time, expressed as INR; the activated partial thromboplastin time; the thrombin time, which measures fibrinogen convergence to fibrin; and platelet function as measured by the Platelet Function Analyzer-100.

TABLE 22. Differential Diagnoses for Patients Experiencing Bleeding

Clotting Assay Abnormality	Differential Diagnoses
Prolonged PT, normal aPTT	Factor VII deficiency
	DIC
	Liver disease
	Vitamin K deficiency
	Warfarin ingestion
Normal PT, prolonged aPTT	Deficiency of factors VIII, IX, XI, or XII
	von Willebrand disease (if severe and factor VIII level is quite low)
	Heparin exposure
Prolonged PT and aPTT	Deficiency of factors V, X, II, or fibrinogen
	Severe liver disease, DIC, vitamin K deficiency, warfarin toxicity
	Heparin overdose
Normal PT and aPTT	Platelet dysfunction (acquired and congenital)
	von Willebrand disease (if mild and factor VIII level is not too low)
	Scurvy
	Ehlers-Danlos syndrome
	Hereditary hemorrhagic telangiectasia
	Deficiency of factor XIII

aPTT = activated partial thromboplastin time; DIC = disseminated intravascular coagulation; PT = prothrombin time.

Congenital Bleeding Disorders

Hemophilia A and B and Other Factor Deficiencies

Hemophilia A and B (deficiency of factors VIII and IX, respectively) are X-linked hereditary bleeding disorders primarily found in male patients. Daughters of men with hemophilia are obligate carriers. Hemophilia A is more common than hemophilia B, but both are rare. They present in a similar fashion, with spontaneous hemarthrosis or bleeding into deep muscles or with excessive or delayed bleeding after trauma. Small cuts do not usually bleed excessively, but patients experience mucocutaneous bleeding. The hemophilias are classified as mild, moderate, or severe according to the circulating factor levels (mild, 5%-40%; moderate, 1%-5%; severe, <1%). Patients with mild disease may not present until adulthood.

Diagnosis requires a prolonged aPTT (that corrects in mixing studies) and a normal PT and complete blood count. Assay of individual factors (VIII and IX) confirms the diagnosis. In hemophilia A, vWF must be measured to rule out type 3 von Willebrand disease (see next section).

Arthropathy of the knees, ankles, and elbows occurs as a late sequela in 50% of patients as a result of recurrent hemarthroses. Inhibitors to infused factors (see Management) develop in up to 25% of patients with hemophilia A, and 3% to 5% of patients with hemophilia B.

Managing bleeding in hemophilia A and B requires using virally inactivated factor concentrates (eliminating the historical risk of hepatitis and HIV). Patients with mild hemophilia A can be treated with desmopressin, which stimulates the release of preformed factor VIII from endothelial cells. Antifibrinolytic agents (such as ε-aminocaproic acid and tranexamic acid) are useful in controlling bleeding from dental procedures.

Factor XI deficiency (also known as hemophilia C) is a rare autosomal hereditary disorder seen predominantly in persons of Ashkenazi Jewish heritage. Bleeding symptoms are variable and cannot be predicted by the level of factor XI alone. Asymptomatic patients do not require intervention (for example, before surgery); symptomatic patients require plasma infusions for bleeding episodes and surgical procedures.

KEY POINTS

- Patients with hemophilia A (factor VIII deficiency) or B (factor IX deficiency) have a prolonged activated partial thromboplastin time with a normal prothrombin time and complete blood count.

- Administration of infused factor concentrates can help prevent and control bleeding in patients with hemophilia A or B; some patients with mild hemophilia A may also be treated with desmopressin to stimulate the release of preformed factor VIII from stores in endothelial cells.

- Patients with factor XI deficiency who are asymptomatic do not require prophylactic intervention for surgery.

HVC

Von Willebrand Disease

Von Willebrand disease (vWD), the most common hereditary bleeding disorder, is caused by either deficiency or ineffectiveness of vWF. vWF promotes platelet adhesion and functions as a protective carrier protein for factor VIII, so a mild secondary decrease in factor VIII levels occurs. vWF deficiency leads to mucocutaneous bleeding symptoms that mimic thrombocytopenia.

Hereditary vWD is subclassified into three broad groups (**Table 23**), with type 1 being the most common. Patients become symptomatic when vWF levels decrease to less than 30%. Clinical features influence vWF levels, including type O blood (decreased levels) and pregnancy or oral contraceptive use (increased levels). Although the aPTT may be prolonged or

TABLE 23.	Types of von Willebrand Disease and Associated Features			
Type of vWD	**Basic Defect**	**Diagnostic Test**	**Symptoms**	**Treatment**
Type 1[a]	Low vWF antigen (<30%) but normal function	RCoF:vWAg 0.6-0.7 PFA-100 prolonged	Mucocutaneous bleeding	Desmopressin
Type 2	Abnormal vWF function	RCoF:vWAg 0.6-0.7	Mucocutaneous bleeding	
Type 2A	From selective deficiency of high-molecular-weight fragments of vWF			Desmopressin vWF concentrates
Type 2B	From increased binding of high-molecular-weight fragments of vWF to platelet receptors			vWF concentrates (desmopressin contraindicated)
Type 3	Severe deficiency	vWAg: unmeasurable RCoF activity: very low Factor VIII activity: 1%-10% of normal	Joint and deep muscle bleeding	vWF concentrates

PFA-100 = Platelet Function Analyzer-100; RCoF = ristocetin cofactor; vWAg = von Willebrand antigen; vWF = von Willebrand factor.

[a]80% of cases.

normal, a prolonged closure time on the PFA-100® would suggest vWD, making this a useful initial evaluation tool. The diagnosis is confirmed by finding a reduction in von Willebrand antigen (quantitative analysis) and reduced vWF ristocetin cofactor activity (a measurement of the functional affect) (see Table 23).

Management of vWD depends on the severity of bleeding, the type of vWD, and the clinical setting. Desmopressin is effective in type 1 vWD, releasing preformed vWF and factor VIII from endothelial cells. It can be given intravenously before a surgical procedure or intranasally as needed in the outpatient setting. Patients with rare type 2B vWD should not receive desmopressin because it induces platelet aggregation, which can cause secondary thrombocytopenia in these patients. Desmopressin is ineffective in patients with type 3 vWD. vWF concentrates are the preferred treatment for these two subgroups; cryoprecipitate is no longer used because virally inactivated vWF concentrates are safer and more effective. Antifibrinolytic therapy (ε-aminocaproic acid and tranexamic acid) is useful after surgical procedures to protect against delayed bleeding and can be used to treat menorrhagia.

KEY POINTS

- Von Willebrand factor deficiency in von Willebrand disease leads to mucocutaneous bleeding symptoms that mimic thrombocytopenia, including bleeding gums, epistaxis, menorrhagia, and easy bruising.

- Desmopressin, which stimulates release of preformed von Willebrand factor and factor VIII, is used to treat minor bleeding in most patients with von Willebrand disease and is given prophylactically before surgery or procedures.

- Von Willebrand factor concentrates are used for major bleeding and to treat patients with rare subtypes 2B and 3.

Acquired Bleeding Disorders

Coagulopathy of Liver Disease

Bleeding in patients with liver disease results from one of many interrelated hemostatic aberrations. The liver is the site of production for procoagulant and fibrinolytic factors. Liver disease is associated with bleeding and thrombosis, but only bleeding manifestations will be discussed here.

Liver disease can result in factor deficiency, hyperfibrinolysis, and mild to moderate thrombocytopenia, leading to PT prolongation, INR elevation, and aPTT prolongation. Distinguishing between liver disease and disseminated intravascular coagulation may be challenging. Measuring factor VIII levels (not affected by liver disease) and factor V levels (not consumed during intravascular coagulation) provides a theoretical means of separating the two disorders. Patients often have components of both liver disease and disseminated

intravascular coagulation, and management rarely differs based on distinguishing the two disorders.

Asymptomatic patients do not require treatment, but vitamin K supplementation should be considered if the INR is elevated. Patients experiencing bleeding may require blood product replacement, with cryoprecipitate to increase fibrinogen levels to greater than 100 mg/dL (1 g/L) and platelet transfusions to maintain a platelet count greater than 75,000/μL (75 × 10⁹/L). Fresh frozen plasma may be given for INRs greater than 2, but the short half-life of plasma components and risk of volume overload limit the effectiveness of plasma administration. Prothrombin complex concentrates are costly and associated with thrombotic complications; they should not be routinely used in managing the coagulopathy of liver disease. Accelerated fibrinolysis also contributes to bleeding, but no laboratory tests reliably measure this condition. Viscoelastic testing may be useful, although the predictive value in documenting accelerated fibrinolysis is debated and the test is not widely available. Antifibrinolytic agents are useful in treating hyperfibrinolysis and should be considered when persistent oozing from mucous membranes or delayed bleeding from procedure sites occurs in the absence of or despite correction of overt coagulopathy.

KEY POINTS

- Although measuring levels of factor VIII (normal in liver disease) and factor V (not consumed during intravascular coagulation) could theoretically distinguish coagulopathy of liver disease from disseminated intravascular coagulation, patients may have components of both disorders, and the management is usually analogous regardless of this distinction.

- Active bleeding in patients with coagulopathy of liver disease should be managed with cryoprecipitate to maintain fibrinogen levels greater than 100 mg/dL (1 g/L) and platelet transfusions to achieve a platelet count greater than 75,000/μL (75 × 10⁹/L).

- Fresh frozen plasma can be administered to patients with coagulopathy of liver disease, active bleeding, and an INR greater than 2, but the short half-life of plasma coagulation factors and risk of volume overload limit its effectiveness.

- Because of their cost and association with prothrombotic complications, prothrombin complex concentrates should not be routinely used to manage the coagulopathy of liver disease.

HVC

Vitamin K Deficiency

Although vitamin K is found in green vegetables, a significant proportion of the daily requirement comes from gut microflora (which may be destroyed by antibiotics); absorption requires biliary and pancreatic function because vitamin K is fat soluble. It acts as a cofactor for carboxylation and activation of certain coagulation factors (see Table 22), as well as for the

CONT.

endogenous anticoagulants, protein C, and protein S. Patients who cannot take anything by mouth, who have poor oral intake while taking long courses of antibiotics, and who have fat malabsorption are especially at risk for vitamin K deficiency. Vitamin K supplements safely and effectively correct the deficiency, so this diagnosis should always be considered when evaluating a patient with a prolonged PT. The response to supplementation occurs within hours because vitamin K acts by converting precursor proteins synthesized in the liver into active factors. Vitamin K can be administered orally for patients who are able to eat. Critically ill patients or those unable to take anything by mouth should receive vitamin K by slow intravenous infusion. Subcutaneous vitamin K is not reliably absorbed and is unlikely to be safer than intravenous vitamin K.

Acquired von Willebrand Disease

Acquired vWD occurs in conditions of high circulatory shear stress (valvular heart disease, hypertrophic cardiomyopathy, circulatory assist devices, and extracorporeal membrane-oxygenation systems) caused by excessive degradation of high-molecular-weight von Willebrand multimers by the proteolytic enzyme ADAMTS13. Affected patients develop bleeding conditions similar to those in hereditary vWD. The prevalence of this disorder is likely to increase as more patients with severe cardiomyopathy are managed with left ventricular assist devices. These patients are routinely managed with warfarin and antiplatelet agents and have a significant incidence of gastrointestinal or other bleeding problems. Desmopressin and vWF concentrates have been used in management.

Acquired Hemophilia

Acquired hemophilia results from an autoantibody directed against factor VIII. Patients present with bleeding symptoms that mimic hereditary hemophilia A. Approximately half of all cases are associated with pregnancy and the postpartum state, malignancy, and other autoimmune disorders, as well as with medications.

Laboratory evaluation shows a normal platelet count and PT with a prolonged aPTT. Mixing studies do not correct the aPTT. Factor analysis shows a low factor VIII level; an inhibitor can be quantified with the Bethesda assay. One Bethesda unit is defined as the reciprocal of the dilution of patient plasma that results in 50% inactivation.

Factor VIII concentrates do not correct the problem. Management of acute bleeding requires activated prothrombin complex concentrates or activated factor VII to overcome the inhibitor. Immunosuppression, using corticosteroids and cyclophosphamide, is required to decrease the formation of inhibitors.

Acquired hemophilia A is just one example of an autoimmune factor deficiency. Acquired inhibitors can occur against any factor and should be considered whenever a patient presents with a new bleeding diathesis and an unexpectedly low factor level.

Disseminated Intravascular Coagulation

Disseminated intravascular coagulation results from the simultaneous stimulation of coagulation and fibrinolysis. It is associated with severe sepsis, usually with septic shock; with disseminated malignancy, most classically with mucin-secreting pancreatic adenocarcinoma; and in pregnancy with various severe complications, including sepsis, placental abruption, and eclampsia. Patients with life-threatening illnesses characterized by systemic immune response syndrome with hypotension and multiorgan dysfunction are also at risk. The initial pathogenesis involves widespread endothelial injury and circulating procoagulants that lead to disseminated microvascular thrombi, with consumption of platelets and clotting factors, and erythrocyte shearing injury leading to hemolysis. Fibrinolysis is accelerated, resulting in dissolution of the microvascular thrombus, usually before thrombotic complications are noted. These factors leave the patient vulnerable to bleeding from thrombocytopenia, clotting factor depletion, and fibrinolysis. Classic laboratory findings include thrombocytopenia, prolonged aPTT and PT, elevated INR, hypofibrinogenemia, and elevated D-dimer levels, although laboratory features are unpredictable from patient to patient. Management is directed primarily at the inciting cause of disseminated intravascular coagulation and supported with platelet transfusions, cryoprecipitate, and fresh frozen plasma as needed.

Transfusion Medicine

Clinical trials supporting the benefits of a more cautious transfusion strategy have dramatically changed transfusion practice. For elective transfusions, ABO and Rh matching based on a properly labeled blood specimen remains the cornerstone of

CONT.

safe transfusion. Approximately 5% to 10% of hospitalized patients have evidence of erythrocyte alloimmunization from previous transfusions, pregnancy, or organ transplantation. These antibodies to non-ABO blood group antigens pose a risk for delayed (as opposed to acute) hemolytic transfusion reaction. Other noninfectious risks of transfusion, such as transfusion-associated circulatory overload, are now better recognized. Although the traditionally feared infectious risks of transfusion, hepatitis C virus and HIV, are now quite rare, transfusions are linked to an evolving spectrum of emerging infectious diseases, such as Zika virus.

Blood Donor Screening

Blood donor screening comprises questions to establish the general health of the donor and exclude high-risk behaviors or potential exposures that increase the risk of transfusion-transmitted infection, followed by selected laboratory testing. The hemoglobin level cutoff is 12.5 g/dL (125 g/L) for women, which excludes a small proportion of otherwise healthy women from donating. Most platelets transfused in the United States are collected from donors by apheresis, which increases platelet yield but is a more time-consuming procedure than whole blood donation. Laboratory testing of whole blood and platelet donations includes screening for hepatitis B and C viruses, HIV, human T-cell lymphotropic virus I/II, and West Nile virus; serologic testing for syphilis; and, in select regions of the country, testing for antibodies to *Trypanosoma cruzi* (agent for Chagas disease), *Babesia*, and most recently, Zika virus. Platelet components are also screened for bacterial contamination before being released for transfusion.

KEY POINT

- Donated whole blood and platelets are screened for hepatitis B and C viruses, HIV, human T-cell lymphotropic virus I/II, and West Nile virus; undergo serologic testing for syphilis; and, in select regions of the country, are tested for antibodies to *Trypanosoma cruzi*, *Babesia*, and most recently, Zika virus.

Blood Group Antigens, Pretransfusion Compatibility Testing, and the Direct Antiglobulin Test

A "type and screen" comprises ABO/Rh blood group determination and a screening test for unexpected (non-ABO) antibodies. A "type and cross" uses patient plasma or serum to crossmatch against a representative sample from a donor erythrocyte unit for transfusion. For procedures in which blood transfusion is not invariably needed, a type and screen showing no unexpected antibodies eliminates the need for specific crossmatching; blood can be quickly crossmatched when and if the decision to transfuse is made. Rh-positive

persons can receive Rh-positive or Rh-negative blood. Rh-negative persons should receive only Rh-negative blood, except in circumstances of massive transfusion (such as gastrointestinal bleeding or traumatic hemorrhage), when Rh-positive blood can be given to preserve the inventory of scarcer Rh-negative units. Rh-positive blood should never be given to persons already sensitized to Rh antigens or to Rh-negative women of childbearing potential because exposure increases their risk for subsequent pregnancies affected by hemolytic disease of the fetus and newborn. Plasma requires ABO but not Rh matching; platelets, with some exceptions, are not ABO or Rh matched.

A direct antiglobulin (Coombs) test is performed to look for IgG or complement coating a patient's erythrocytes and is part of the investigation for suspected hemolytic transfusion reactions (acute or delayed), autoimmune hemolytic anemia, and hemolytic disease of the newborn.

KEY POINTS

- Women of childbearing age or younger and patients previously sensitized to Rh antigens should never receive Rh-positive blood.

- For procedures in which blood transfusion is not invariably needed, a type and screen showing no unexpected antibodies eliminates the need for specific crossmatching of individual units.

Blood Components
Packed Red Blood Cells

Packed red blood cells (PRBCs), which contain a small amount of residual plasma, are suspended in anticoagulant-preservative solution at a hematocrit level of 55% to 65%. Transfusion of one unit of PRBCs to an average-sized nonbleeding adult raises the hematocrit level by 3% and the hemoglobin level by 1 g/dL (10 g/L). Erythrocyte transfusion to patients with anemia increases oxygen-carrying capacity; the threshold for transfusion varies according to the chronicity of the anemia and the patient's comorbidities.

Plasma

Plasma contains coagulation factors, albumin, immunoglobulins, and other plasma proteins. Plasma transfusion is indicated to restore coagulation factors for which specific factor concentrates are not available or in the setting of multiple acquired deficiencies, as in disseminated intravascular coagulation. If frozen within 6 hours of collection, the product is called "fresh frozen plasma" and has a shelf life of 1 year at −20 °C (−4 °F), or 24 hours after it is thawed at 37 °C (98.6 °F). Thawed fresh frozen plasma can be relabeled as thawed plasma, extending its shelf life to 5 days of storage. Although thawed plasma has lower levels of labile factors, such as factors V and VIII, the difference is not clinically significant in most transfusion situations, particularly because factor VIII is an acute phase reactant.

Cryoprecipitate

Cryoprecipitate is the small fraction of plasma that precipitates when fresh frozen plasma is thawed at 1 to 4 °C (33.8-39.2 °F). It contains mostly fibrinogen and factor VIII and is most often used in conditions associated with hypofibrinogenemia, such as disseminated intravascular coagulation. It is also sometimes used empirically in uremic bleeding, but the mechanism of action is poorly understood. For adult patients who require fibrinogen replacement, multiple (8-10) units of cryoprecipitate (from 8-10 donors) must be pooled together.

Platelets

A unit of platelets is suspended in plasma and has a short shelf life of 5 days at 20 to 24 °C (68-75.2 °F). Platelets can be made from a whole blood donation (a platelet concentrate) or collected by apheresis. A bag of apheresis platelets provides a platelet dose equivalent to 4 to 6 units of platelet concentrate and raises the platelet count of an average-sized adult by 20,000 to 25,000/µL (20-25 × 10^9/L) (for example, from a platelet count of 10,000/µL to 30,000/µL). Platelets are not generally indicated in patients with thrombocytopenia in the absence of trauma, surgery, or bleeding until the platelet count decreases to less than 10,000 to 20,000/µL (10-20 × 10^9/L); the lower platelet count is more applicable to patients with chronic thrombocytopenia who are otherwise stable. The transfusion threshold for patients with bleeding, trauma, or both, is approximately 50,000/µL (50 × 10^9/L).

PRBCs and platelet components can be modified through processes such as leukoreduction, irradiation, and washing, which are indicated in special transfusion circumstances (**Table 24**).

- Transfusion of one unit of packed red blood cells to an average-sized nonbleeding adult raises the hematocrit level by 3% and the hemoglobin level by 1 g/dL (10 g/L); transfusion to patients with anemia increases oxygen-carrying capacity.

- Cryoprecipitate contains a concentrated amount of fibrinogen and is used to treat hypofibrinogenemia seen in disseminated intravascular coagulation.

- Platelets are not generally indicated in otherwise stable patients with chronic thrombocytopenia until the platelet count decreases to less than 10,000 to 20,000/µL (10-20 × 10^9/L).

Plasma Derivatives

Plasma pooled together from thousands of donors is fractionated into derivatives such as albumin (used for oncotic pressure in hypotensive patients or after large volume paracentesis cirrhotic patients), intravenous immune globulin (for patients who have humoral immunodeficiencies), Rh immune globulins (for Rh-negative pregnant women to prevent sensitization from an Rh-positive fetus), or coagulation factor concentrates (such as factor VIII concentrate for von Willebrand disease) (**Table 25**). Plasma derivatives are processed to reduce the risk of infectious disease transmission. Recombinant factor concentrates (not containing any donor plasma) have become the standard of care for younger patients with hemophilia A and B (factor VIII and IX deficiency, respectively).

TABLE 24. Cellular Transfusion Product Modifications	
Modification	**Notes**
Leukoreduction[a]: decreases number of leukocytes present in transfused erythrocytes or platelets	Reduces class I HLA alloantibody production and subsequent platelet transfusion refractoriness.
	Decreases febrile nonhemolytic transfusion reactions.
	Decreases transmission of CMV.
	Leukoreduction cannot be relied on to prevent transfusion-associated GVHD.
Irradiation: prevents replication of lymphocytes and circulating stem cells present in erythrocyte or platelet products	Prevents transfusion-associated GVHD, which is mediated by donor lymphocytes.
	Indicated in patients with severe immunodeficiency, whether inherited or acquired or following chemotherapy.
	Indicated in immunocompetent patients receiving HLA-matched platelets or transfusions from relatives.
Washing: removes proteins remaining in the plasma of erythrocyte and platelet products	Used in patients with a history of severe/recurrent allergic reactions, IgA deficiency (when IgA-deficient donors are unavailable).
	May be indicated for patients with complement-dependent autoimmune hemolytic anemia.
	Reduces the amount of potassium transfused for patients who are at high risk for hyperkalemia.

CMV = cytomegalovirus; GVHD = graft-versus-host disease.

[a]More than 80% of blood banks in the United States adhere to universal leukoreduction. For those that do not, leukoreduction should be performed for chronically transfused patients, those with a history of a febrile hemolytic transfusion reaction, patients who are potential candidates for or recipients of a solid-organ or hematopoietic stem cell transplant, and immunocompromised recipients who are CMV seronegative.

FOUR FACTOR PROTHROMBIN — FACTOR II, VII, IX, X IN A POWDER
COMPLEX CONCENTRATE — GIVEN IN SMALL VOLUME
※ USED FOR URGENT WARFARIN REVERSAL
— AVOID IN HX OF HIT
— THROMBOEMBOLISM RISK

TABLE 25. Plasma-Derived Therapeutic Products

Product	Indication(s) for Use
Fresh frozen plasma	Replacement fluid for plasma exchange in thrombotic thrombocytopenic purpura
	Prevention and treatment of coagulopathy from massive transfusion
	Treatment of bleeding associated with multiple acquired clotting factor deficiencies (liver disease, disseminated intravascular coagulation, nonemergent warfarin toxicity)
Cryoprecipitate	Congenital or acquired fibrinogen deficiency FIBRINOGEN
	Dysfibrinogenemia
	Factor XIII deficiency
	Treatment of hemophilia A and von Willebrand disease when a specific factor concentrate is not available
Intravenous immune globulin	Acquired or congenital hypogammaglobulinemia
	Autoimmune disorders
Albumin	Replacement fluid for plasma exchange
	Large-volume paracentesis
Prothrombin complex concentrates[a]	Major warfarin-associated hemorrhage
Factor VIII[b]	Hemophilia A, treatment and prevention of bleeding
von Willebrand protein–rich factor VIII[b,c]	von Willebrand disease, treatment and prevention of bleeding
Factor IX[b]	Hemophilia B, treatment and prevention of bleeding
Fibrinogen concentrate	Congenital fibrinogen deficiency, treatment of bleeding
Thrombin[b]	Topical application for small vessel bleeding despite standard surgical techniques or when surgical intervention is not feasible
Protein C concentrate	Severe congenital protein C deficiency (prevention and treatment of venous thrombosis and purpura fulminans)
Antithrombin[b]	Hereditary antithrombin deficiency (perisurgical and obstetric procedure prophylaxis and treatment of established venous thrombosis)
α_1-antitrypsin	Congenital α_1-antitrypsin deficiency (high-risk phenotype, α_1-antitrypsin level <11 µmol/L, ≥18 years of age, and airflow obstruction by spirometry)
C1-esterase inhibitor	Hereditary angioedema, acute attacks

[a]Four-factor prothrombin complex concentrate (containing factors II, VII, IX, and X) is preferred over three-factor prothrombin complex concentrates in which factor VII is missing.

[b]Recombinant product available and preferred as a way of reducing the risk of transmissible infections.

[c]Select plasma-derived factor VIII products are rich in von Willebrand protein.

Prothrombin complex concentrates (PCCs), specifically the newer generation of four-factor PCC, which contains factors II, VII, IX, and X, are the preferred product for patients experiencing life-threatening bleeding while taking warfarin anticoagulation. Previously, plasma transfusion with or without vitamin K supplementation was used with the attendant risks of volume overload and allergic reactions. Inappropriate use of PCCs carries a thrombotic risk, so they should not be used in patients who have elevated INRs from warfarin without life-threatening bleeding or before elective invasive procedures in patients receiving anticoagulation or patients with chronic liver disease. A recent multicenter trial demonstrated the safety and efficacy of PCCs compared with plasma transfusion in patients requiring urgent surgical interventions. PCCs contain residual heparin and are contraindicated in patients with heparin-induced thrombocytopenia. H

KEY POINTS

- Recombinant factor concentrates (not containing any donor plasma) are the standard of care for younger patients with hemophilia A and B.

- The newer generation of four-factor prothrombin complex concentrates is the preferred product for patients experiencing life-threatening bleeding while taking warfarin anticoagulation.

Blood Management

Patient-centered blood management uses allogeneic blood components to achieve a clinically relevant goal rather than to correct an abnormal laboratory finding; identifies and corrects specific causes of anemia that eliminate the need for transfusion; and reduces iatrogenic blood loss by eliminating unnecessary phlebotomy for routine laboratory testing.

CONT. In the previous 2 decades, several large, randomized controlled trials have demonstrated the safety of a restrictive transfusion threshold (hemoglobin level <7-8 g/dL [70-80 g/L]) compared with a more liberal threshold (hemoglobin level <9-10 g/dL [90-100 g/L]) in common clinical settings in which blood is transfused, such as in critically ill patients in the ICU, patients with gastrointestinal bleeding, and older adult patients after hip fracture surgery. With the exception of the "TITRe" trial in cardiac surgery, all the trials found that a restrictive transfusion threshold produced equivalent, and in some cases superior, outcomes, such as in patients with upper gastrointestinal bleeding. Incorporating restrictive transfusion guidelines in computerized physician order entry pathways increases adherence to these thresholds. Although a restrictive transfusion threshold has proven beneficial in many clinical scenarios, emergent transfusion at more liberal transfusion thresholds will remain important in specific instances, such as in patients with anemia and acute coronary syndrome or acute stroke and patients who are actively bleeding and hemodynamically unstable. ▣

KEY POINT

- A restrictive transfusion threshold (hemoglobin level <7-8 g/dL [70-80 g/L]) provides equivalent outcomes as a more liberal threshold (hemoglobin level <9-10 g/dL [90-100 g/L]) in managing critically ill patients in the ICU, patients with acute gastrointestinal bleeding, and older patients after hip fracture.

Transfusion Complications

Transfusion reactions occur in approximately 1% of transfusions. They are best classified according to the main presenting symptoms, such as fever and chills, respiratory distress, and allergic manifestations. Although fatal reactions are rare (incidence of 1:200,000-400,000 units), the leading causes are hemolysis, transfusion-related acute lung injury, and transfusion-associated circulatory overload.

Hemolytic Reactions
Acute Hemolytic Transfusion Reactions
Acute hemolytic transfusion reactions result from clerical errors at the time of specimen collection or blood administration. Electronic barcode systems that print a specimen label from the patient's wristband on demand or verify patient-unit compatibility at the time of bedside transfusion reduce such errors but are not yet widely adopted. Patient and specimen identification can be particularly problematic in high turnover areas such as the emergency department or in mass-casualty incidents. Patients develop fever and flank pain and appear anxious and distressed. Hypotension and diffuse bleeding may be signs that acute hemolysis has triggered disseminated intravascular coagulation. Hemoglobinuria and hemoglobinemia may be noted. Platelets, because of their short shelf life, are administered in adult transfusion practice

without regard to ABO compatibility, and, rarely, high-titer ABO antibodies in the plasma of group O platelets may mediate less extensive hemolytic transfusion reactions, which are more subtle and harder to recognize, such as an unexplained drop in hematocrit level or a newly positive direct antiglobulin test result. The most important step in managing signs or symptoms consistent with an acute hemolytic transfusion reaction is to stop the transfusion; outcomes worsen as more incompatible blood is transfused. Clerical review and blood bank notification should follow. Laboratory tests include the direct antiglobulin test, haptoglobin and plasma free hemoglobin measurements, and urinalysis to assess hemoglobinuria. Volume expansion and supportive care for associated complications (disseminated intravascular coagulation, acute kidney injury) are required.

Delayed Hemolytic Transfusion Reaction
Antibodies to non-ABO blood group antigens (so-called "minor" antigens) develop in some persons after transfusion or pregnancy but may be not be detectable when subsequent transfusion is needed years later. When re-exposed to transfused cells with the same antigen, an anamnestic antibody response leads to delayed hemolysis of the transfused antigen-positive erythrocytes, typically 7 to 14 days after the transfusion. The causative association between a hematocrit level decrease, often accompanied by low-grade fever, and a transfusion 1 to 2 weeks beforehand is not always appreciated, particularly in postoperative patients or patients discharged from the hospital. Investigation of a suspected delayed hemolytic transfusion reaction should include a direct antiglobulin test (and blood bank notification) and evaluation of markers of hemolysis, such as lactate dehydrogenase and bilirubin levels and reticulocyte count. Patients should be informed regarding their alloimmunization status so they can communicate this information to other health care providers for subsequent surgery or other care. Some jurisdictions outside the United States have transfusion "antibody registries" for this purpose. ▣

KEY POINTS

- Acute hemolytic transfusion reactions manifest with fever, flank pain, hypotension, hemoglobinemia, and hemoglobinuria; discontinuing the transfusion is the most important step in treatment.

- A delayed hemolytic transfusion reaction, with low-grade fever and worsening anemia, occurs 1 to 2 weeks after transfusion and should be evaluated measuring direct antiglobulin, haptoglobin, lactate dehydrogenase, bilirubin, and reticulocyte count.

Nonhemolytic Transfusion Reactions

Transfusion-Associated Circulatory Overload
Transfusion-associated circulatory overload (TACO) is an underrecognized problem and may be the most common serious complication of blood transfusion, affecting 1% to 8% of transfusion recipients. Risk factors include older age, pre-existing

CONT.

cardiovascular or kidney disease, and rapid administration rate. Signs and symptoms include respiratory distress within 6 hours of transfusion, positive fluid balance, elevated central venous pressure, elevated B-type natriuretic peptide, and compatible radiographic findings of pulmonary edema. Therapy consists of diuretics and a slower rate of blood administration.

Transfusion-Related Acute Lung Injury

Transfusion-related acute lung injury (TRALI) is defined as noncardiogenic pulmonary edema that occurs within 6 hours of transfusion. These patients are more likely to present with fever and hypotension and less likely to have overt signs of volume overload as in patients with TACO. Radiographic findings usually suggest a noncardiac pulmonary edema or adult respiratory distress syndrome but may resemble those seen in TACO. Most cases of TRALI occur because of HLA or neutrophil-specific antibodies in multiparous donors that bind to and activate recipient leukocytes in the pulmonary vasculature. The incidence of this complication has been significantly reduced by screening donors for these antibodies. Management is supportive and includes supplemental oxygen or mechanical ventilatory support as needed. This management is analogous to that used for other causes of adult respiratory distress syndrome, although the prognosis is better and the recovery quicker. TRALI is unlikely to recur in subsequent transfusions for individual patients.

Febrile Nonhemolytic Transfusion Reaction

Febrile nonhemolytic transfusion reaction (FNHTR) is common, occurring in about 1% of transfusion episodes, and is mediated by proinflammatory cytokines elaborated by donor leukocytes during storage. Symptoms encompass a temperature increase of 1 °C (1.8 °F) to greater than 38 °C (100.4 °F) within 4 hours of transfusion or chills and rigors even in the absence of a fever. The differential diagnosis of fever occurring in association with transfusion includes hemolysis and septic transfusion reaction. Investigation consists of a direct antiglobulin test, visual inspection of patient plasma for hemolysis, and a clerical check and, if warranted, obtaining a blood bag culture and blood cultures from the patient. Although antipyretics are appropriate as therapy, no studies have shown that they prevent FNHTR, so routine prophylaxis with antipyretics is not warranted. Prestorage leukocyte reduction of whole blood by filtration at the blood center or at the time of platelet apheresis collection can prevent FNHTR. ⬚

KEY POINTS

- Signs and symptoms of transfusion-associated circulatory overload include respiratory distress within 6 hours of transfusion, positive fluid balance, elevated central venous pressure, elevated B-type natriuretic peptide, and compatible radiographic findings of pulmonary edema.

(Continued)

KEY POINTS *(continued)*

- Transfusion-related acute lung injury is defined as noncardiogenic pulmonary edema that occurs within 6 hours of transfusion and is managed similarly to other causes of acute respiratory distress syndrome.

Infectious Complications

PLTS → GP&⊕
RBCs → GN ⊖

⬚

Bacterial contamination of blood components occurs from inadequate cleansing of the donor's skin before phlebotomy or from occult (asymptomatic) bacteremia in the blood donor. Platelet components are screened for bacterial contamination before release for transfusion, but residual risk remains, typically for gram-positive organisms that are part of skin flora. Erythrocyte components, when contaminated, tend to contain gram-negative organisms such as *Yersinia*, which thrive in a cold and iron-rich environment. Infectious complications include the transmission of agents not routinely tested for, such as *Babesia*. The clinical features may include fever with or without hypotension.

Allergic Reactions and Anaphylaxis

Mild allergic reactions with pruritus and urticaria occur in 1% to 5% of recipients, during or after the transfusion of plasma-rich components (including platelets). If symptoms resolve after the administration of antihistamines, transfusion can be restarted with the same unit under close observation. The transfusion must be discontinued if symptoms recur or progress beyond urticaria. No evidence supports the routine use of antihistamine or glucocorticoid prophylaxis in patients with previous mild allergic transfusion reactions.

Anaphylactic or anaphylactoid reactions are rare. Manifestations include angioedema, stridor, abdominal symptoms, and hypotension. In addition to antihistamines (H_1 and H_2 blockers), patients may require bronchodilators, fluid resuscitation, and epinephrine. Investigation of possible underlying protein deficiency (IgA or haptoglobin) should be undertaken in a patient with an anaphylactic transfusion reaction. The documentation of severe IgA deficiency with anti-IgA antibodies necessitates the future use of washed cellular blood components or plasma components from IgA-deficient donors. ⬚

KEY POINTS

- No evidence supports the routine use of antihistamine or glucocorticoid prophylaxis in patients with a history of mild allergic transfusion reactions.

- Manifestations of anaphylactic or anaphylactoid transfusion reactions include angioedema, stridor, abdominal symptoms, and hypotension and should prompt an investigation for an underlying protein deficiency (IgA or haptoglobin).

Transfusion-Associated Graft-versus-Host Disease

Transfusion-associated graft-versus-host disease is a rare but fatal complication in which donor lymphocytes in a cellular

CONT.

blood product (erythrocytes or platelets) engraft in an immunocompromised recipient and cause toxic effects in the bone marrow, skin, liver, and gastrointestinal tract. Patients at risk include those receiving chemotherapy for autoimmune disorders or malignancy, recipients of blood components from first-degree relatives, and premature infants. Prevention involves γ irradiation of cellular blood components intended for recipients at risk. Patients who have undergone stem cell transplantation typically require irradiated blood components indefinitely; this should be communicated from the transplant center at the time of discharge from the transplant program.

KEY POINT

- Patients who have undergone stem cell transplantation typically require γ-irradiated blood products to prevent transfusion-associated graft-versus-host disease.

Transfusion in Special Circumstances

Massive transfusion refers to the transfusion of one total blood volume, which is equivalent to 8 to 10 units of blood, within a 24-hour period. Conditions requiring massive transfusion include trauma, ruptured aortic aneurysm, and severe gastrointestinal bleeding. When whole blood is lost and replaced with crystalloid and PRBCs, a dilutional coagulopathy develops that is often exacerbated by hypothermia, acidosis, and liver injury as well as concomitant disseminated intravascular coagulation. Contemporary practice is to transfuse plasma and platelets concurrently with PRBCs to avert the development of dilutional coagulopathy. During resuscitation, patients must be monitored for electrolyte disturbances such as hypocalcemia (because the citrate in the anticoagulant used for all blood components binds free calcium, which lowers the serum calcium concentration), hyperkalemia or hypokalemia, and metabolic alkalosis (from citrate metabolism).

Autoimmune hemolytic anemia presents a unique transfusion challenge. Warm reactive autoantibodies are usually polyclonal IgG antibodies directed against erythrocytes (the patient's own, reagent, and donor erythrocytes). The clinical significance of warm autoantibodies derives from their hemolytic potential and their interference with routine pretransfusion compatibility testing, specifically the detection of alloantibodies and the provision of crossmatch-compatible blood. The urgency of the transfusion, particularly the presence of acute cardiopulmonary or central nervous system symptoms, must be considered along with the risk for hidden alloantibodies, which are rare in patients without previous pregnancy or transfusion. Transfused units should be matched for ABO and Rh. Care of these patients should be closely coordinated between the hospitalist, hematologist, and blood bank specialist.

KEY POINTS

- As patients requiring massive transfusion are resuscitated, they must be monitored for electrolyte disturbances such as hypocalcemia, hyperkalemia or hypokalemia, and metabolic alkalosis.
- Patients with warm autoimmune hemolytic anemia have autoantibodies that react against all erythrocytes, including donor erythrocytes, so a completely crossmatch-compatible unit may be impossible to find; these patients should be transfused with ABO and Rh type-specific, crossmatch-incompatible blood.

Therapeutic Apheresis

Apheresis procedures use an automated blood cell separator to collect whole blood, separate it into the plasma and cellular components, remove the component contributing to disease, and return the other blood components to the patient combined with replacement fluids. Plasmapheresis for patients suspected of having Guillain-Barré syndrome is a classic example. Crystalloid and colloid fluids are used for replacement, and plasma components are typically avoided. Therapy for thrombotic thrombocytopenic purpura is more appropriately characterized as plasma exchange because fresh frozen plasma is provided as the replacement fluid. The same cell separators can be used to perform plateletpheresis, erythrocyte exchange transfusion, and other procedures in patients with specific indications (**Table 26**).

Thrombotic Disorders

The burden of venous thromboembolic disease continues to increase despite increased awareness of risk factors and prevention options. The incidence of a first episode of venous thromboembolism (VTE) is approximately 1 to 2 per 1000 person/years.

VTE most commonly manifests as lower extremity deep venous thrombosis (DVT) or pulmonary embolism (PE). Many nosocomial VTEs are preventable, although thromboprophylaxis continues to be underused. D-dimer testing and imaging for VTE diagnosis should be used within the context of appropriate clinical algorithms.

Opinions differ regarding the relevance of thrombophilia testing, and results usually do not affect the length of anticoagulation. The landscape of treatment options continues to evolve.

Pathophysiology of Thrombosis

Alterations in three primary mechanisms of thrombosis predispose persons to VTE. Described by the German pathologist Rudolph Virchow more than 150 years ago, reduced or otherwise turbulent blood flow, alterations or injury to the vessel

TABLE 26. Indications for Therapeutic Apheresis[a]

Plasmapheresis/Plasma Exchange

Thrombotic thrombocytopenic purpura

Hyperviscosity syndrome (Waldenström macroglobulinemia and multiple myeloma)

Paraproteinemic polyneuropathies

Guillain-Barré syndrome (acute inflammatory demyelinating polyneuropathy)

Chronic inflammatory demyelinating polyradiculoneuropathy

Myasthenia gravis

ANCA-associated rapidly progressive glomerulonephritis

Anti–glomerular basement membrane disease

Recurrent focal segmental glomerulosclerosis

Severe, symptomatic cryoglobulinemia

Antibody-mediated renal allograft rejection

Fulminant Wilson disease

Erythrocyte Exchange

Severe babesiosis[b]

Sickle cell disease with acute cerebral infarct

Sickle cell disease with severe acute chest syndrome[c]

Leukapheresis

Hyperleukocytosis syndrome

Plateletpheresis

Symptomatic extreme thrombocytosis[d]

Extracorporeal Photopheresis

Cardiac allograft rejection, prophylaxis

Erythrodermic cutaneous T-cell lymphoma/Sézary syndrome

Selective Blood Component Removal

LDL cholesterol for familial hypercholesterolemia

[a]This list includes diseases for which apheresis is an accepted part of front-line therapy for a particular indication, either as the sole therapeutic modality or in combination with other therapy. It is not an all-inclusive list.

[b]Erythrocyte exchange for severe malaria is a category II indication (accepted second-line therapy).

[c]Erythrocyte exchange for acute chest syndrome is a category II indication but recommended by many as first-line therapy for those severely affected.

[d]The use of plateletpheresis is a category II indication for patients with life-threatening thrombosis or hemorrhage associated with thrombocytosis (for example, in a patient with essential thrombocytosis).

Data from Szczepiorkowski ZM, Winters JL, Bandarenko N, Kim HC, Linenberger ML, Marques MB, et al; Apheresis Applications Committee of the American Society for Apheresis. Guidelines on the use of therapeutic apheresis in clinical practice—evidence-based approach from the Apheresis Applications Committee of the American Society for Apheresis. J Clin Apher. 2010;25:83-177. [PMID: 20568098] doi:10.1002/jca.20240

CONT.

wall, and changes in blood components that are prothrombotic or that inhibit fibrinolysis (or both) compose the Virchow triad. VTE usually develops as a result of the synergistic effect of multiple risk factors, which may be inherited, acquired, or a combination of both.

Thrombophilia

Thrombophilia Testing

One aspect of the Virchow triad is blood hypercoagulability, or thrombophilia. Thrombophilia can be inherited or acquired. Thrombophilia testing should not be routinely pursued in all patients presenting with DVT or PE. Although guidelines differ, most experts agree that thrombophilia evaluation should be considered only in certain populations, including patients with thromboses at unusual sites or recurrent idiopathic thrombosis, patients younger than 45 years with unprovoked thrombosis, patients with a clear family history of thrombosis in one or more first-degree relatives, and patients with warfarin-induced skin necrosis.

Additionally, many variables can affect outcomes of thrombophilia testing, including acute thrombosis and anticoagulant use, which may lead to false-positive test results. For this reason, and because a known thrombophilia will not change immediate management, testing should not be pursued in the acute setting. Asymptomatic patients with a family history of thrombosis should not undergo thrombophilia testing. **H**

KEY POINTS

- Thrombophilia evaluation should not be performed in most patients with acute venous thromboembolism. **HVC**

- Thrombophilia testing should be considered in patients with thromboses at unusual sites or recurrent idiopathic thrombosis, patients younger than 45 years with unprovoked thrombosis, patients with a clear family history of thrombosis in one or more first-degree relatives, and patients with warfarin-induced skin necrosis.

- Thrombophilia testing is less accurate during episodes of acute venous thromboembolism, and test results would not change immediate management; if indicated, testing should be performed after anticoagulation has been discontinued. **HVC**

Inherited Thrombophilias

Inherited thrombophilias typically affect components of the coagulation cascade (see Figure 2 in Bleeding Disorders) that keep the hemostatic system in balance, either causing the prothrombotic system to continue unsuppressed or inhibiting clot lysis. All known inherited thrombophilias are autosomal dominant, meaning that most affected patients are heterozygous for the disorder. The two most common inherited causes are factor V Leiden and prothrombin *G20210A* gene mutation. Less common mutations involve antithrombin deficiency and protein C and S deficiency, although these latter disorders seem to be more significant risk factors for VTE.

Failure to identify a thrombophilia does not mean a thrombophilia does not exist. Studies have shown that even when an inherited disorder is not identified, a family history of thrombosis remains an independent risk factor for VTE. It is also possible for two thrombophilic defects to coexist, such as protein S deficiency and factor V Leiden.

CONT.

Although identification of the inherited thrombophilias has advanced our understanding of the pathophysiology of VTE, it has had less influence on clinical management. The acute management of patients with VTE does not differ based on the presence of an inherited thrombophilia. Management duration is typically determined by whether the VTE event was provoked by a reversible or self-limited insult and is not often influenced by the presence of an underlying inherited thrombophilia, especially the more common disorders. Even if a patient with VTE is found to have an inherited thrombophilia, no evidence indicates asymptomatic family members should be screened to determine whether they also have the mutation.

Factor V Leiden

Factor V Leiden is the most common inherited thrombophilia. When factor V is activated, it combines with factor X to produce thrombin, which leads to clot formation. This process is regulated by activated protein C, which inactivates factor V to stop the process of ongoing clot formation. Factor V Leiden is resistant to cleavage by activated protein C, leading to predisposition of thrombus formation. Although persons who are heterozygous are at a fourfold to eightfold increased risk for developing a first VTE, most remain asymptomatic. Heterozygous factor V Leiden is found in about 5% of whites, whereas the homozygous form is found in less than 1%. Factor V Leiden is rare in Asian, African, African American, and Native American populations. It does not appear to be associated with arterial thrombosis. Factor V Leiden genetic testing or activated protein C resistance testing can be used to diagnose this condition.

Prothrombin *G20210A* Gene Mutation

The prothrombin *G20210A* gene mutation occurs in approximately 2% of whites and 0.5% of blacks and causes increased production of prothrombin (factor II) through a mutation at nucleotide 20210 from guanine to adenine. Persons with this mutation are at a twofold to fourfold increased risk for developing a first VTE, although, as with factor V Leiden, most patients with this mutation do not experience VTE events. Data are unclear regarding risks with the homozygous state, which is rare.

Antithrombin Deficiency

Antithrombin III (ATIII) and proteins C and S serve as natural anticoagulants in the body. Mutations that lead to loss of function of these components contribute to a tendency to develop VTE.

ATIII deficiency, although rare, with a prevalence of 1 in 3000 to 5000 persons, is a more significant thrombophilic risk factor than factor V Leiden or the prothrombin *G20210A* gene mutation. The main role of ATIII is to inhibit thrombin and activated factors IX and X (IXa and Xa). VTE-related pregnancy loss and pregnancy morbidity is common. Acquired ATIII deficiency is much more common than the congenital version (**Table 27**),

TABLE 27. Conditions Associated with Acquired Decreased Coagulation Factor Levels	
Coagulation Factor	**Acquired Condition**
Protein C	Acute thrombosis
	Warfarin therapy
	Liver disease
	Protein-losing enteropathy
Protein S	Acute thrombosis
	Warfarin therapy
	Liver disease
	Inflammatory states
	Estrogens (contraceptives, pregnancy, postpartum state, hormone replacement therapy)
	Protein-losing enteropathy
Antithrombin	Acute thrombosis
	Heparin therapy
	Liver disease
	Nephrotic syndrome
	Protein-losing enteropathy

and repeat testing is typically required to determine whether the deficiency is persistent.

For patients in whom heparin is initiated and titration to a therapeutic range is difficult, ATIII deficiency should be considered because heparin requires ATIII to be effective. ATIII concentrate can be used to treat this condition.

Protein C Deficiency

Protein C is a vitamin K–dependent protein that degrades activated factors V and VIII. Heterozygous protein C deficiency is uncommon, with a prevalence of 2 to 5 per 1000 persons. Many persons with this deficiency will experience a thrombotic event or pregnancy morbidity before 50 years of age, with a strong family history of thrombosis. Patients can also develop warfarin-induced skin necrosis because of further rapid depletion of protein C, which proceeds more rapidly than depletion of the coagulation factors. Homozygous deficiency is rare and causes neonatal purpura fulminans. If protein C deficiency is found, acquired causes should be ruled out (see Table 27). Repeat testing is often necessary to confirm a hereditary deficiency. Patients should not be tested during acute VTE events or while receiving warfarin. Protein C functional testing can be ordered to evaluate for evidence of deficiency.

Protein S Deficiency

Protein S is a cofactor for protein C to degrade activated factors V and VIII. Deficiency is uncommon and bears many similarities to protein C deficiency. Patients who are heterozygous for protein S deficiency typically experience VTE at a younger age

CONT.

(<50 years). Protein S is a vitamin K–dependent factor synthesized by the liver; it circulates in a free form and bound to a complement-binding protein. Although rare case reports show patients with a functional protein S deficiency, immunoassay of the free form of protein S is usually sufficient to make the diagnosis. Protein S deficiency is likely the most difficult hereditary thrombophilia to confirm because multiple laboratory assays for protein S are available, with cutoffs between normal and deficient that may be imprecise.

Other Inherited Disorders
Methylene tetrahydrofolate reductase (*MTHFR*) gene polymorphisms cause mild elevations in homocysteine levels, which are associated with a mildly increased risk of cardiovascular and thrombotic disease. The heterozygous mutation is found in 20% of whites and 2% of blacks. Vitamin B_6 and B_{12} supplementation can lower homocysteine levels without lowering thrombotic risk, which suggests the mutation may be a marker of thrombotic risk rather than a cause of thrombosis. Testing for the *MTHFR* mutation and measuring homocysteine levels should not be done in the evaluation of thrombophilia.

Factor VIII levels and plasminogen activator inhibitor activity should not be part of the standard thrombophilia evaluation because clinical trials regarding their importance have been inconclusive and results do not influence management. H

> **KEY POINTS**
>
> - Although the risk of venous thromboembolism is increased in patients who are heterozygous for factor V Leiden or prothrombin *G20210A* gene mutation, most patients are asymptomatic.
>
> **HVC** - Methylene tetrahydrofolate reductase (*MTHFR*) gene mutations are associated with an elevated homocysteine level and a modest increased risk of venous thrombosis; no treatment is available, and *MTHFR* mutation testing and homocysteine level measurement should not be performed.
>
> **HVC** - Measurement of homocysteine, factor VIII levels, and plasminogen activator inhibitor activity should not be part of the standard thrombophilia evaluation because results do not influence management.

Acquired Thrombophilias
VTE is more likely to occur in the setting of an acquired rather than an inherited thrombophilia. Many conditions predispose patients to the development of thrombosis.

Surgery, Trauma, Hospitalization, and Immobility
Surgery, trauma, hospitalization, and immobilization are some of the most significant risk factors for VTE. VTE occurs frequently in medical and surgical patients. Approximately half of all new VTEs are diagnosed during or within 3 months of a hospital stay or surgical procedure. If prophylaxis is not used,

the risk of DVT in the general surgical patient is 15% to 30%. In the orthopedic patient, the risk of DVT is approximately 60% after hip fracture surgery. Patients with cancer who undergo surgery and those undergoing orthopedic procedures, including knee arthroplasty, hip fracture repair, or hip replacement, are at particularly high risk. Nosocomial VTE risk is also increased for nonsurgical hospitalized patients, more so for immobilized patients, patients with acute neurologic illness, and patients in the medical ICU.

Certain medical conditions, including inflammatory conditions, nephrotic syndrome, and inflammatory bowel disease, have also been associated with increased thrombotic risk. In nephrotic syndrome, this risk is attributed to loss of antithrombin and proteins C and S in the urine. Obesity is also associated with increased thrombotic risk.

Cancer
Thrombosis remains a leading cause of death in patients with cancer and is a significant source of morbidity. Increased thrombotic risk has been associated with numerous malignancies, including prostate and breast cancer.

Cancer is diagnosed in 10% of patients within 1 year of an unprovoked VTE occurrence. Cancer of the ovary, pancreas, and liver are most often found. The only randomized controlled clinical trial that compared routine age- and gender-indicated screening with extensive malignancy screening using CT of the thorax, abdomen, and pelvis showed that extensive malignancy screening provided no survival benefit. Extensive cancer screening should not be performed beyond recommendations for gender and age, independent of the VTE event.

In addition, other factors, such as hormonal therapy, can further increase risk.

Medication
Hormones used in oral contraceptives and in the treatment of menopause increase the risk of VTE. The risk in women using oral contraceptives is increased approximately threefold, but the absolute number of patients affected in this young healthy population remains small. VTE risk correlates with the specific progestin agent and is somewhat higher in oral contraceptives containing desogestrel and gestodene and somewhat lower with levonorgestrel. Injectable progestin agents do not increase the risk. Regardless of the type of contraceptive, VTE risk tends to be greater in obese women and those who are older than 39 years. Women with a previous VTE event and a known inherited thrombophilia should not take oral contraceptives because the thrombotic risk is further increased. However, experts do not recommend routine thrombophilia screening before beginning contraceptive therapy because many women would need to be screened to prevent one adverse event from pulmonary embolism (PE). VTE risk is also increased by approximately twofold in menopausal women taking conjugated estrogen-medroxyprogesterone hormone replacement therapy, but the absolute risk remains small. The VTE risk in

CONT.

menopausal women seems lower in those taking estrogen only and in those using transdermal hormone replacement.

The antiestrogen, tamoxifen, also increases VTE risk in women with estrogen receptor-positive breast cancer, and the risk increases further, approximately three times baseline, in women receiving tamoxifen with systemic chemotherapy. The risk for VTE with aromatase inhibitors, such as anastrozole, is lower than that seen with tamoxifen.

Patients with multiple myeloma receiving thalidomide and its analogs as part of combination chemotherapy have a significant risk of VTE that warrants prophylaxis. The vascular endothelial growth factor inhibitor bevacizumab and newer multitargeted tyrosine kinase inhibitors, such as sunitinib and sorafenib, also increase VTE risk.

Glucocorticoid therapy has also been identified to increase the risk for VTE.

Antiphospholipid Antibody Syndrome

The antiphospholipid antibody syndrome is an autoimmune disorder in which thrombosis and fetal demise (in pregnancy) may occur. Patients with antiphospholipid antibody syndrome are at risk for arterial and venous thrombosis.

Antiphospholipid antibodies are the anticardiolipin antibodies and the lupus anticoagulant. The diagnosis of antiphospholipid antibody syndrome is based on the clinical criteria of thromboembolism or pregnancy morbidity and laboratory findings of medium or high titer antiphospholipid antibodies present on two or more occasions at least 12 weeks apart (**Table 28**). A clue to the presence of the lupus anticoagulant is activated partial thromboplastin time prolongation.

↑ aPTT

Typically, patients who are diagnosed with antiphospholipid antibody syndrome require long-term anticoagulation owing to the risk of recurrent thrombosis.

Other Acquired Thrombophilic Conditions

The myeloproliferative neoplasms have been found to carry a particularly increased risk of thrombosis; although these thromboses include PE and DVT, portal vein thrombosis and Budd-Chiari syndrome (hepatic venous outflow obstruction) (see MKSAP 18 Gastroenterology and Hepatology) are often found. Evidence of a myeloproliferative neoplasm is found in approximately 50% of patients with Budd-Chiari syndrome, even when the complete blood count is normal. In the setting of splanchnic vein thrombosis (which includes Budd-Chiari syndrome and portal vein thrombosis), evaluation for evidence of a myeloproliferative neoplasm should be considered, including evaluation for the *JAK2* tyrosine kinase mutation.

Paroxysmal nocturnal hemoglobinuria is another acquired stem cell disorder associated with hemolytic anemia, bone marrow failure, and thrombosis (see Erythrocyte Disorders).

A previous VTE event is one of the most powerful predictors of a subsequent VTE, regardless of whether an additional inherited or acquired thrombophilic risk factor is identified. H

KEY POINTS

- Approximately half of all new VTEs are diagnosed during or within 3 months of a hospital stay or surgical procedure.

- Patients with cancer undergoing extensive surgery and those undergoing knee arthroplasty, hip fracture repair, or hip replacement surgery are at especially high risk for postoperative venous thromboembolism.

- The diagnosis of antiphospholipid antibody syndrome is based on the clinical criteria of thromboembolism or pregnancy morbidity and laboratory findings of medium or high titer antiphospholipid antibodies present on two or more occasions at least 12 weeks apart.

- Evidence of a myeloproliferative neoplasm is found in approximately 50% of patients with Budd-Chiari syndrome, and *JAK2* tyrosine kinase mutation testing should be performed even if blood counts are normal.

TABLE 28. Diagnosis of Antiphospholipid Antibody Syndrome[a]		
Vascular Thrombosis	**Pregnancy Morbidity**	**Laboratory Criteria**
One or more objectively confirmed episodes of arterial, venous, or small vessel thrombosis occurring in any tissue or organ	One or more unexplained deaths of a morphologically normal fetus at or beyond the 10th week of gestation; or	Lupus anticoagulant, detected according to the guidelines of the International Society on Thrombosis and Haemostasis
	One or more premature births of a morphologically normal neonate before the 34th week of gestation because of eclampsia, pre-eclampsia, or placental insufficiency; or	Anticardiolipin antibody of IgG and/or IgM isotype, present in medium or high titer (greater than 40 GPL or MPL, or greater than the 99th percentile), measured by a standardized ELISA
	Three or more unexplained consecutive spontaneous abortions before the 10th week of gestation	Anti-β_2-glycoprotein-1 antibody of IgG and/or IgM isotype, present in titer greater than the 99th percentile, measured by a standardized ELISA

ELISA = enzyme-linked immunosorbent assay; GPL = specificity for IgG phospholipid antigens; MPL = specificity for IgM phospholipid antigens.

[a]Diagnosis is based on the presence of vascular thrombosis OR pregnancy morbidity PLUS relevant laboratory criteria.

Deep Venous Thrombosis and Pulmonary Embolism

Prevention

All hospitalized patients should be assessed for the risk of developing a VTE and treated with appropriate prophylaxis (see MKSAP 18 General Internal Medicine) because VTE is a major preventable cause of hospital morbidity and mortality. Generally, unless a clear contraindication to prophylaxis exists, pharmacologic treatment is indicated as opposed to mechanical prophylaxis. In acutely ill patients with risk for thrombosis, low-molecular-weight heparin, low-dose unfractionated heparin, or fondaparinux is advised for prophylaxis. Patients with cancer or stroke and those in the ICU have a particularly high risk for VTE. Despite the well-recognized risks of VTE, the rate of appropriate prophylaxis remains low in general hospitalized patients. Most patients do not require continued pharmacologic VTE prevention after discharge. However, patients with cancer who are undergoing major surgical procedures, patients undergoing knee arthroplasty, and those with hip fracture repair or hip replacement require VTE prophylaxis for as long as 4 weeks after discharge.

Diagnosis

DVT and PE cause significant morbidity and require efficient evaluation and diagnosis. Previous VTE, immobilization, and other thrombophilia risk factors, especially cancer, should be assessed. History pertinent to other potential causes of leg or respiratory symptoms should be elicited. The typical clinical presentation of DVT involves unilateral swelling, pain, warmth, and erythema of the extremity. Patients with PE may present with chest pain, dyspnea, and tachypnea. Less commonly, symptoms may include cough, fever, cyanosis, syncope, or shock.

CT angiography has significantly improved the accuracy of evaluating PE, generally replacing ventilation-perfusion scanning, which lacks specificity, and avoiding the need for more invasive pulmonary arteriography. However, the overuse of CT angiography and D-dimer measurement in patients at low risk for PE has needlessly exposed patients to the additional radiation and expense of these procedures. For patients who present with symptoms suspicious for an acute VTE, validated prediction rules have been developed that use D-dimer testing to help effectively evaluate this condition. The Wells criteria for diagnosis of DVT (**Table 29**) and PE (**Table 30**) and the Geneva Score (**Table 31**) for diagnosis of PE are well-studied tools in this setting. Based on these criteria, patients with low pretest probability and low D-dimer levels do not require imaging because a VTE diagnosis is unlikely. Recent studies suggest that a subset of patients at very low risk can be identified using the Pulmonary Embolism Rule-Out Criteria (PERC) (**Table 32**); these patients do not require D-dimer testing to eliminate the need for additional imaging. American College of Physicians guidelines published in 2015 recommend using the PERC as the initial step in evaluating patients at low risk. If the PERC score

is zero, no D-dimer testing is needed, and no CT angiography should be performed. In a recent meta-analysis of 12 studies, it was found that if the PERC were applied, only 0.3% of PEs

TABLE 29.	Wells Criteria for Deep Venous Thrombosis	
Variables		**Points**
Leg Symptoms and Findings		
Calf swelling ≥3 cm		+1
Swollen unilateral superficial veins (nonvaricose)		+1
Unilateral pitting edema		+1
Swelling of the entire leg		+1
Localized tenderness along the deep venous system		+1
History		
Previously documented DVT		+1
Active cancer or treatment in previous 6 months		+1
Paralysis, paresis, recent cast immobilization of legs		+1
Recently bedridden for ≥3 days; major surgery		+1
Alternative explanation for leg symptoms at least as likely		−2

DVT = deep venous thrombosis.

0-1 points = DVT unlikely; obtain D-dimer assay. If the result is negative, no further evaluation; if the result is positive, obtain Doppler ultrasonography.

>1 point = DVT likely; obtain Doppler ultrasonography.

From Wells PS, Anderson DR, Rodger M, Forgie M, Kearon C, Dreyer J, et al. Evaluation of D-dimer in the diagnosis of suspected deep-vein thrombosis. N Engl J Med. 2003;349:1227-35. [PMID: 14507948] Reprinted with permission from Massachusetts Medical Society.

TABLE 30.	Wells Criteria for Pulmonary Embolism	
Variables		**Points**
Symptoms and Signs		
Hemoptysis		1
Heart rate >100/min		1.5
Clinical signs and symptoms of DVT		3
History		
Previously documented DVT or PE		1.5
Active cancer		1
Bedridden ≥3 days or major surgery in previous 4 weeks		1.5
Other		
PE is most likely diagnosis		3

DVT = deep venous thrombosis; PE = pulmonary embolism.

≤4 points = PE unlikely; obtain D-dimer.

4-6 points = moderate possibility of PE.

>6 points = high probability of PE.

Republished with permission of Schattauer, from Wells PS, Anderson DR, Rodger M, Ginsberg JS, Kearon C, Gent M, et al. Derivation of a simple clinical model to categorize patients probability of pulmonary embolism: increasing the models utility with the SimpliRED D-dimer. Thromb Haemost. 2000;83:416-20. [PMID: 10744147]

TABLE 31.	Revised Geneva Score
Clinical Characteristic	**Score**
Age >65 y	1
Previous PE or DVT	1
Heart rate 75-94/min	1
Heart rate ≥94/min	2
Active cancer	1
Unilateral lower limb pain	1
Hemoptysis	1
Surgery or fracture within last month	1
Pain on lower limb deep venous palpation	1

DVT = deep venous thrombosis; PE = pulmonary embolism.

<2 points: low probability of PE.

2-4 points: intermediate probability.

≥5 points: high probability.

TABLE 32. Pulmonary Embolism Rule-Out Criteria for Predicting Probability of Pulmonary Embolism in Patients with Low Pretest Probability		
Clinical Characteristic	**Meets Criterion**	**Does Not Meet Criterion**
Age <50 y	0	1
Initial heart rate <100 beats/min	0	1
Initial oxygen saturation >94% on room air	0	1
No unilateral leg swelling	0	1
No hemoptysis	0	1
No surgery or trauma within 4 wk	0	1
No history of venous thromboembolism	0	1
No estrogen use	0	1

Pretest probability with score of 0 is <1%.

Reprinted with permission from Raja AS, Greenberg JO, Qaseem A, Denberg TD, Fitterman N, Schuur JD; Clinical Guidelines Committee of the American College of Physicians. Evaluation of patients with suspected acute pulmonary embolism: best practice advice from the clinical guidelines committee of the American College of Physicians. Ann Intern Med. 2015;163:701-11. [PMID: 26414967] doi:10.7326/M14-1772. Copyright 2015 American College of Physicians.

Duplex ultrasonography is the imaging modality of choice for suspected DVT. Lower extremity DVT is considered proximal if the popliteal veins are involved and is considered distal if only the calf veins are involved. CT angiography is the study of choice for suspected PE.

In patients with kidney disease or in whom intravenous contrast is contraindicated, a ventilation-perfusion lung scan can be pursued. A normal ventilation-perfusion scan result effectively rules out PE, and a high probability study result in a patient with a high likelihood of disease has a strong positive predictive value. The sensitivity and specificity of low probability or intermediate probability study results may not be accurate enough to establish or rule out the diagnosis. MRI can visualize intraluminal filling defects in the pulmonary vasculature, but not as well as CT, and avoids the ionizing radiation of CT. New MRI techniques are being evaluated that may enhance its role in diagnosis. CT is still considered standard of care for evaluation of PE.

Patients with study results that establish the diagnosis of PE do not require routine duplex imaging of the lower extremities, and patients with acute DVT in the absence of respiratory symptoms do not require CT angiography. Patients with established PE should undergo cardiac ultrasonography to evaluate acute pulmonary artery hypertension and right ventricular strain that may signify a more massive PE. Serum troponin and B-type natriuretic peptide measurements also help stratify risk in patients with PE. An elevated serum troponin level is associated with increased mortality. **H**

KEY POINTS

- Patients with a Pulmonary Embolism Rule-Out Criteria score of zero do not require further testing with D-dimer or imaging. **HVC**

- Patients with a low probability Wells criteria score for DVT or PE should undergo D-dimer testing; if the results are normal, no further imaging is necessary. **HVC**

- Patients with moderate or high probability Wells criteria do not require D-dimer testing but should undergo duplex imaging of the lower extremities for symptoms suggesting deep venous thrombosis or CT angiography for symptoms suggesting pulmonary embolism.

Treatment

Most patients with DVT can be efficiently and safely diagnosed and treated without hospitalization. More recent literature has shown a subset of patients with PE with an excellent prognosis who can also avoid inpatient care. Clinical predication models have been developed to help determine the outcome of patients with acute PE, such as the Pulmonary Embolism Severity Index (PESI), which predicts clinical severity and outcome of patients with PE using 11 clinical criteria. In a multicenter, prospective, open-label, randomized trial of patients with low-risk PE as determined by the PESI score, no difference was found between outpatient and inpatient management

CONT.

would have been missed, and 22% of D-dimer testing would have been safely avoided. PERC will help eliminate unnecessary D-dimer testing in patients at low risk.

In patients at low risk but who have a PERC score greater than zero, D-dimer testing should be pursued. If the result is negative, no imaging is warranted. If the result is positive, further evaluation is merited. If a patient has a moderate or high pretest probability, imaging studies are indicated. D-dimer testing should not be pursued in patients with moderate or high pretest probability because results would not change the need for imaging.

CONT.

in recurrent VTE, major bleeding, or 90-day mortality. A simplified version of the PESI defines patients who are younger than 80 years, who are without significant comorbidity, and who have a pulse rate less than 110/min, systolic blood pressure greater than 100 mm Hg, and oxygen saturation greater than 90% breathing ambient air as low risk for adverse outcomes.

For most patients, anticoagulation is the primary treatment for VTE. Anticoagulant options for acute VTE include unfractionated heparin, which usually requires hospitalization, low-molecular-weight heparin (LMWH), fondaparinux, or one of the non–vitamin K oral anticoagulants, all of which are safe and effective for immediate outpatient management, although patients must learn injection technique for LMWH and fondaparinux. Traditional vitamin K antagonists are not effective without at least 5 days of concomitant parenteral heparin therapy, and dabigatran and edoxaban have not been evaluated in acute VTE without previous parenteral heparin therapy. Apixaban and rivaroxaban are safe and effective as monotherapy. Patients who require hospitalization should avoid initial treatment with unfractionated heparin because of its unpredictable bioavailability compared with LMWH; however, unfractionated heparin, with a short half-life of residual anticoagulation after the infusion is stopped, may be preferred in patients who are not stable and who may need emergent surgery or transition to thrombolytic therapy.

Duration of therapy varies based on the clinical scenario surrounding the event (**Table 33**). In provoked thrombosis with reversible risk factors, 3 months of anticoagulation is adequate. Extended therapy should be considered in patients at low bleeding risk with unprovoked VTE or with irreversible

risk factors for recurrent VTE, such as underlying heart failure or stroke with long-term ambulatory dysfunction. If extended therapy is chosen, the risks, benefits, and choice of anticoagulant should be re-evaluated yearly.

In patients with unprovoked VTE in whom anticoagulation is discontinued, initiating aspirin is associated with approximately a 30% to 40% risk reduction in recurrent VTE. The American College of Chest Physicians (ACCP) guidelines published in 2016 recommend aspirin if a patient with unprovoked VTE does not continue long-term anticoagulation.

[handwritten note: ASA ONCE AC IS D/C'd IF UNPROVOKED]

In patients with malignancy, LMWH remains preferable to warfarin; the CLOT trial, in which patients were randomly assigned to LMWH or warfarin, found that 15% of patients treated with warfarin developed recurrent VTE compared with 7.9% of patients treated with LMWH. Anticoagulation should be continued as long as the cancer is active.

The role of non–vitamin K antagonist oral anticoagulants compared with LMWH has not been studied in patients with cancer. Although 6 months of anticoagulation was studied in clinical trials, anticoagulation is recommended for the duration of cancer activity.

Thrombolytic therapy is necessary to treat patients with massive PE and shock from low cardiac output. Growing data, including meta-analyses, support thrombolytic therapy as superior to traditional anticoagulation in select patients with submassive PE who remain normotensive but have poor prognostic features on cardiac ultrasonography and elevated serum troponin and B-type natriuretic peptide levels. For acute DVT, thrombolysis is indicated for massive thrombus leading to impaired venous drainage, severe edema, and acute limb

TABLE 33.	Duration of Anticoagulant Therapy for Venous Thromboembolism[a]
Type of Thrombotic Event	**Duration of Anticoagulant Therapy**
Distal leg DVT	
Provoked or unprovoked, mild symptoms	No anticoagulation suggested, but monitor with serial duplex ultrasonography for 2 weeks
Provoked or unprovoked, moderate-severe symptoms	3 months
Proximal leg DVT or PE	
Provoked (by surgery, trauma, immobility)	3 months
Unprovoked	Extended[b]
Recurrent	Duration of therapy depends on whether VTE events were provoked or unprovoked
Upper extremity DVT, proximal	At least 3 months
Cancer-associated DVT or PE	As long as the cancer is active or being treated
	LMWH is the preferred anticoagulant
Chronic thromboembolic pulmonary hypertension	Extended[b]

DVT = deep venous thrombosis; LMWH = low-molecular-weight heparin; PE = pulmonary embolism; VTE = venous thromboembolism.

[a]Decisions regarding duration of anticoagulation must always weigh the risk of VTE recurrence, risk of bleeding, and patient preference.

[b]Indicates long-term anticoagulation therapy with periodic (such as once per year) re-evaluation of the risks, benefits, and burdens of long-term therapy and discussion of new clinical study results and new anticoagulant drugs.

Data from Kearon C, Akl EA, Ornelas J, Blaivas A, Jimenez D, Bounameaux H, et al. Antithrombotic therapy for VTE disease: CHEST Guideline and Expert Panel Report. Chest. 2016;149:315-52. [PMID: 26867832] doi:10.1016/j.chest.2015.11.026

CONT.

ischemia. The main function of an inferior vena cava (IVC) filter is to prevent death from PE. In 2012, the ACCP recommended IVC filters for those with a contraindication to anticoagulation who either have acute PE or acute proximal (above the knee) DVT. If an IVC filter is placed, a temporary filter should be used.

Distal DVT does not usually require anticoagulation. Isolated distal DVT can be monitored with serial Doppler ultrasonography performed 5 to 7 days after the initial event in otherwise healthy, asymptomatic patients. According to ACCP guidelines, anticoagulation similar to that for proximal DVT is suggested in patients with certain risk factors for extension, including a positive D-dimer test result, extensive thrombosis or proximity to proximal veins, no reversible provoking factor for DVT, active cancer, history of VTE, and inpatient status. **H**

KEY POINTS

HVC
- Most patients with deep venous thrombosis and those with pulmonary embolism who have a good prognosis (defined as age <80 years, no significant comorbidity, and stable vital signs) can be safely managed without hospitalization.

- If patients with deep venous thrombosis or pulmonary embolism require hospitalization, they should be treated initially with low-molecular-weight heparin, fondaparinux, or the non–vitamin K antagonist oral anticoagulants (apixaban or rivaroxaban) instead of unfractionated heparin, unless they are unstable and at risk for requiring emergent surgery or thrombolytic therapy.

- In patients with a provoked thrombosis with reversible risk factors, 3 months of anticoagulation is adequate, but in patients at low bleeding risk with unprovoked VTE or with irreversible risk factors, extended therapy should be considered.

H **Long-term Complications**

Patients with DVT or PE can develop long-term complications affecting function and quality of life. Approximately 25% to 40% of patients with symptomatic DVT can develop aspects of postthrombotic syndrome (PTS) and chronic venous insufficiency, which often develop within 2 years of diagnosis. Symptoms of postthrombotic syndrome include pain in the affected limb, heaviness, swelling, stasis dermatitis, and ulceration. It often leads to poor quality of life and contributes to work disability. Treatment includes leg exercises, avoiding dependent positions for lengthy periods, and using compression stockings. Skin moisturizers and a low-moderate potency topical glucocorticoid may be used for stasis dermatitis (see MKSAP 18 Dermatology).

Patients with PE can also develop chronic thromboembolic pulmonary hypertension (see Pulmonary and Critical Care Medicine), cardiopulmonary dysfunction, or decreased exercise tolerance.

Other Sites of Thrombosis
Superficial Vein Thrombosis and Thrombophlebitis

Superficial thrombophlebitis describes thrombus in a vein located near the skin's surface; it is a common inflammatory-thrombotic disorder that does not usually cause significant morbidity or progress to PE. It typically is treated with supportive care, analgesia, warm compresses, and NSAIDs. Imaging is indicated if symptoms progress or swelling occurs. Cannulated veins of the hands and arms often thrombose after infusions and intravenous catheter placement; this condition does not require anticoagulant therapy.

Superficial vein thrombosis (SVT) often affects the lower extremities and is thought to account for 10% of lower extremity thromboses. When affecting the great saphenous vein (also referred to as the greater or long saphenous vein), SVT may progress into the deep venous system. In a randomized trial of fondaparinux versus placebo for lower extremity SVT, it was found that fondaparinux was safe and effective in preventing PE. In patients with lower extremity SVT of at least 5 cm in length or close to the deep venous system, fondaparinux or an alternate anticoagulant is recommended. Anticoagulation may also be indicated for patients with SVT and other thrombophilic risk factors, including cancer or previous DVT. Patients with lower extremity SVT who are not treated initially with anticoagulants should undergo follow-up evaluation in 1 week to assess signs of thrombus progression. Imaging is necessary for persistent or worsening symptoms. **H**

KEY POINTS

- Patients with lower extremity superficial vein thrombosis managed conservatively with warm compresses, analgesics, and NSAIDs require follow-up evaluation after 1 week to determine whether symptoms have resolved; duplex imaging is indicated for symptoms that persist or worsen.

- In patients with lower extremity superficial vein thrombosis of at least 5 cm in length or close to the deep venous system, or in patients with other thrombophilic risk factors, including cancer or previous venous thromboembolism, therapy with fondaparinux or an alternate anticoagulant is recommended.

Unexplained Arterial Thrombosis

Thrombophilias do not play a significant role in arterial thrombosis. The primary causes of arterial thrombosis are arteriosclerosis and atrial fibrillation with systemic arterial embolism. Patients with arterial thrombosis due to arteriosclerosis are typically treated with antiplatelet therapy. It is unknown whether patients with arterial clots in whom a strong thrombophilia is found are more effectively treated with antiplatelet therapy or anticoagulants. **H**

- Patients with arterial thrombosis due to arteriosclerosis are typically treated with antiplatelet therapy.

Upper Extremity Deep Venous Thrombosis

Upper extremity DVT accounts for 10% all DVT occurrences. Secondary DVT of the upper extremity is much more common than primary (two thirds versus one third). Secondary upper extremity DVT usually occurs with central venous catheter use or malignancy; treatment consists of 3 months of anticoagulation. However, if the catheter will not be removed in the setting of a proximal DVT, anticoagulation should continue as long as the catheter remains in place.

Primary upper extremity DVT is uncommon and usually caused by anatomic abnormalities of the thoracic outlet system leading to axillosubclavian compression and thrombosis (venous thoracic outlet syndrome). Patients are usually young, and thrombus occurs with strenuous upper extremity activity. Expert recommendations vary regarding the use of thrombolysis or thoracic outlet decompression surgery in addition to anticoagulation. ACCP guidelines recommend that treatment of primary and secondary upper extremity DVT follow similar guidelines as lower extremity DVT. Provoked upper extremity DVT should be treated for 3 months.

- Provoked upper extremity deep venous thrombosis (DVT) should be managed with 3 months of anticoagulation; however, in patients with catheter-associated DVT in whom the catheter will not be removed, anticoagulation should continue for as long as the catheter remains in place.

Anticoagulants

Unfractionated Heparin

Unfractionated heparin works by binding to antithrombin, which leads to activation and potentiation of its action, resulting in inactivation of thrombin and factor Xa.

The activated partial thromboplastin time (aPTT) is used in monitoring patients receiving heparin therapy. In the setting of lupus anticoagulant (which prolongs the aPTT), heparin resistance, or markedly elevated factor VIII, antifactor Xa monitoring can be used. Although ideal dosing has been controversial, a weight-based nomogram is usually used, and most hospitals follow a specific heparin dosing algorithm. Typically, an initial bolus dose of 80 to 100 U/kg is given.

Heparin is available in intravenous and subcutaneous preparations for the treatment of VTE, although the intravenous form is typically used. A parenteral agent should be overlapped with warfarin for 5 days and until the INR is 2 or greater for at least 24 hours.

The rate of heparin-associated major bleeding is approximately 3%. Failure to follow a dosage adjustment algorithm is associated with increased bleeding risk. When major bleeding occurs, protamine sulfate can be administered to reverse anticoagulation. A dose of 1 mg of protamine per 100 units of heparin is recommended. Protamine has its own significant adverse effects, which include allergic reactions, hypotension, bradycardia, and respiratory toxicity.

Although weight-based nomograms for instituting heparin therapy and specific algorithms for adjusting dose based on aPTT results have enhanced the safety and efficacy of unfractionated heparin, variations in bioavailability and potential delay in arriving at a therapeutic dose are still more likely than in patients treated with LMWH. Unfractionated heparin should generally be reserved for patients for whom LMWH is contraindicated or in those who require anticoagulation that can be stopped quickly, generally in anticipation of an invasive procedure or surgery.

Heparin-induced thrombocytopenia is a paradoxical adverse effect of heparin that can result in life-threatening thrombosis (see Platelet Disorders).

- A weight-based nomogram is usually used to determine the initial dose of unfractionated heparin, and algorithms are used to calculate subsequent dose modifications based on the activated partial thromboplastin time.

- Protamine sulfate can be administered to reverse the anticoagulant effects of unfractionated heparin.

- Variations in bioavailability of unfractionated heparin lead to an increased likelihood of delay in achieving a steady-state therapeutic dose compared with treatment with low-molecular-weight heparin.

Low-Molecular-Weight Heparin

LMWH is derived from unfractionated heparin through a chemical depolymerization producing smaller fragments that are one third the size of heparin.

LMWH does not affect the aPTT because the smaller fragment size does not bind as readily to thrombin but retains the ability to inactivate factor Xa. Dosing is more predictable and laboratory testing is generally unnecessary. LMWH is cleared through the kidney, and the biological half-life is increased in patients with kidney disease. In obese patients, twice daily dosing is suggested. Although laboratory monitoring is typically unnecessary, it is required when treating patients with stage V chronic kidney disease or severe obesity; anti-Xa levels should be obtained 3 to 4 hours after dosing.

LMWH is preferred to unfractionated heparin. In a meta-analysis of DVT treatment comparing LMWH with unfractionated heparin, LMWH was associated with less major bleeding, decreased mortality, and decreased thrombotic recurrence.

Protamine does not fully reverse the anti-Xa effect of LMWH but provides some benefit in restoring hemostasis; it should be given at a dose of 0.5 to 1 mg of protamine per 1 mg of enoxaparin.

- Low-molecular-weight heparin typically does not require laboratory monitoring and is associated with less bleeding, decreased recurrent thrombosis, and improved mortality compared with unfractionated heparin.
- Patients with severe obesity or stage V chronic kidney disease who are treated with low-molecular-weight heparin should have factor Xa levels measured 3 to 4 hours after a dose is administered to assess the adequacy of anticoagulation.

Fondaparinux

In a clinical trial, fondaparinux, dose adjusted based on patients' weights, was noninferior to enoxaparin with respect to the primary endpoint of recurrent VTE at 3 months (3.9% vs. 4.1%). Fondaparinux is also cleared through the kidney and should be avoided in patients with creatinine clearance less than 30 mL/min. As with LMWH or unfractionated heparin, treatment with fondaparinux and warfarin should overlap for 5 days.

Fondaparinux has no reversal agent. Caution should be used in patients at risk for bleeding because the half-life is 17 hours. Prothrombin complex concentrates (PCCs) and fresh frozen plasma (FFP) have been administered with positive outcomes in patients experiencing bleeding. ▪

- Because fondaparinux is cleared through the kidney, it should be avoided in patients with a creatinine clearance less than 30 mL/min.

Warfarin

Warfarin is a vitamin K antagonist. It inhibits vitamin K epoxide reductase, which leads to inhibition of γ carboxylation of precursor coagulation factors II, VII, IX, and X and proteins C and S. Laboratory monitoring involves the prothrombin time and INR.

Because warfarin lowers protein C levels before inducing its anticoagulant effect, it can initially cause a prothrombotic state. For this reason, for the treatment of acute VTE, it must be administered initially with a parenteral anticoagulant. Warfarin should be initiated as soon as possible after diagnosis of VTE. Typically, unfractionated heparin or LMWH is used with warfarin. As noted previously, the parenteral agent should be given for at least 5 days, and the INR can be measured on day 3; heparin is continued until the INR is 2 or greater for at least 24 hours.

Although non–vitamin K antagonist oral anticoagulants have changed the landscape of treatment for patients with VTE, warfarin remains a reasonable anticoagulant for some patients. This may include patients with known kidney disease and obesity or patients with a mechanical heart valve, for whom alternate oral anticoagulants have not been approved.

Patients must have access to continued outpatient INR monitoring. Studies evaluating the use of cytochrome 2C9 and vitamin K epoxide reductase (VKORC1) pharmacogenetics to guide warfarin therapy have not shown benefit. Common reasons for fluctuations in INR include changes in vitamin K intake, medications, and nonadherence. Studies attempting to decrease INR variability with low-dose daily vitamin K supplementation were unsuccessful, so this supplementation is not indicated.

Bleeding is the most significant complication in patients treated with warfarin, occurring in 1% to 3% of patients per year. The risk is higher when warfarin therapy is initiated and during episodes of concurrent acute illness. Bleeding risk increases further in patients with an INR greater than 5. Independent of INR, bleeding risk is increased in patients older than 75 years or in those with previous stroke, gastrointestinal bleeding, or most other chronic comorbidities. Concomitant aspirin, clopidogrel, and NSAID use increases the bleeding risk. The indication for antiplatelet agents for patients taking warfarin should be carefully reviewed, and dual antiplatelet therapy avoided if possible. Acetaminophen should be used instead of NSAIDs when feasible.

Concern is often expressed when older adults begin oral anticoagulation, often for atrial fibrillation, because age is an important risk factor for stroke and bleeding complications associated with warfarin. Oral anticoagulation may be prematurely excluded as a therapeutic option in these patients because of concerns regarding a "falls risk." The true risk of serious bleeding related to a fall while taking an anticoagulant is unclear, although small studies have not shown an increased risk of major bleeding in patients taking oral anticoagulants who were considered at high risk for falls. Risk factors for falls should be thoroughly evaluated and appropriate steps employed for prevention (see MKSAP 18 General Internal Medicine). Recommendations suggest that neither age nor a risk of falls is reason to withhold warfarin anticoagulation from a patient who has clinical criteria warranting such therapy for VTE or stroke prevention.

Patients with asymptomatic INR elevation between 4.5 and 10 can often be managed by simply withholding warfarin. For INRs greater than 10 in patients without bleeding, oral vitamin K, 2.5 mg, should be given. In patients experiencing bleeding, in addition to vitamin K, three- or four-factor PCCs should be given rather than FFP. Although FFP contains the appropriate clotting factors, it requires thawing and large volumes to correct the INR. Three- and four-factor PCCs contain proteins C and S and factors II, IX, and X; four-factor PCC also contains factor VII. In a clinical trial of vitamin K antagonist–related bleeding, four-factor PCC was found to be noninferior to FFP for hemostatic efficacy. Four-factor PCC is preferred because of its rapid reversal of INR, rapid infusion and administration, and lack of volume overload. Recombinant factor VIIa is not recommended for warfarin reversal.

Bridging therapy, which uses heparin or LMWH for patients in whom warfarin has been stopped for an invasive

CONT.

procedure and will be resumed, is not necessary for most patients and is associated with more bleeding complications without additional anticoagulant benefit. The exception to this may be patients with recent VTE (within the past 4 weeks), history of VTE during anticoagulant interruption for surgery, or a procedure with very high VTE risk, such as orthopedic surgery. Bridging is also indicated in patients with atrial fibrillation who have had a stroke or transient ischemic attack in the preceding year, in patients who have multiple risk factors for stroke (CHADS$_2$ score of 5-6), and in most patients with a mechanical heart valve. **H**

KEY POINTS

- Warfarin must be administered initially with at least 5 days of a parenteral anticoagulant (usually unfractionated or low-molecular-weight heparin) for the treatment of venous thromboembolism.

HVC
- Bridging therapy, which uses unfractionated heparin or low-molecular-weight heparin during warfarin discontinuation before an invasive procedure, is not indicated for most patients because it is associated with more bleeding complications without any reduction in thrombotic events.

Non-Vitamin K Antagonist Oral Anticoagulants

The non–vitamin K antagonist oral anticoagulants (NOACs) have emerged as a safe and effective treatment for certain patients with VTE. In the 2016 CHEST guidelines for DVT and PE treatment, NOACs are suggested as the treatment of choice for anticoagulation in patients without cancer. The NOACs available for use in the United States are dabigatran, rivaroxaban, apixaban, edoxaban, and betrixaban. In clinical trials of patients with VTE, patients were initially treated with a parenteral agent and transitioned to dabigatran or edoxaban. Rivaroxaban and apixaban were studied without concomitant parenteral therapy and were approved as monotherapy for DVT and PE. Dabigatran functions as a direct thrombin inhibitor, whereas the other agents are factor Xa inhibitors. Betrixaban is only approved for DVT prophylaxis (**Table 34**).

Routine coagulation studies do not reliably measure the degree of coagulation activity. However, the thrombin time is quite sensitive to the presence of dabigatran and, if normal, indicates that the anticoagulant effect of dabigatran is no longer significant.

Advantages of the NOACs include no need for routine monitoring, rapid onset of action and short half-life, fixed dosing, and fewer drug-drug interactions. These drugs are as effective as warfarin in the prevention of VTE; although the overall bleeding risk was comparable, less central nervous system bleeding, fatal bleeding, and use of blood product support among patients taking NOACs was seen than with warfarin. The bleeding risk is higher in patients taking aspirin or clopidogrel with a NOAC and is further increased in patients taking dual antiplatelet drugs plus NOACs. These qualities must be considered when choosing the appropriate patient for

these therapies. No head-to-head trials have been performed comparing the various NOACs. It must be noted that certain patient groups were excluded from the major trials of the NOACs, including patients with severe obesity (BMI >40), pregnant patients, and those with mechanical heart valves. Nonadherent patients should not be treated with NOACs, and the additional cost of these drugs compared with warfarin may be a barrier for some patients. Few patients with cancer were included in clinical trials, and LMWH is still considered standard of care for VTE in these patients. In patients with antiphospholipid antibody syndrome, the role of NOACs remains unclear, although clinical trials are ongoing. Treatment failures with the use of NOACs in patients with antiphospholipid antibody syndrome have been reported. Dyspepsia and gastrointestinal bleeding were seen more frequently with dabigatran compared with warfarin in clinical trials. In patients with concern for gastrointestinal bleeding, dabigatran may not be the preferred option.

All of the NOACs are at least partially eliminated through the kidney (see Table 34), and the dose must be reduced in patients with advanced chronic kidney disease. Apixaban has the lowest renal elimination, so it is approved for patients undergoing dialysis; however, many physicians still prefer warfarin in patients with kidney disease, and caution should be used.

Bridging therapy is typically unnecessary in patients taking NOACs. Discontinuation of the NOAC depends on the half-life of the drug, the type of procedure, and the patient's kidney function. NOACs should be stopped 24 to 48 hours before surgery with moderate bleeding risk and 72 hours before surgery with higher bleeding risk. In patients with impaired kidney function, NOACs should be stopped earlier. For procedures with low bleeding risk, NOACs can be resumed promptly when effective hemostasis is secured. For procedures with higher rates of bleeding, reinstitution is usually delayed 2 to 3 days.

The standard approach to patients experiencing bleeding involves hemodynamic monitoring and resuscitation with fluid and blood products. Activated charcoal can be considered if the NOAC was ingested recently (<6 hours). Hemodialysis can be considered with dabigatran therapy if new kidney disease is found. No specific antidote is available for bleeding associated with rivaroxaban, apixaban, or edoxaban. For patients experiencing major bleeding while taking these agents, fibrinolytic agents such as tranexamic acid or ε-aminocaproic acid may be used. Although three- and four-factor PCCs and recombinant factor VIIa have been used in NOAC-associated bleeding, their benefit has not been confirmed in randomized trials, and the data remain unclear. Idarucizumab, a monoclonal antibody fragment, binds free and thrombin-bound dabigatran and neutralizes its activity. In a phase 3, multicenter, prospective, cohort trial, idarucizumab was found to be safe and effective in reversing the anticoagulant effects of dabigatran in patients who either experienced serious, overt, life-threatening bleeding determined to require

TABLE 34. Key Features of the Non-Vitamin K Antagonist Oral Anticoagulants

	Dabigatran	Rivaroxaban	Apixaban	Edoxaban	Betrixaban
Class of anticoagulant	Direct factor IIa inhibitor	Direct factor Xa inhibitor	Direct factor Xa inhibitor	Direct factor Xa inhibitor	Direct factor Xa inhibitor
T_{max} (h)	2	3	3	1-2	3-4
Half-life (h)	12-17	7-11	9-14	9-11	20
Protein binding	35%	95%	87%	54%	60%
Renal elimination	80%	66% (33% as active metabolite)	25%	35%	5%
FDA-approved indications	Atrial fibrillation VTE treatment	Atrial fibrillation VTE treatment[a] VTE prevention	Atrial fibrillation VTE treatment[a] VTE prevention	Atrial fibrillation VTE treatment	Extended VTE prophylaxis
Reversal agent	Idarucizumab	No	No	No	No
Dosing					
Atrial fibrillation	CrCl >30 mL/min: 150 mg twice daily CrCl 15-30 mL/min: 75 mg twice daily CrCl ≤15 mL/min: do not use	CrCl >50 mL/min: 20 mg once daily CrCl 15-50 mL/min: 15 mg once daily CrCl ≤15 mL/min: do not use	5 mg twice daily 2.5 mg twice daily if ≥2 criteria present: (a) ≥80 years of age (b) Weight ≤60 kg (132 lb) (c) Creatinine ≥1.5 mg/dL (133 µmol/L)	60 mg once daily CrCl 15-50 mL/min: 30 mg once daily CrCl >95 mL/min: do not use	NA
VTE prevention	NA	10 mg once daily	2.5 mg twice daily	NA	160 mg day 1; 80 mg/d for 35-42 days
VTE treatment	CrCl >30 mL/min: 150 mg twice daily CrCl <30 mL/min: do not use	CrCl >30 mL/min: 15 mg twice daily × 3 wk, then 20 mg once daily CrCl ≤30 mL/min: do not use	VTE treatment: 10 mg twice daily × 1 wk, then 5 mg twice daily Reduction in VTE recurrence: 2.5 mg twice daily	60 mg once daily 30 mg once daily with the following criteria: CrCl 30-50 mL/min Weight ≤60 kg (132 lb) Concomitant p-glycoprotein inhibitor use	NA

CrCl = creatinine clearance; h = hour; NA = not applicable; T_{max} = time to maximum concentration; VTE = venous thromboembolism.

[a]Approved as monotherapy for VTE.

CONT.

a reversal agent or who required an urgent invasive procedure that could not be delayed. Idarucizumab was FDA approved for this indication in October 2015. Specific antidotes for this class of agents continue to be developed. **H**

KEY POINTS

- The non–vitamin K antagonist oral anticoagulants dabigatran, rivaroxaban, apixaban, edoxaban, and betrixaban have a rapid onset of activity, no need for laboratory monitoring, and therapeutic effect that is less likely than warfarin to be influenced by changes in diet or medications.

(Continued)

KEY POINTS (continued)

- Non–vitamin K antagonist oral anticoagulants (NOACs) are as effective as warfarin in preventing and treating venous thromboembolism; although the overall rate of bleeding is comparable, patients taking a NOAC have less central nervous system bleeding and less fatal bleeding.

- The non–vitamin K antagonist oral anticoagulants should not be used in patients with valvular heart disease or severe obesity, or in those who are pregnant or nonadherent; patients with active cancer are better treated with low-molecular-weight or unfractionated heparin.

Hematologic Issues in Pregnancy

Gestational Anemia

During pregnancy, an increase in plasma volume occurs that is greater than the increase in erythrocyte mass, resulting in a physiologic decrease in measured hemoglobin level, although it typically remains greater than 10.5 g/dL (105 g/L). If the hemoglobin level decreases further, additional evaluation of the anemia is warranted. Iron, vitamin B_{12}, and folate levels should be tested.

Sickle Cell Disease

The physiologic stresses of pregnancy are especially challenging for women with sickle cell disease (SCD). Patients are unable to produce the expected increase in erythrocyte mass, and folate requirements increase because of the rapid turnover of erythrocytes, requiring additional folate supplementation. Iron and vitamin B_{12} stores must also be monitored. Although expert opinion is not uniform, recent guidelines from the National Institutes of Health did not recommend prophylactic transfusions in pregnancy for women with sickle cell anemia. Other experts disagree, suggesting prophylactic transfusion in pregnant women during the third trimester to achieve a hemoglobin level of 9 g/dL (90 g/L) or reserving such transfusions for women with previous fetal loss, more severe anemia, frequent acute painful events, or history of acute chest syndrome. However, frequent transfusions may lead to alloimmunization, increasing the risk of hemolytic disease of the newborn. Although routine use of prophylactic transfusion is debatable, pregnant women with more severe and symptomatic anemia should be transfused as should any woman with acute chest syndrome or stroke. Pregnant women with SCD should be monitored closely with monthly complete blood counts in collaboration with a hematologist.

In women with SCD, pregnancy affects multiple organ systems in addition to causing anemia. The risk of venous thromboembolism is increased, and prophylactic anticoagulation should be administered in hospitalized patients. The increased cardiopulmonary demands of pregnancy increase the risk of pulmonary hypertension, with an associated 16% mortality risk. Suggestive clinical features should be evaluated by echocardiography.

Medications used to control SCD, such as hydroxyurea and chelating agents, must be discontinued during pregnancy. Painful vaso-occlusive crises increase during pregnancy; pain should be managed with narcotic analgesics, and NSAIDs should be avoided after the 30th week of gestation.

Pregnant patients with SCD are also at increased risk for complications of the pregnancy itself, including intrauterine growth restriction, eclampsia, preterm labor, placental abruption, and stillbirth. **H**

KEY POINTS

- Although the use of routine prophylactic transfusion in pregnant women with sickle cell anemia remains controversial, transfusions should be given to those patients with more severe and symptomatic anemia or those who develop additional complications such as acute chest syndrome or stroke.

- Medications used to control sickle cell disease, such as hydroxyurea and chelating agents, must be discontinued during pregnancy.

Thrombocytopenia in Pregnancy

Gestational Thrombocytopenia

Gestational thrombocytopenia affects approximately 5% of pregnant women. The cause is uncertain, but it may be a milder form of immune thrombocytopenic purpura. Most patients are asymptomatic, with platelet counts greater than 100,000/μL (100 × 10⁹/L), although platelet counts may reach a nadir of 70,000/μL (70 × 10⁹/L). Patients with gestational thrombocytopenia have no history of thrombocytopenia, and the platelet count does not decrease until late in gestation. The fetus is unaffected, intervention is unnecessary, and platelet counts spontaneously return to normal after delivery.

KEY POINT

- Patients with gestational thrombocytopenia have no history of thrombocytopenia, and because the thrombocytopenia is not severe, without predisposition to bleeding, and platelet counts resolve spontaneously, no treatment is necessary.

HVC

Immune Thrombocytopenic Purpura

Immune thrombocytopenic purpura (ITP) (see Platelet Disorders) can occur in women of childbearing age and may present during pregnancy. Differentiating ITP from gestational thrombocytopenia may be difficult, but features suggesting ITP include earlier presentation (first trimester), lower platelet count nadir (<70,000/μL [70 × 10⁹/L]), and history of thrombocytopenia before pregnancy (even if it was only mild). If the platelet count remains greater than 30,000/μL (30 × 10⁹/L), the pregnancy is not at risk. Patients should receive intravenous immune globulin or glucocorticoids at any time during pregnancy if the platelet count decreases below 30,000/μL (30 × 10⁹/L). The target platelet count for delivery (vaginal or cesarean section) is 50,000/μL (50 × 10⁹/L), and therapy should begin approximately 1 week before the expected delivery date to achieve that goal. Neuraxial anesthesia requires a platelet count greater than approximately 80,000/μL (80 × 10⁹/L).

ITP autoantibodies can cross the placenta and affect the fetus; 20% to 30% of neonates are reported to have platelet counts less than 50,000/μL (50 × 10⁹/L) (especially if an older sibling was born with thrombocytopenia). Fetal platelet counts can continue to decrease for 2 to 5 days after delivery. Fetal thrombocytopenia is not influenced by maternal treatment with either glucocorticoids or intravenous immune globulin. Despite the increased likelihood of neonatal thrombocytopenia, the risk of intracerebral hemorrhage is less than 1% and is unaffected by delivery by cesarean section.

KEY POINTS

- Differentiating immune thrombocytopenic purpura from gestational thrombocytopenia may be difficult, but suggestive features include earlier presentation (first trimester), lower platelet count nadir (<70,000/µL [70 × 10⁹/L]), and history of thrombocytopenia before pregnancy.

- Women should receive intravenous immune globulin or glucocorticoids to treat immune thrombocytopenic purpura if the platelet count decreases below 30,000/µL (30 × 10⁹/L) at any time during the pregnancy as well as 1 week before delivery to achieve a platelet count of at least 50,000/µL (50 × 10⁹/L) for delivery or 80,000/µL (80 × 10⁹/L) if neuraxial anesthesia is anticipated.

Microangiopathy of Pregnancy

The thrombotic microangiopathies of pregnancy encompass a spectrum of disorders presenting with clinical features of microangiopathic hemolytic anemia and thrombocytopenia. The differentiating features of these disorders are noted in **Table 35**.

The distinction between HELLP (Hemolysis, Elevated Liver enzymes, Low Platelets) syndrome, pre-eclampsia, and acute fatty liver of pregnancy may be difficult but is not crucial because management for all of these is supportive and focused on early delivery. Thrombotic thrombocytopenic purpura and hemolytic uremic syndrome (see Platelet Disorders) can also occur during pregnancy (see Table 35) and may require additional therapy, including plasma exchange or the anticomplement agent eculizumab.

KEY POINTS

- HELLP (Hemolysis, Elevated Liver enzymes, Low Platelets) syndrome, pre-eclampsia, and acute fatty liver of pregnancy present with microangiopathic hemolysis and, usually, thrombocytopenia; although distinguishing among these disorders may be difficult, the management of each is supportive and involves early delivery.

- Thrombotic thrombocytopenic purpura and hemolytic uremic syndrome may present during pregnancy and are important to distinguish from other causes of microangiopathic hemolysis and thrombocytopenia because more specific therapy, such as plasma exchange, may be indicated.

Thrombophilia and Venous Thromboembolism in Pregnancy
Epidemiology, Pathophysiology, and Risk Factors

The risk of venous thromboembolism (VTE) in pregnancy is higher than in the general population, but the absolute risk is still low (<1%). Nevertheless, pulmonary emboli account for about 9% of maternal deaths. The increased risk is a result of venous stasis caused by uterine compression and increased venous capacitance, increased circulating procoagulant factors,

TABLE 35. Clinical and Laboratory Features of the Thrombotic Microangiopathies of Pregnancy

Feature	Pre-eclampsia	HELLP	AFLP	TTP	HUS
Hypertension	+++	+++	+	+/−	+
Proteinuria	+++	++	+/−	+	+
Abdominal pain	+/−	++	++	+/−	+/−
Jaundice	+/−	+/−	++	+/−	+/−
Neurologic findings	+/−	+/−	+/−	++	+/−
Thrombocytopenia	+	+++	+	+++	++
Hemolysis	+/−	+++	+	+++	++
Kidney disease	+	+	+/−	+	+++
Disseminated intravascular coagulation	+/−	++	+++	+/−	+/−
Elevated liver chemistry test results	+	+++	+++	+/−	+/−
Hypoglycemia	+/−	+/−	+++	+/−	+/−

AFLP = acute fatty liver of pregnancy; HELLP = Hemolysis, Elevated Liver enzymes, and Low Platelets; HUS = hemolytic uremic syndrome; TTP = thrombotic thrombocytopenic purpura.

+++ = always present.

++ = usually present.

+ = likely to be present.

+/− = may or may not be present.

and decreased circulating protein S. VTE risk increases further in the postpartum period after endothelial injury during delivery and an additional increase in the procoagulant factors. Factors that further increase VTE risk include multiple births, advanced maternal age, obesity, smoking, cesarean section, and varicose veins.

The possibility of VTE is increased in patients with inherited thrombophilias. However, testing for these disorders in pregnancy is complicated and is not routinely recommended. Deep venous thrombosis most often occurs in the left lower extremity.

Prevention

Patients with a history of an idiopathic VTE, VTE associated with pregnancy or oral contraceptives, or a hereditary thrombophilia require antenatal and postpartum anticoagulation continuing for 6 weeks following delivery. Low-molecular-weight heparin (LMWH) should be used in the antenatal setting because warfarin is teratogenic and the non–vitamin K antagonist oral anticoagulants have not been studied in pregnancy. LMWH can be transitioned to unfractionated heparin (for its shorter duration of action) around the time of delivery.

Diagnosis

Diagnosing a deep venous thrombosis requires evaluation by Doppler ultrasonography. Pulmonary embolism diagnosis in pregnancy presents a challenge because concerns about fetal radiation exposure may limit use of CT angiography, which is the definitive diagnostic test. Although D-dimer levels rise during pregnancy, patients at low risk (Wells score ≤4) who have a normal D-dimer level do not require further evaluation (see Thrombotic Disorders). In women for whom the risk remains moderate or high, a ventilation-perfusion lung scan should be performed. If the ventilation-perfusion scan result is normal, pulmonary embolism is ruled out, and if marked perfusion defects unmatched by ventilation abnormalities are noted, the diagnosis is likely. If the ventilation-perfusion scan result remains indeterminate, the patient should undergo CT angiographic imaging.

Treatment

LMWH is the treatment of choice for pregnant women with VTE. Therapy should begin with the standard recommended dose and then be titrated to the anti-Xa level because weight-based dosing algorithms that customarily eliminate the need for anti-Xa monitoring may not be reliable during pregnancy. Warfarin is teratogenic and must be avoided in the first trimester, but it is safe to resume after delivery and with breastfeeding. The non–vitamin K antagonist oral anticoagulants have not been evaluated in this setting, so they cannot be recommended. Thrombolytic therapy raises the risk of maternal hemorrhage and should be reserved for life-threatening situations. LMWH must be interrupted at least 24 hours before delivery; unfractionated heparin can be used instead and

discontinued as labor progresses or several hours before cesarean section. Postpartum treatment is begun as soon as hemostasis is achieved. Postpartum anticoagulation should continue for at least 6 weeks. The goal is for a total anticoagulation period of 3 to 6 months. **H**

KEY POINTS

- Patients with a history of idiopathic venous thromboembolism (VTE), VTE associated with pregnancy or oral contraceptives, or a hereditary thrombophilia require antenatal and postpartum anticoagulation continuing for 6 weeks after delivery.

- Unfractionated or low-molecular-weight heparin should be used for anticoagulation during pregnancy in patients with venous thromboembolism because warfarin is teratogenic and the non–vitamin K antagonist oral anticoagulants have not been studied in pregnancy; warfarin is safe to resume postpartum and while breastfeeding.

Issues in Oncology

Introduction

Technological advances are changing the field of medical oncology at a rapid rate. The successful incorporation of immune checkpoint inhibitors and other immunologic strategies to facilitate activation of the patient's own immune system as part of the standard treatment of many malignancies has been a major advance. Other changes include expanded routine use of molecular profiling in several tumor types and the resultant application of precision therapeutics, which are selected on the basis of specific mutations within a person's tumor. "Precision medicine," or "precision therapeutics," is a term often used interchangeably with "personalized medicine," but rather than denoting therapeutic approaches tailored to individual patients, precision medicine focuses on identifying effective approaches for patients based on genetic, environmental, and lifestyle factors. However, many aspects of oncology, including the use of traditional histologic diagnosis and clinical staging, as well as extensive use of cytotoxic chemotherapy, radiation therapy, and surgery, remain central to current oncologic practice.

Despite the many technological advances, careful clinical evaluation and staging, understanding and communicating realistic goals of care, and recognizing and promoting patient preferences remain central to the practice of oncology. Meaningful progress has been made in many cancers. However, most cancers, once metastasized, are treatable but still incurable. Oncology has also become the focus of concerns regarding unsustainable costs in care, specifically in terms of the costs of new drugs, and the impact of financial toxicity has become an important consideration in oncologic care.

Staging

In order to plan a proper treatment strategy, a clinician must first determine the stage, or extent, of the cancer. Early-stage cancers often can be cured by local therapy, such as surgery or radiation, whereas more advanced-stage cancers require a more systemic approach. With the use of the TNM cancer staging system, most solid tumors are staged on a scale of 1 to 4. In the TNM system, *T* (T1-T4) refers to the size or extent of local invasion of the primary tumor, *N* (N0-N3) indicates locoregional lymph node involvement, and *M* indicates the absence (M0) or presence (M1) of distant metastases. If the main tumor, cancer in nearby lymph nodes, or metastasis cannot be measured, this is denoted with X (for example, TXNXMX). Some hematologic tumors have unique tumor-specific staging systems.

The required studies and imaging techniques will be dependent on the expected behavior pattern of each cancer type and will differ from one tumor to the next. Therefore, a proper cancer evaluation requires knowledge of the specific disease entity so that the necessary tests can be done. Tests with a very low yield should not be ordered in the absence of specific directing symptoms. For example, bone and brain imaging is appropriate in the staging of patients with lung cancer because bone and brain metastases are common in the early course of this disease. However, patients with presumed locoregional colorectal cancer rarely present with bone or brain metastases; consequently, routine imaging of these sites as part of staging in the absence of specific symptoms is not necessary. Thoughtfully performed staging is generally the most accurate prognostic indicator and largely dictates the therapeutic strategy for patients with cancer.

KEY POINTS

- Most solid tumors are staged using the TNM cancer staging system, in which *T* represents the size or extent of local invasion of the primary tumor (T1-T4), *N* indicates locoregional lymph node involvement (N0-N3), and *M* indicates the absence (M0) or presence (M1) of distant metastases.
- **HVC** Diagnostic imaging may be crucial in determining the accurate stage of a tumor, but patients with localized tumors that have a low likelihood of distant metastases to certain sites, such as bone or brain, should not have routine imaging of those sites.
- Thoughtfully performed staging is generally the most accurate prognostic indicator and largely dictates the therapeutic strategy for patients with cancer.

Performance Status

Performance status is a means of quantifying how medically fit a patient is overall. A good performance status predicts favorable tolerance and response to treatment. Patients with a poor performance status are much more likely to experience serious or life-threatening toxicity and much less likely to benefit from treatment.

It is important to differentiate patients with a poor performance status who are debilitated due to chronic comorbidities from patients who would otherwise be medically fit but are acutely debilitated by their disease. The latter situation may warrant an attempt at aggressive treatment, because reversing the cancer process is the only thing that will improve the patient's overall condition, whereas the former may need to be treated with less aggressive treatment or possibly no specific anticancer treatment. Cancer drug approvals are based on clinical trials, virtually all of which limit participants to patients with good performance status, so the degree to which the results of these trials are relevant to patients with poor performance status is questionable.

In addition, age alone should not be regarded as a reason to avoid aggressive treatment. Elderly patients who are otherwise medically fit and healthy and hence have a good performance status may tolerate aggressive therapy well, whereas younger patients with several medical comorbidities resulting in a poor performance status may be unable to tolerate aggressive treatment.

The two most commonly used performance status scales are the Karnofsky score and the Eastern Cooperative Oncology Group/World Health Organization system (also called the Zubrod score). These are outlined and contrasted in **Table 36**.

KEY POINTS

- Patients with poor performance status may be conceptualized as composing two groups: patients who are debilitated by chronic comorbidities and may need less aggressive treatment and patients who are debilitated by the cancer but are otherwise medically fit and might benefit from aggressive treatment.
- Most clinical trials used to determine treatment efficacy are based on patients with good performance status.

Goals of Therapy

Clear and candid communication between clinician and patient is essential for good oncologic care. When communicating treatment options and recommendations, clinicians must work to establish realistic treatment goals. When cure is not realistically possible, goals such as lengthening survival, shrinking a tumor, controlling disease growth, palliation or prevention of disease-related symptoms, and maintaining quality of life at a level acceptable to the patient should be considered. The potential benefits of treatment have to be weighed and discussed along with their risks and toxicities. Patients with incurable cancer face choices of more aggressive therapy associated with more unpleasant and potentially dangerous side effects that are designed to prolong their life. The gravity of those side effects is weighed against the duration of prolonged survival, but all patients have a unique perspective on how they interpret this equation. Similarly, more aggressive initial therapy may result in prolonged remission or disease-free survival but no change in overall survival. Some patients would gladly accept the increased

TABLE 36.	Oncology Performance Status Systems
ECOG/WHO Performance Status[a]	
0 - Fully active; no restrictions on activities	
1 - Unable to do strenuous activities, but able to carry out office work, light housework, or sedentary activities	
2 - Able to walk and manage self-care, but unable to work; out of bed or chair >50% of waking hours	
3 - Confined to bed or chair >50% of waking hours; capable of limited self-care	
4 - Moribund. Fully confined to a bed or chair; unable to do any self-care	
5 - Death	
Karnofsky Performance Status	
100 - Normal; no symptoms or evidence of disease	
90 - Minor symptoms, but able to carry on normal activities	
80 - Some symptoms; normal activity requires effort	
70 - Unable to carry on normal activities, but able to care for self	
60 - Needs frequent care for most needs; some occasional assistance with self-care	
50 - Needs considerable assistance with self-care and frequent medical care	
40 - Disabled; needs special care and assistance	
30 - Severely disabled; hospitalized	
20 - Very ill; significant supportive care is needed	
10 - Actively dying	
0 - Death	

ECOG = Eastern Cooperative Oncology Group; WHO = World Health Organization.

[a]Also called the Zubrod score.

toxicity of such therapy for a prolonged period without cancer, whereas others would not.

More recently, as costs of anticancer treatments have increased astronomically, the concept of financial toxicity—the impact that the cancer diagnosis will have on the patient's financial stability and overall well-being—has received greater attention. A diagnosis of cancer has been shown to be a leading cause of personal bankruptcy, and studies show financial worries contribute to the anxiety of many patients with cancer. Inability to meet copays or coinsurance requirements, especially for expensive oral anticancer medications, is a leading cause of failure to properly receive therapy. A clear understanding of the goals of care and the toxicities, including financial toxicity, is necessary for patients and physicians to make informed choices in treatment options. This concept of financial toxicity goes beyond individual patients in affecting the overall health care economy. Quantifying the overall benefit of extending a patient's life by relatively short periods (less than 2 months' median benefit) and contrasting that benefit by the financial cost of care require complex ethical, economic, and public health decisions.

Early-stage cancers often have a high chance of cure. With increasing cancer stage, however, the possibility of cure diminishes. Most metastatic cancers are treatable but not curable. This is especially true for patients with poor performance status due to chronic medical comorbidities or those who have not been able to tolerate initial treatment attempts. For such patients or for those who have exhausted standard treatment options, supportive, comfort-oriented care may be most appropriate. Use of adequate analgesia, as well as support from palliative medicine specialists, is important throughout the continuum of care but particularly so in patients with pain or with symptoms from either disease or therapy. Recent studies suggest that such palliative care, when instituted as part of early aggressive therapy, helps patients better tolerate their cancer care and should not be delayed to the point at which no more active cancer therapy is considered.

KEY POINTS

- The potential benefits of treatment must be weighed and discussed along with their risks and toxicities, including financial toxicity, as the costs of anticancer treatments have increased significantly.

- Palliative care should be instituted early on in the management of patients with cancer and not reserved for the time when they are no longer receiving cancer therapy.

Understanding Cancer Terminology

The field of oncology has its own language and terminology that is often misunderstood. A clear understanding of this terminology is necessary to facilitate informed discussions and develop realistic treatment goals.

The one pure and simple term is *cure*. *Cure* means, as one would expect, that the cancer is gone, no further treatment is required, and the patient will live out his or her life without seeing that type of cancer again. This should not be confused with *overall survival*, which is defined as the amount of time from initiation of a treatment until death. Overall survival is often misunderstood by patients to be synonymous with *cure*. Median survival benefits that are reported in studies are typically offered to patients as indicators of how long they will live, but it must be understood that medians of studies are meaningful for populations but not for individual patients. This can be further compounded by the frequent use of the phrase *significant improvement in survival*, in which *significant* refers to the statistical certainty of the finding but is often misinterpreted as a *substantial* improvement in survival. Many drugs have been approved with *significant* improvements in survival that are limited to less than 2 or 3 months, a quantity that most would agree is not substantial. Furthermore, one must be cautious about interpreting nonrandomized comparisons of older versus newer survival data, because screening and surveillance techniques are leading to more accurate staging and earlier recognition of smaller volumes of cancer recurrence, creating a lead-time bias that may appear to amplify the benefits of a newer treatment compared with an older one. Thus, randomized controlled trials are the optimal means of comparing one treatment with another.

One of the most misrepresented and misunderstood terms is *progression-free survival*. It is the time from when a treatment is started until that treatment is no longer controlling the tumor. Because the duration of progression-free survival is defined by cancer progression or death, whichever occurs first, the word *survival* is maintained in the term; however it has little to do with overall survival and is often, and sometimes deliberately, confused with it. *Progression-free interval* would more accurately describe what is referred to as progression-free survival.

Response rate is the percentage of patients in a clinical trial whose tumor shrinks to a prespecified degree with treatment as indicated on imaging studies, such as CT or MRI. Response rate has not been shown to correlate with other metrics, such as overall survival, but there is a strong emotional benefit to patients when the tumor is regressing, and in symptomatic patients, such shrinkage is likely to alleviate, prevent, or delay symptoms.

KEY POINT

- The terminology used in oncology is often misunderstood and can affect patients' understanding of their disease; an increase in overall survival is not synonymous with cure, median survival is only relevant to populations (not individuals), and significant improvements seen in clinical trials do not necessarily mean substantial improvements.

Treatment Approaches

The classic cancer treatment modalities are surgery, radiation, and chemotherapy. As current technology has advanced, chemotherapy is best subdivided into the more classic cytotoxic chemotherapies, targeted or precision therapies, and immunotherapies.

Traditional Cancer Therapies

For tumors that are localized, surgical resection remains at the center of treatment. Following resection, the patient is never at risk for harm from the tumor that has been removed but rather from microscopic tumors that may still remain in the patient. Neoadjuvant (preoperative) or adjuvant (postoperative) treatment with radiation, chemotherapy, or both, may be used to eradicate residual microscopic disease and increase the chance for cure. The nature of the treatment, in terms of chemotherapy, radiation, or both, will depend on the type of tumor and its characteristic pattern of spread. Neoadjuvant and adjuvant therapy acknowledge the fact that some patients being treated would be cured with surgery alone and are therefore exposed to needless additional toxicity. Randomized trials are crucial in determining whether, for any given population of patients, neoadjuvant or adjuvant therapy improves some important outcome, such as cure, overall survival, or disease-free survival, without unacceptable toxicity. Conversion therapy seeks to convert an unresectable tumor to a resectable one by shrinking it away from critical structures and creating a plane for resection that previously was lacking; this differs from neoadjuvant chemotherapy, which is used for micrometastases of an already resectable tumor.

Balancing therapy efficacy and toxicity—in particular, the need for adjuvant or neoadjuvant therapy or the desired aggressiveness of the primary chemotherapy, radiation therapy, or surgical therapy for populations of patients—has traditionally been based on stage, pathology, and understanding of the overall behavior of that tumor. Currently available imaging and laboratory studies are somewhat limited in terms of their ability to identify which patients will or will not be at risk for recurrence of cancer after definitive surgery. Numerous tumor markers, gene panels, and other technologies are available, but few are definitive. The preferred assay would be predictive, meaning that it could identify the subset of those patients who are at risk for recurrence and who will benefit from an intervention such as adjuvant chemotherapy to delay or prevent such recurrence. An example of this is a commercially available 21-gene assay for breast cancer that identifies a patient population who is at risk for recurrence and will have that risk lowered by chemotherapy. Such predictive tools are highly useful because they provide actionable information in terms of who to treat and who not to treat. Unfortunately, attempts to develop such predictive assays have rarely been successful. A similar multigene assay in colorectal cancer is prognostic in that it can quantitate a patient's risk of recurrence, but fails to identify which patients, if any, will have their risk lowered by chemotherapy. Therefore, it does not provide information that is definitive for decision making. Such prognostic tests are of much less value than risk factors that can be used to define better therapy, but these tests still may be of value to individual patients who may rely on that statistical information to better plan their lives.

Cancer Treatment During Pregnancy

According to the International Network on Cancer, Infertility, and Pregnancy (INCIP), prenatal exposure of children to maternal cancer with or without treatment has not been shown to impair physical or mental development in early childhood.

> **KEY POINTS**
>
> - Treatment with radiation, chemotherapy, or both, in addition to definitive surgery is called neoadjuvant if administered preoperatively or adjuvant if administered postoperatively.
> - Predictive assays can identify the subset of patients who will or will not benefit from an intervention, whereas prognostic assays can identify the subset of patients at higher or lower risk but not those who will or will not benefit from an intervention.

Precision Medicine

Current developments in chemotherapy are centered on creating agents that target specific aspects of a tumor cell. Although in theory these agents should be more selective and have fewer toxicities than older, conventional chemotherapies, this has not always turned out to be the case. Many of the signaling pathways that are hyperactive in tumor cells remain at least somewhat active in normal cells, and so disruption of these pathways can produce considerable side effects.

The goal of precision medicine is to identify specific aspects of the tumor that can guide clinicians in deciding which therapies are or are not appropriate for a particular patient. Markers can be either inclusionary, in that they include a patient in a therapy that otherwise might not be considered, or exclusionary, in that they exclude a patient from a treatment that otherwise might have been used.

An example of an inclusionary marker is the V600 *BRAF* mutation in melanoma. Specific *BRAF* inhibitors, such as vemurafenib and dabrafenib, would only be appropriate for use in melanomas that harbor this specific mutation. Melanomas lacking this mutation would not be treated with these agents. Trastuzumab, a monoclonal antibody against the human epidermal growth factor receptor 2 (*HER2*) on the cell surface, is only active in those breast or gastroesophageal tumors that overexpress *HER2*. In short, targeted therapy only works if the target is both present and clinically relevant.

Examples of exclusionary markers are *RAS* mutations. The anti–epidermal growth factor receptor (EGFR) monoclonal antibodies cetuximab and panitumumab were initially thought to be appropriate for treatment of all colorectal cancers. Subsequently, it was determined that any tumors harboring mutations in either the *KRAS* or *NRAS* gene were not only highly resistant to responding to these agents, but in fact the growth of the *RAS*-mutated tumors may even be accelerated by these agents. All metastatic colorectal cancers now require tumor genotyping for *KRAS* and *NRAS* mutations, and only those tumors lacking the mutations are appropriate for treatment with cetuximab or panitumumab.

> **KEY POINT**
>
> - Precision medicine refers to agents that target specific aspects of a tumor cell; inclusionary markers include patients in a therapy that otherwise might not be considered, and exclusionary markers exclude patients from a treatment that might otherwise be used.

Immunotherapy

Immunotherapy agents are drugs that do not attack the cancer directly but rather mobilize the patient's own immune system to do so. This has become possible through the identification of "immune checkpoints," which serve as "brakes" on the immune system in order to prevent the immune system from attacking itself and causing autoimmune diseases. Antibodies that block these checkpoints release the brakes on the immune system and allow it to aggressively attack the tumor. Side effects are related to resultant autoimmunity from the less-regulated immune system. The first immune checkpoint identified was the antigen-4 (A-4) molecule on the surface of the cytotoxic lymphocyte (T cell), hence its designation cytotoxic T-lymphocyte antigen-4 (CTLA-4). Antibodies that block CTLA-4, such as ipilimumab, have been successful in mobilizing the immune system against melanoma, renal cell carcinoma, and other malignancies. The other immune checkpoint that has been successfully exploited is the programmed death 1 (PD-1) receptor. Anti–PD-1 agents, such as nivolumab or pembrolizumab, have shown substantial and durable activity against melanoma and non-small cell lung cancers, as well as other tumors. Agents against the ligand of PD-1 have also shown important clinical activity. Combinations of these agents are showing further effectiveness but with increased toxicity and also considerable expense. Many other checkpoints in the immune system are now being exploited by numerous drugs in development, and it is possible that immunotherapy will substantially change the outlook for patients with many different types of cancer in the foreseeable future.

> **KEY POINT**
>
> - Immune checkpoints prevent the immune system from attacking normal tissues (self), but immunotherapy can take advantage of this by inhibiting the checkpoints and allowing the immune system to be more aggressive and so attack cancer cells.

Breast Cancer

Introduction

Breast cancer is the most common type of cancer in women in the United States, excluding skin cancers. In 2015, there were an estimated 231,840 new invasive breast cancer cases and 60,290 in situ cases diagnosed. The lifetime risk of developing invasive breast cancer is 12.4% (about 1 in 8) for U.S. women. There were an estimated 40,290 deaths from breast cancer in the United States in 2015: it remains the second leading cause of cancer death in women. The lifetime risk of dying from breast cancer for U.S. women is 2.76%. Breast cancer is rare in men.

Epidemiology and Risk Factors

Breast cancer incidence increases with age. The incidence per decade of life is listed in **Table 37**. The median age of diagnosis in women is 61 years. Incidence rates are highest in non-Hispanic white and black women. Other risk factors for breast cancer are listed in **Table 38**.

Patients with deleterious *BRCA1* or *BRCA2* gene mutations have a 50% to 85% lifetime risk of breast cancer. Patients who received chest wall irradiation between ages 10 and 30 years for treatment of Hodgkin lymphoma have a 30% to 50% risk of breast cancer. Atypical breast lesions, such as atypical hyperplasia or lobular carcinoma in situ, result in a cumulative 30-year breast cancer risk of up to 35%.

Patients with possible hereditary breast cancer syndromes should be referred to a genetic counselor for assessment and possible genetic testing. The criteria for genetic testing are outlined in **Table 39**.

KEY POINTS

- Breast cancer incidence increases with age, with the highest incidence in non-Hispanic white women and second highest in black women.
- Women with possible hereditary breast cancer syndromes should be referred to a genetic counselor for possible genetic testing for breast cancer susceptibility genes, such as *BRCA1* and *BRCA2*.

Chemoprevention and Other Risk Reduction Strategies

Breast cancer screening for average-risk women is discussed in MKSAP 18 General Internal Medicine. The American Cancer Society recommends screening certain women at high risk using annual mammography and breast MRI (**Table 40**).

Women with a 5-year risk of breast cancer of 1.67% or greater are candidates for breast cancer chemoprevention

TABLE 37. Breast Cancer Risk per Decade of Life for U.S. Women[a]

Decade of Life	Fractional Risk for Being Diagnosed with Breast Cancer in the Next 10 Years
20s	1 in 1674
30s	1 in 225
40s	1 in 68
50s	1 in 42
60s	1 in 28
70s	1 in 26
80s	1 in 33

[a]All Races.

Data from Howlader N, Noone AM, Krapcho M, Garshell J, Miller D, Altekruse SF, et al. SEER Cancer Statistics Review, 1975-2012, National Cancer Institute. Bethesda, MD. http://seer.cancer.gov/csr/1975_2012/. Based on November 2014 SEER data submission. The Surveillance, Epidemiology, and End Results Program (SEER) Website. Updated November 18, 2015. Accessed February 7, 2018.

with antiestrogens. A recommended tool for estimating 5-year and lifetime risks of breast cancer is the Gail Model Risk Assessment Tool (www.cancer.gov/bcrisktool/). All patients with atypical hyperplasia or lobular carcinoma in situ (LCIS) are candidates for chemoprophylaxis. At present, there is insufficient evidence to recommend for or against screening with breast MRI in patients with atypical hyperplasia or LCIS.

Tamoxifen and raloxifene are selective estrogen receptor modifiers (SERMs) that block estrogen uptake in breast tissue. Exemestane and anastrozole are aromatase inhibitors that prevent the conversion of androgens into estrogens. These agents proportionally decrease the risk of breast cancer by 28% to 65% and are given for 5 years. **Table 41** summarizes these chemoprophylaxis options.

For women with *BRCA1* or *BRCA2* mutations, breast cancer screening with breast MRI should start at age 25 years and with mammography at age 30 years. The benefit of tamoxifen prophylaxis in *BRCA1* and *BRCA2* mutation carriers is not clear, although limited retrospective data suggest a benefit. Surgical prophylaxis options for *BRCA1* and *BRCA2* mutation carriers include prophylactic bilateral mastectomies, which decrease the risk of breast cancer by greater than 90%, and prophylactic bilateral salpingo-oophorectomy (BSO), which decreases the risk of ovarian, fallopian tube, and primary peritoneal cancers by greater than 80% and all-cause mortality to age 70 years by 77%. If done while a woman is premenopausal, prophylactic bilateral salpingo-oophorectomy also decreases the risk of breast cancer by 50% and is recommended between ages 35 and 40 years, after completion of childbearing. Because *BRCA2* mutation carriers on average develop ovarian cancer 8 to 10 years later than *BRCA1* carriers, bilateral salpingo-oophorectomy can be delayed until age 40 to 45 years in women who have had prophylactic mastectomies.

TABLE 38. Breast Cancer Risk Factors

Breast Cancer Risk Factor Category	Breast Cancer Risk Factors	Increase in Breast Cancer Risk or Lifetime Breast Cancer Risk
Reproductive factors	Early menarche, late menopause, first full-term pregnancy after age 30 years, or nulliparous	RR 1.2-3.5
Lifestyle	Obesity (BMI ≥30), lack of regular exercise, vitamin D deficiency, alcohol intake	RR 1.2-1.6 Obesity: RR, 1.6 for BMI >30.7 versus BMI <22.9 in postmenopausal women[a] Regular exercise: RR decreased by 25% in physically active women compared with the least active women[b] Vitamin D deficiency: Postmenopausal breast cancer risk decreased by 12% for each 5 ng/mL (12.5 nmol/L) increase in 25(OH)D levels between 27 and 35 ng/mL[c] (67.4 and 87.4 nmol/L) Alcohol intake: mildly increased risk (RR 1.05) with 2 to 3 drinks per week. RR 1.41 for women consuming 2 to 5 drinks per day[d]
Treatment related: radiation	Prior chest wall radiation in patients younger than age 30 years (e.g., mantle radiation for Hodgkin lymphoma)	RR 5.0, with highest risk for younger age at radiation therapy; risk remains increased for at least 40 years after radiation therapy, with 30% to 50% lifetime risk of breast cancer[e]
Treatment related: HRT	Combination estrogen and progesterone HRT after menopause	RR 1.2-1.4; increased risk begins after 3 years of therapy[a]
Breast density[f]	Increased breast density	Risk increases with each category of breast density; for ≥75% density, RR is 4.7 compared with <10% density[g]
Atypical breast lesions	Atypical ductal or lobular hyperplasia, LCIS	RR 3.8-5.3 for atypical hyperplasia[h] and RR 5.4-8.0 for LCIS[i]; 30% to 35% lifetime risk of breast cancer (bilateral risk)[h,i]
Family history of breast cancer and familial breast cancer syndromes	*BRCA1/2* mutation represents the most common familial breast cancer syndrome (5% to 10% of all breast cancer tumors); others are rare	*BRCA1/2* mutations (RR 3.0 to 7.0) confer a 50% to 87% lifetime risk of breast cancer and a 20% to 45% lifetime risk of ovarian cancer

25(OH)D = 25-hydroxyvitamin D; *BRCA1/2* = breast cancer susceptibility 1 or breast cancer susceptibility 2 genes; HRT = hormone replacement therapy; LCIS = lobular carcinoma in situ; RR = relative risk.

[a]Data from Clemons M, Goss P. Estrogen and the risk of breast cancer. N Engl J Med. 2001 Jan 25;344 (4):276-85. Erratum in: N Engl J Med. 2001 Jun 7;344(23):1804. [PMID: 11172156]

[b]Data from Lynch BM, Neilson HK, Friedenreich CM. Physical activity and breast cancer prevention. Recent Results Cancer Res. 2011;186:13-42. [PMID: 21113759]

[c]Data from Bauer SR, Hankinson SE, Bertone-Johnson ER, Ding EL. Plasma vitamin D levels, menopause, and risk of breast cancer: dose-response meta-analysis of prospective studies. Medicine (Baltimore). 2013 May;92(3):123-31. [PMID: 23625163]

[d]Data from Bagnardi V, Rota M, Botteri E, et al. Light alcohol drinking and cancer: a meta-analysis. Ann Oncol. 2013 Feb;24(2):301-8. [PMID: 22910838] and Smith-Warner SA, Spiegelman D, Yaun SS, et al. Alcohol and breast cancer in women: a pooled analysis of cohort studies. JAMA. 1998 Feb 18;279(7):535-40. [PMID: 9480365]

[e]Data from Swerdlow AJ, Cooke R, Bates A, et al. Breast cancer risk after supradiaphragmatic radiotherapy for Hodgkin's lymphoma in England and Wales: a National Cohort Study. J Clin Oncol. 2012 Aug 1;30(22):2745-52. [PMID: 22734026]

[f]Breast density refers to the amount of radiologically dense breast tissue appearing on a mammogram.

[g]Data from Boyd NF, Guo H, Martin LJ, et al. Mammographic density and the risk and detection of breast cancer. N Engl J Med. 2007 Jan 18;356(3):227-36. [PMID: 17229950]

[h]Data from Degnim AC, Cisscher DW, Berman HK, et al. Stratifications of breast cancer risk in women with atypia: a Mayo cohort study. J Clin Oncol. 2007 Jul 1;25(19):2671-7. [PMID: 17563394] and Marshall LM, Hunter DJ, Connolly JL, et al. Risk of breast cancer associated with atypical hyperplasia of lobular and ductal types. Cancer Epidemiol Biomarkers Prev. 1997 May;6(5):297-301. [PMID: 9149887]

[i]Data from Bodian CA, Perzin KH, Lattes R. Lobular neoplasia. Long term risk of breast cancer and relation to other factors. Cancer. 1996 Sep 1;78(5):1024-34. [PMID: 8780540]

KEY POINTS

- Women at high risk for breast cancer should be screened with annual mammography and breast MRI; this includes women with a *BRCA1* or *BRCA2* gene mutation or with a first-degree relative with a *BRCA1* or *BRCA2* mutation, women with a strong family history of breast cancer, those with a history of chest radiation at a young age, and those with a rare hereditary breast cancer syndrome.

(Continued)

KEY POINTS (continued)

- Women with a 5-year risk of breast cancer of 1.67% or greater or with lobular carcinoma in situ or atypical hyperplasia are candidates for breast cancer chemoprophylaxis.

- Surgical prophylaxis options for *BRCA1* and *BRCA2* mutation carriers include prophylactic bilateral mastectomy and prophylactic bilateral salpingo-oophorectomy.

TABLE 39. Highlights of NCCN[a] and USPSTF[b] Recommendations for Breast and Ovarian Cancer Syndrome Genetic Testing

Individuals with a Personal History of Breast or Ovarian Cancer

Breast cancer diagnosed at or before age 45 years

Breast cancer diagnosed at or before age 50 years with one or more relatives[c] with breast cancer, pancreatic cancer, or prostate cancer with Gleason score ≥7 at any age

Women with two primary breast cancers, with the first diagnosed at or before age 50

Breast cancer diagnosed at any age with one or more relatives[c] diagnosed with ovarian cancer

Triple negative breast cancer[d] diagnosed at or before age 60 years

Breast cancer in women of Ashkenazi (Eastern European) Jewish ancestry

Men with breast cancer diagnosed at any age

Ovarian cancer diagnosed at any age

Individuals without a Personal History of Breast or Ovarian Cancer

Family history of a known deleterious *BRCA1/2* mutation

Two first-degree relatives with breast cancer, one of whom received the diagnosis at age 50 years or younger

Three or more first- or second-degree relatives with breast cancer regardless of age at diagnosis

More than three family members[c] with breast cancer, ovarian cancer, pancreatic cancer, and/or aggressive prostate cancer

A combination of both breast and ovarian cancer among first- and second-degree relatives

A first-degree relative with bilateral breast cancer

A combination of two or more first- or second-degree relatives with ovarian cancer regardless of age at diagnosis

A first- or second-degree relative with both breast and ovarian cancer at any age

A history of breast cancer in a male relative

Women of Ashkenazi (Eastern European) Jewish ancestry with a first-degree relative (or two second-degree relatives on the same side of the family) with breast or ovarian cancer

BRCA1/2 = breast cancer susceptibility 1 or breast cancer susceptibility 2 genes; NCCN = National Comprehensive Cancer Network; USPSTF = U.S. Preventive Services Task Force.

[a]Full testing guidelines can be accessed at www.nccn.org/professionals/physician_gls/f_guidelines.asp.

[b]Full testing guidelines can be accessed at www.uspreventiveservicestaskforce.org/Page/Document/RecommendationStatementFinal/brca-related-cancer-risk-assessment-genetic-counseling-and-genetic-testing.

[c]First-degree, second-degree, or third-degree relatives on the same side of the family.

[d]Negative for estrogen and progesterone receptors and *HER2* amplification.

TABLE 40. American Cancer Society Recommendations for MRI Breast Cancer Screening

Women with *BRCA1/2* mutations

Women who are a first-degree relative of a *BRCA1/2* carrier but are untested[a]

Women with a strong family history of breast cancer with a lifetime breast cancer risk of ≥20% to 25% as calculated by models[b] largely dependent on family history

Women who had radiation to the chest wall between ages 10 and 30 years (e.g., mantle radiation therapy for Hodgkin lymphoma)

Women with a history of other rare familial breast cancer syndromes

BRCA1/2 = breast cancer susceptibility 1 or breast cancer susceptibility 2 genes.

[a]Testing for the *BRCA1* or *BRCA2* mutation that is present in the family is strongly recommended, but some patients decide to defer testing. In this situation where their carrier status is unknown, breast MRI screening is recommended. If they are later tested and do not carry the mutation, MRI screening should be stopped.

[b]Models that can be used to estimate lifetime risk of breast cancer to determine if MRI screening is appropriate (please note that the Gail Model is not recommended for this use):

- BRCAPRO: www4.utsouthwestern.edu/breasthealth/cagene/default.asp

- Claus model: Claus EB, Risch N, Thompson WD. The calculation of breast cancer risk for women with a first degree family history of ovarian cancer. Breast Cancer Res Treat. 1993 Nov;28(2):115-20. [PMID: 8173064]

- Tyrer-Cuzik (also called IBIS Breast Cancer Risk Evaluation Tool): www.ems-trials.org/riskevaluator/

TABLE 41. Primary Chemoprevention for Breast Cancer

Considerations	Tamoxifen	Raloxifene	Exemestane	Anastrozole
Mechanism of action	SERM	SERM	Aromatase inhibitor	Aromatase inhibitor
Breast cancer risk reduction	43% at 7 years[a] 28% at 10 years[b]	As effective as tamoxifen at reducing the risk of invasive cancers, but less effective at reducing noninvasive cancers[c]	65% at 3 years[d]	53% at 5 years[e]
Important toxicities	Vasomotor symptoms, cataracts, vascular events (stroke, TIA, DVT/PE), and endometrial cancer and uterine sarcoma in postmenopausal women	Vasomotor symptoms, cataracts, vascular events (25% lower risk of vascular events than with tamoxifen)	Vasomotor symptoms, arthralgia, headaches, and insomnia	Vasomotor symptoms, arthralgia, carpal tunnel syndrome, dry eyes, and hypertension
Indicated for use in premenopausal women	Yes	Not studied; should not be used unless part of a clinical trial	Not effective in premenopausal women	Not effective in premenopausal women
Other	Contraindicated in women with prior thromboembolic events; 32% reduction in osteoporotic fractures[a]	Contraindicated in women with prior thromboembolic events	At 3-year follow-up, no increase in osteoporosis, fractures, endometrial cancer, vascular events, or cardiac disease	At 5-year follow-up, no increase in thromboembolic events, fractures, cerebrovascular events, or myocardial infarction

DVT = deep venous thrombosis; PE = pulmonary embolism; SERM = selective estrogen receptor modulator; TIA = transient ischemic attack.

[a]Fisher B, Constantino JP, Wickerham DL, et al. Tamoxifen for the prevention of breast cancer: current status of the National Surgical Adjuvant Breast and Bowel Project P-1 study. J Natl Cancer Inst. 2005 Nov 16;97(22):1652-62. [PMID: 16288118]

[b]Cuzick J, Sestak I, Cawthorn S, et al; IBIS-I Investigators. Tamoxifen for prevention of breast cancer: extended long-term follow-up of the IBIS-I breast cancer prevention trial. Lancet Oncol. 2015 Jan;16(1):67-75. [PMID: 25497694]

[c]Vogel VG, Costantino JP, Wickerham DL, et al; National Surgical Adjuvant Breast and Bowel Project (NSABP). Effects of tamoxifen vs raloxifene on the risk of developing invasive breast cancer and other disease outcomes: the NSABP study of tamoxifen and raloxifene (STAR) P-2 trial. JAMA. 2006 Jun 21;295(23):2727-41. Erratum in: JAMA. 2006 Dec 27;296(24):2926. [PMID: 16754727]

[d]Goss PE, Ingle JN, Alés-Martínez JE, et al; NCIC CTG MAP.3 Study Investigators. Exemestane for breast-cancer prevention in postmenopausal women. N Engl J Med. 2011 Jun 23;364(25):2381-91. Erratum in: N Engl J Med. 2011 Oct 6;365(14):1361. [PMID: 21639806]

[e]Cuzick J, Sestak I, Forbes JF, et al; IBIS-II Investigators. Anastrozole for prevention of breast cancer in high-risk postmenopausal women (IBIS-II): an international, double-blind, randomised placebo-controlled trial. Lancet. 2014 Mar 22;383(9922):1041-8. Erratum in: Lancet. 2014 Mar 22;383(9922):1040. [PMID: 24333009]

Staging and Prognosis of Early-Stage Breast Cancer

Breast cancer is most commonly staged by the TNM system. Breast cancer staging and prognosis are presented in **Table 42**. In addition to the excellent prognosis for small tumors with neither lymph node involvement nor distant metastases, the presence of hormone receptors, absence of human epidermal growth factor 2 (*HER2*) overexpression, and absence of lymphovascular invasion also favorably affect prognosis. Estrogen receptors, when detected, imply a better differentiated tumor and suggest response to hormone antagonist therapy. Tumors with a genetic mutation that leads to *HER2* overexpression imply an unfavorable prognosis, although monoclonal antibodies such as trastuzumab that block those receptors are effective therapy and have markedly improved the prognosis for these women.

For asymptomatic patients with newly diagnosed stage 0 to II (early-stage) breast cancer, current guidelines recommend against using imaging studies such as PET, CT, or bone scan, or measuring serum markers such as CA15-3 or CA27-29, for staging. These studies have little diagnostic yield for patients with stage I to II breast cancer who do not have symptoms, findings on examination,

or laboratory evidence of metastases. One large series showed that the incidence of bone metastases in stage I to III breast cancer was 5% to 6% for stage I to II and 14% for stage III; for liver metastases, the incidence was 0% in stage I to II and 0.7% in stage III; and for lung metastases, incidence was 0% in stage I to II and 7% in stage III. Imaging studies for staging are recommended in patients with stage III disease or in patients with earlier-stage disease who have signs or symptoms suggestive of metastatic disease.

Advances in breast cancer diagnosis and treatment have led to markedly improved survival rates during the past 40 years. Surveillance, Epidemiology, and End Results (SEER) data from 1975 to 2013 show a 34% decrease in deaths from breast cancer. The 5-year relative survival for all invasive breast cancer stages in patients diagnosed from 2006 to 2012 is 90.8%.

KEY POINTS

- Clinical features associated with a more favorable prognosis of early-stage breast cancer include hormone receptor–positive cancer, absence of *HER2* overexpression, small tumor size, low tumor grade, and negative lymph nodes.

(Continued)

TABLE 42. Staging and Prognosis of Invasive Breast Cancer

Stage	Definition	5-Year Relative Survival[a] Rates
0	Ductal carcinoma in situ (negative lymph nodes)	99%
I	IA: Tumor ≤2 cm and negative lymph nodes	95%
	IB: Tumor ≤2 cm and 1 to 3 micrometastatic positive lymph nodes (0.2-2 mm)	
IIA	Tumor ≤2 cm with 1 to 3 positive lymph nodes (>2 mm) OR	85%
	Tumor 2-5 cm with negative lymph nodes	
IIB	Tumor 2-5 cm with 1 to 3 positive lymph nodes OR	70%
	Tumor >5 cm with negative lymph nodes	
IIIA	Tumor ≤5 cm with 4 to 9 positive lymph nodes OR	52%
	Tumor >5 cm with 1 to 9 positive lymph nodes	
IIIB	Tumors with skin or chest wall involvement with 0 to 9 positive lymph nodes	48%
IIIC	Tumors with 10 or more positive lymph nodes	Not stated
IV	Distant metastatic disease	22%

[a]Relative survival is an estimate of the percentage of patients who would be expected to survive the effects of their cancer.

Data from Howlader N, Noone AM, Krapcho M, Garshell J, Miller D, Altekruse SF, et al. SEER Cancer Statistics Review, 1975-2012, National Cancer Institute. Bethesda, MD. http://seer.cancer.gov/csr/1975_2012/. Based on November 2014 SEER data submission. The Surveillance, Epidemiology, and End Results Program (SEER) Website. Updated November 18, 2015. Accessed February 7, 2018.

KEY POINTS *(continued)*

HVC • Imaging studies such as PET, CT, or bone scan for staging are not recommended in asymptomatic patients with newly diagnosed stage 0 to II breast cancer.

Primary Breast Cancer Therapy

Ductal Carcinoma in Situ

Ductal carcinoma in situ (DCIS), classified as stage 0 breast cancer, is a noninvasive breast cancer that usually presents as calcifications on mammography (see **Figure 19**). Its incidence has increased greatly, from 3% of breast cancers before the era of mammographic screening to 20% to 25% of breast cancers today. Infrequently, DCIS presents as a palpable mass.

Because more than half of local recurrences of DCIS are invasive cancers, the goal of treatment has been to eradicate the area of DCIS and decrease the risks of local recurrence and deaths from breast cancer. Surgical treatment has traditionally been either wide excision (lumpectomy), often followed by breast radiation or mastectomy. Radiation may be omitted in some cases of low-grade or intermediate-grade DCIS. Mastectomy is usually recommended if the DCIS is more extensive and cannot be fully removed by a wide excision.

Recent studies have questioned the benefit of these approaches. An observational study of more than 100,000 women with DCIS showed that although adding radiation to wide excision decreased the risk of local recurrence from 4.9% to 2.5%, it did not decrease the 10-year breast cancer–specific mortality of 0.9%. Similarly, patients who had mastectomies had a lower risk of local recurrence than patients who had lumpectomies but no decrease in the risk of death from breast cancer. Women younger than 35 years, black women, women younger than 40 years presenting with a palpable mass, and women with DCIS that is either estrogen receptor negative or *HER2* positive have a worse prognosis.

In women with estrogen receptor–positive DCIS, tamoxifen and aromatase inhibitors decrease the risks of local recurrence and contralateral breast cancers. Tamoxifen is the

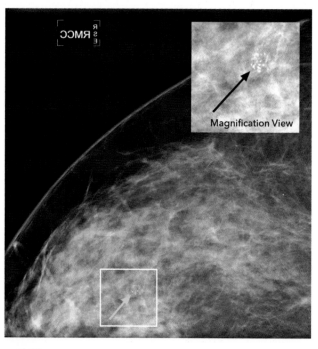

FIGURE 19. Ductal carcinoma in situ presenting as calcifications on mammography.

appropriate treatment in premenopausal women. For post-menopausal women, both tamoxifen and anastrozole are effective options, with anastrozole being superior in women younger than age 60 years. Both hormonal therapies are equally effective in women age 60 years or older. Unlike with hormone receptor–positive invasive cancers, antiestrogen treatment of DCIS does not have a survival benefit.

Patients with DCIS should have annual mammography starting 6 to 12 months after radiation therapy, if given, and follow-up visits every 6 to 12 months for 5 years after diagnosis.

KEY POINTS

- Although mastectomy or postlumpectomy radiation decreases the risk for local recurrence when compared to wide excision in women with ductal carcinoma in situ, neither improves overall 10-year survival.

- In estrogen receptor–positive DCIS, tamoxifen and aromatase inhibitors further decrease the risks of local recurrence and contralateral breast cancer but do not improve overall survival.

Invasive Breast Cancer

Most early-stage invasive breast cancers are treated with initial excision, followed by radiation and systemic adjuvant therapy. There are two surgical options for invasive breast cancer. Breast conservation therapy involves wide excision followed by breast radiation and is typically used in patients with cancers 5 cm or less in size, without skin involvement, and with clear margins after excision. Mastectomy is recommended for larger cancers, cancers with skin involvement, and inflammatory breast cancers. Mastectomy may also be chosen in situations where radiation is contraindicated, or in women with *BRCA1* or *BRCA2* mutations or strong family histories of breast cancer where there is a high risk of subsequent breast cancers. For some patients with large tumors, neoadjuvant chemotherapy or endocrine therapy can be given before surgery to decrease the cancer to a size that allows for breast conservation.

In patients with clinically negative axillary lymph nodes, a sentinel node biopsy is done at the time of breast surgery. In patients having breast conservation surgery who will receive chemotherapy or antiestrogen therapy as well as whole breast radiation, axillary dissection is not required if no more than two sentinel nodes are involved. For patients with clinically involved axillary nodes or three or more positive sentinel nodes, an axillary dissection is recommended. The sentinel node procedure has a lower risk of lymphedema, sensory loss, and shoulder abduction defects than axillary dissection.

Primary breast radiation usually consists of radiation to the whole breast, although partial breast radiation is an option in some patients. Postmastectomy radiation is recommended for cancers greater than 5 cm in size, inadequate or positive margins or skin involvement, inflammatory breast cancers, or four or more positive axillary nodes. Depending on other risk factors, it may be recommended in women with one to three

positive axillary nodes. Postmastectomy radiation decreases both the risk of local recurrence and the risk of distant metastases and increases overall survival.

For women older than age 70 years with cancers less than 2 cm in size, no clinically involved lymph nodes, and estrogen receptor–positive breast cancer, wide excision followed by antiestrogen therapy alone is an acceptable treatment option. Whole breast radiation in this situation decreases the risk of local recurrence from 9% to 2% at 12 years, but has no impact on the risk of distant metastases, breast cancer–specific survival, or overall survival.

KEY POINTS

- Breast-conserving therapy is effective for patients with tumors 5 cm or less in size, without skin involvement, and with clear margins after excision in women who do not have hereditary syndromes that place them at high risk for subsequent breast cancer.

- For patients undergoing breast conservation surgery followed by chemotherapy or antiestrogen therapy and whole breast radiation, axillary node dissection is not required if no more than two sentinel nodes are involved. **HVC**

- Postmastectomy radiation is recommended for cancers greater than 5 cm in size, positive margins or skin involvement, inflammatory breast cancers, and many patients with positive axillary lymph nodes.

Adjuvant Systemic Therapy for Nonmetastatic Breast Cancer

Patients with stage I to III (potentially curable) breast cancer receive adjuvant systemic therapy to eradicate occult microscopic foci of breast cancer and decrease the risk of local and distant recurrence. The type of adjuvant therapy used depends on the biology and stage of the breast cancer. Antiestrogen therapy has the additional benefit of decreasing the risk of contralateral breast cancer.

Adjuvant Endocrine Therapy

Approximately 75% of breast cancers are hormone receptor positive (positive for the estrogen receptor, progesterone receptor, or both). Patients with hormone receptor–positive breast cancers are recommended to receive adjuvant antiestrogen therapy for at least 5 years. The Early Breast Cancer Trialists Collaborative Group meta-analysis of adjuvant tamoxifen showed a 39% proportional reduction in breast cancer recurrence at 15 years and a 30% proportional reduction in breast cancer mortality. In postmenopausal women, aromatase inhibitors compared to tamoxifen resulted in a further 29% proportional decrease in breast cancer recurrence. Both tamoxifen and aromatase inhibitors also decrease the risk of contralateral breast cancer.

Tamoxifen is a selective estrogen receptor modulator that blocks estrogen uptake by breast cancer cells. It is effective in both premenopausal and postmenopausal women. The aromatase inhibitors letrozole, anastrozole, and exemestane have similar efficacy and prevent conversion of adrenal androgens to estrogen but do not inhibit ovarian estrogen production. They are thus not effective in premenopausal women unless ovarian suppression is given concomitantly.

For postmenopausal women, aromatase inhibitor therapy provides superior results to using tamoxifen alone. Patients may take tamoxifen for 2 years and then change to an aromatase inhibitor for at least 3 to 5 years, or they can take 5 years of an aromatase inhibitor. A 2016 study showed the benefit of extending aromatase inhibitor use to a total of 10 years, whether or not tamoxifen was given initially, with an improvement in disease-free survival at 5 years from 91% to 95% but no difference in overall survival. Recommending extended aromatase inhibitor treatment will depend on a patient's quality of life, the toxic effects of treatment, and the risk of recurrence.

For premenopausal women with low-risk breast cancer who do not require adjuvant chemotherapy, tamoxifen for at least 5 years and preferably 10 years is recommended. Extending tamoxifen use to 10 years decreased the absolute risk of recurrences between 5 and 14 years after diagnosis from 25% to 21.4% and reduced the risk of breast cancer mortality from 15% to 12.5%. Patients who become postmenopausal while taking tamoxifen may be changed to an aromatase inhibitor.

For premenopausal women who receive adjuvant chemotherapy for higher-risk hormone-positive breast cancer and who remain premenopausal, ovarian suppression achieved by surgical oophorectomy or pelvic irradiation in addition to either tamoxifen or an aromatase inhibitor is superior to tamoxifen alone. In the Suppression of Ovarian Function Trial (SOFT), adding ovarian suppression to tamoxifen improved absolute 5-year breast cancer–free survival by 4.5%. Breast cancer–free survival was improved by 7.7% with the use of ovarian suppression and exemestane compared to tamoxifen alone. The benefit was particularly dramatic in patients younger than age 35 years. Patients treated with ovarian suppression had more hot flushes, vaginal dryness, decreased libido, insomnia, depression, arthralgia, hypertension, glucose intolerance, and osteoporosis.

Tamoxifen side effects include endometrial cancer in women older than age 55 years, hot flushes, vaginal discharge, sexual dysfunction, venous thromboembolic events, and stroke.

Aromatase inhibitor side effects include arthralgia; vaginal dryness; sexual dysfunction; and higher risks of osteoporosis, fractures, cardiovascular events, and hyperlipidemia. Compared to tamoxifen, they have a lower risk of venous thrombosis and endometrial cancer. Up to one third of women develop aromatase inhibitor–associated symmetric arthralgia, joint stiffness, and bone pain. This musculoskeletal syndrome is managed with NSAIDs, a treatment break and change to an alternate aromatase inhibitor, or a change to tamoxifen.

KEY POINTS

- Premenopausal women with low-risk breast cancer who do not require adjuvant chemotherapy should receive tamoxifen for at least 5 years and preferably 10 years.

- Premenopausal women with higher-risk hormone-positive breast cancer who receive adjuvant chemotherapy should also receive ovarian suppression in addition to either tamoxifen or an aromatase inhibitor.

- Postmenopausal women should receive an aromatase inhibitor for 5 years and preferably 10 years, whether or not tamoxifen was given initially.

Adjuvant Chemotherapy

Increasingly, the use of adjuvant chemotherapy for early breast cancer is based more on tumor biology rather than on stage. The behavior of hormone receptor–negative and of HER2-positive cancers is more aggressive and there is benefit to adjuvant chemotherapy for cancers that are greater than 5 mm in size, lymph node positive, or both.

For hormone receptor–positive, HER2-negative breast cancers with zero to three positive axillary nodes, the use of multigene assays that predict the risk of recurrence with antiestrogen therapy alone has significantly decreased the use of adjuvant chemotherapy. The most commonly used molecular prognostic profile in the United States is the 21-gene recurrence score. Tumors with low-risk scores have a favorable prognosis with antiestrogen therapy alone and do not benefit from the addition of chemotherapy.

Clinicopathologic factors that suggest benefit to adjuvant chemotherapy include high tumor grade, extensive lymphatic invasion, very large primary tumor size, skin or chest wall involvement, and involvement of more than four axillary nodes.

Women with hormone receptor–negative, HER2-negative cancers (triple-negative breast cancer) have a 50% proportional reduction in the risk of recurrence and of breast cancer mortality with adjuvant chemotherapy. Adjuvant chemotherapy is recommended for triple-negative cancers larger than 5 mm in size or with positive lymph nodes.

When adjuvant chemotherapy is given for high-risk hormone receptor positive cancers or triple-negative cancers, typically two or three agents are given for four to eight cycles. The most common chemotherapies used for adjuvant treatment are anthracyclines (doxorubicin or epirubicin), cyclophosphamide, and the taxanes (paclitaxel or docetaxel).

Adjuvant chemotherapy combined with HER2-targeted treatment such as the monoclonal antibody trastuzumab or the combination of trastuzumab and pertuzumab is recommended for HER2-positive cancers that are greater than 5 mm in size, node positive, or both. Chemotherapy with trastuzumab decreases the risk of cancer recurrence by 53% and the risk of death by 34%. The main toxicities of trastuzumab are infusion reactions such as fever, chills, and cardiomyopathy. The addition of pertuzumab in treatment of cancers that are greater than 2 cm in size, node positive, or both, improves 5-year disease-free survival from 81% to 86%. For *HER2*-positive breast cancers that are smaller than 3 cm in size and node negative, treatment with paclitaxel and trastuzumab is a less toxic option, with a 3-year disease-free survival rate of 98.5%.

Acute side effects of adjuvant chemotherapy include bone marrow suppression with anemia and neutropenia, alopecia, allergic reactions, neuropathy, nausea, and premature menopause and infertility in premenopausal women (see Effects of Cancer Therapy and Survivorship). Women of childbearing age who wish to preserve fertility should meet with a fertility specialist before chemotherapy. Serious long-term toxicities include cardiomyopathy, neuropathy, myelodysplasia, and acute myelocytic leukemia. The risk of cardiomyopathy after four cycles of an anthracycline is 1.5%. The risk of acute leukemia after regimens containing an anthracycline or cyclophosphamide is 0.5%.

For women of advanced age with higher-risk early breast cancer, it is important to consider estimated life expectancy, functional status, and medical comorbidities before administering adjuvant chemotherapy. There is a higher risk of cardiotoxicity in older women.

KEY POINTS

- Patients with hormone receptor–positive tumors, zero to three positive axillary lymph nodes, and low-risk scores on the 21-gene recurrence assay have a favorable prognosis with antiestrogen therapy alone and do not benefit from the addition of chemotherapy.
- Adjuvant chemotherapy is most appropriate for patients with triple-negative tumors greater than 5 mm in size, skin involvement, or positive axillary lymph nodes.
- **HVC** • For women of advanced age with higher-risk early stage breast cancer, consider life expectancy, functional status, and medical comorbidities before administering adjuvant chemotherapy.

Locally Advanced and Inflammatory Breast Cancer

Locally advanced breast cancer includes a subset of clinical stage IIB cancers (T3N0M0), as well as stages IIIA to IIIC cancers. These cancers have high-risk characteristics such as skin involvement, chest wall involvement, extensive lymph node involvement, or inflammatory changes.

Inflammatory breast cancer is a type of locally advanced breast cancer that presents with swelling, thickening, and erythema of the skin overlying the breast, classically with a peau d'orange (orange peel) appearance (**Figure 20**). Patients often present with breast enlargement or swelling developed during a few weeks or months and may have been treated for presumed mastitis. It is important to consider that inflammatory breast cancer may be the underlying cause in patients who do not respond to antibiotics for an apparent mastitis. A palpable breast mass may be present. The skin changes are due to the obstruction of dermal lymphatic vessels by cancer cells,

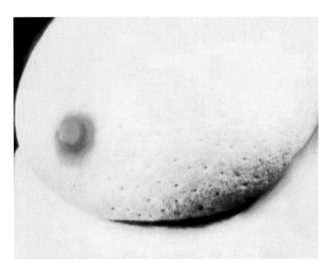

FIGURE 20. Inflammatory breast cancer often has a characteristic "p'eau d'orange" (orange peel) appearance of the skin, due to tumor emboli in the dermal lymphatics. Erythema is often present as well.

although demonstrating dermal lymphatic invasion on biopsy is not necessary for the diagnosis. One third of patients have distant metastases at diagnosis, and nearly all have lymph node involvement. For this reason, these patients should have routine CT and bone scan imaging, even in the absence of symptoms of metastatic disease.

Locally advanced cancers are usually treated initially with neoadjuvant chemotherapy, followed by surgery, and then radiation. In some situations, neoadjuvant antiestrogen therapy can be used instead of chemotherapy, although this is typically limited to postmenopausal women who are not candidates for chemotherapy. Tumors with skin involvement or inflammatory cancers require mastectomy, but in other cases, neoadjuvant therapy will often decrease the size of the primary breast cancer to allow for breast-conserving lumpectomy. All patients should have an axillary dissection at the time of mastectomy or lumpectomy and should receive radiation therapy afterward. The amount of residual cancer after neoadjuvant chemotherapy has prognostic significance, particularly in triple-negative or hormone-negative, *HER2*-positive cancers. Patients with complete pathologic responses have the lowest risk of recurrence.

Patients with hormone receptor–positive cancers should receive at least 5 years and ideally 10 years of antiestrogen therapy. Patients with *HER2*-positive cancers should complete one year of trastuzumab therapy.

KEY POINTS

- Inflammatory breast cancer, characterized by swelling, thickening, and erythema of the skin overlying the breast, classically with a peau d'orange (orange peel) appearance, may be mistaken for infectious mastitis and delay evaluation and treatment of the underlying malignancy.
- Locally advanced cancers are usually treated with neoadjuvant chemotherapy, surgery, and radiation.

Breast Cancer Follow-up and Survivorship

In 2016, there were more than 2.8 million women alive in the United States with a previous or current diagnosis of breast cancer. Once patients with nonmetastatic breast cancer complete surgery, radiation, and chemotherapy, they are monitored for local recurrence, distant recurrence, second primary cancers, and physical and psychosocial long-term effects of breast cancer and treatment. Patients with hormone receptor–positive breast cancer remain on antiestrogen treatment for at least 5 years and up to 10 years and require management of menopausal symptoms and other toxicities during that time. Guidelines recommend that patients be evaluated for a detailed cancer-related history and physical examination every 3 to 6 months for the first 3 years, every 6 to 12 months for the next 2 years, and then annually.

Patients should have annual mammograms of remaining breast tissue. Screening breast MRIs are needed only if patients meet criteria for screening MRIs (see Chemoprevention and other Risk Reduction Strategies). Patients should not have routine blood tests at follow-up visits or other routine imaging studies as these are not helpful for diagnosing recurrences earlier. Laboratory and imaging studies other than breast imaging should be guided by a patient's symptoms or findings on examination that raise concern for recurrence.

Patients should be evaluated at each visit for changes in family history of cancers and referred for genetic counseling as appropriate. Patients on tamoxifen should have annual gynecologic examinations and be evaluated by a gynecologist for any abnormal vaginal bleeding. Patients on aromatase inhibitors should have bone density studies every 2 years and should receive treatment of osteoporosis, ideally with a bisphosphonate, if their T score is -2.5 or lower.

For patients with breast asymmetry, reconstruction options can be offered and are often fully covered by insurance. Patients should receive physical therapy for lymphedema or decreased arm mobility after surgery or radiation to axillary nodes. Menopausal symptoms should be managed with nonhormonal options, such as gabapentin for nocturnal hot flushes. Depression, anxiety, and sexual dysfunction are not uncommon in this population and should be appropriately assessed and managed. For patients taking tamoxifen, it is important to avoid medications with strong CYP2D6 inhibition, such as bupropion or fluoxetine, as these may decrease tamoxifen activation.

KEY POINTS

- After completion of treatment, follow-up monitoring should be every 3 to 6 months for the first 3 years, every 6 to 12 months for the next 2 years, and then annually, with annual mammography for all survivors, and breast MRI for those at high risk of recurrence.

(Continued)

KEY POINTS *(continued)*

- Patients with hormone receptor–positive breast cancer remain on antiestrogen treatment for at least 5 years and up to 10 years.
- Surveillance blood tests and other imaging tests for breast cancer should not be routinely performed and should be guided by a patient's symptoms or findings on examination that raise concern for recurrence.
- Breast cancer survivors should be monitored and treated for the side effects of treatment.

HVC

Metastatic Breast Cancer

Approximately 5% of patients with breast cancer present with initial stage IV disease and up to 30% with early-stage disease develop metastases. Metastatic breast cancer is not curable, but systemic therapy can improve survival, relieve symptoms, and maintain quality of life. Treatment and prognosis are related to whether visceral metastases are present, the number of sites involved, the interval between initial diagnosis and metastases (intervals of less than 2 years have a poorer prognosis), the patient's performance status, and tumor biology. The median overall survival for patients with metastatic breast cancer is 2 years but is longer for women with hormone receptor–positive cancer or *HER2*-positive cancer some of whom may have prolonged survival, in part related to more treatment options.

It is important to biopsy a site of initial metastasis both to confirm the diagnosis and to assess hormone receptor and *HER2* status. Because there may be discordance in the receptors in the metastatic lesion compared to the primary breast cancer in 10% to 15% of patients, the selection of systemic therapy might be altered.

In postmenopausal women with hormone receptor-positive, *HER2*-negative breast cancer, initial treatment is usually hormonal therapy; aromatase inhibitors are superior to other agents as first-line treatment. Fulvestrant, which inhibits estrogen receptor function, and tamoxifen are other options. Premenopausal women can receive tamoxifen, ovarian suppression alone, or ovarian suppression combined with either tamoxifen or aromatase inhibitors as initial treatment. Patients who respond are usually treated with sequential hormonal therapies. In patients with rapidly progressive disease or extensive visceral metastases, initial chemotherapy may be used because of its higher response rate.

Combining targeted agents such as the CDK4/6 inhibitor palbociclib or the mammalian target of rapamycin (mTOR) inhibitor everolimus with antiestrogens improves the response rate and duration of response to hormonal therapy. In patients who develop metastatic breast cancer during adjuvant therapy with an aromatase inhibitor, palbociclib plus fulvestrant is usually the recommended first-line therapy. For women who develop metastatic breast cancer after having completed adjuvant therapy with an aromatase inhibitor, palbociclib plus an aromatase inhibitor is usually given as the initial systemic therapy.

In *HER2*-positive advanced breast cancer, treatment should include *HER2*-directed therapy such as trastuzumab given with either chemotherapy or antiestrogen therapy, depending on the hormone receptor status of the cancer and the sites of disease. First-line treatment with dual *HER2*-targeted therapy with trastuzumab and pertuzumab added to the taxane docetaxel has been shown to improve overall survival, with median overall survival of 56 months in a phase 3 clinical trial. Ado-trastuzumab emtansine is an innovative antibody-drug conjugate that links trastuzumab to the microtubule inhibitor emtansine, delivering chemotherapy more specifically to *HER2*-overexpressing cells.

Triple-negative breast cancers have a higher relapse rate than hormone receptor–positive cancers; recur earlier, with a peak at 3 years after diagnosis and a very low risk of relapse after 5 years; and have a higher risk of locoregional recurrence and brain and lung metastases. Advanced triple-negative breast cancer is treated with chemotherapy. These cancers may be particularly responsive to platinum agents, particularly in *BRCA1* mutation carriers.

Chemotherapy agents used in patients with advanced breast cancer include taxanes, capecitabine, eribulin, gemcitabine, ixabepilone, and liposomal doxorubicin. Single-agent chemotherapy is usually given, with combination chemotherapy reserved for patients with extensive visceral metastases where a higher response rate is important.

In patients with *BRCA1* or *BRCA2* mutations, poly (ADP-ribose) polymerase (PARP) inhibitors have shown encouraging results. These agents cause "synthetic lethality" by producing an increase in double-strand DNA breaks that would usually be repaired by the *BRCA* pathway.

For all subtypes of metastatic breast cancer, bone-modifying agents such as zoledronic acid or denosumab are recommended for patients with bone metastases to decrease skeletal-related events (fractures, pain, and need for radiation). Palliative radiation can be used to treat painful bone metastases as well as other sites of tumor-related pain or obstruction. Triple-negative breast cancers and *HER2*-positive cancers have a higher risk of brain metastases, which are treated with whole brain radiation, stereotactic radiation, or surgery. Palliative care teams can be helpful for managing symptoms of pain, nausea, anorexia, and fatigue. Throughout the course of advanced breast cancer, discussions with patients about their goals of care should take place, focusing on their values and preferences as they are treated for an incurable illness.

KEY POINTS

- Metastatic breast cancer is not curable, but it can be treated with systemic therapy with the goals of improved survival, palliation of symptoms, and maintaining quality of life.

- The site of initial metastasis should be biopsied to confirm the diagnosis and to assess hormone receptor and *HER2* status, which can be discordant from the primary breast cancer.

Ovarian Cancer

Epidemiology and Risk Factors

Ovarian cancer, the leading cause of gynecologic cancer deaths, will be newly diagnosed in approximately 22,000 women in 2016 in the United States, with an estimated 14,000 deaths. This chapter will focus on the 95% of ovarian cancers that are of epithelial origin.

Risk factors for ovarian epithelial cancer include inheritance of ovarian cancer susceptibility genes, increasing age, infertility, nulliparity, endometriosis, polycystic ovary syndrome, use of an intrauterine device, and cigarette smoking.

The most common ovarian cancer susceptibility genes are *BRCA1*, *BRCA2*, and the mismatch repair (MMR) genes associated with hereditary nonpolyposis colon cancer (HNPCC), also known as Lynch syndrome. Approximately 10% to 15% of women with ovarian cancer carry a mutation in one of these genes, and all women with epithelial ovarian cancer should be offered genetic testing for *BRCA1* and *BRCA2* mutations. In patients with a personal or family history of other HNPCC-related cancers (colorectal, small bowel or endometrial cancers or transitional cell cancers of the renal pelvis or ureter), HNPCC testing is recommended as well. There are different criteria for HNPCC genetic testing, including criteria and prediction models based on the number of affected relatives and age of onset, as well as tumor-based strategies often used in colorectal and endometrial cancers involving testing for microsatellite instability (MSI) or immunohistochemistry staining for mismatch repair proteins. The cumulative lifetime risk of ovarian cancer is 1.4% in patients without a susceptibility gene, 45% in *BRCA1* carriers, 12% in *BRCA2* carriers, and 3% to 13.5% in MMR gene mutation carriers.

KEY POINT

- Genetic testing for *BRCA1*, *BRCA2*, and mismatch repair gene mutations is recommended for all women with ovarian cancer.

Screening and Risk-Reduction Strategies

Ovarian cancer screening with transvaginal ultrasonography or serum CA-125 testing is not effective and is not recommended for patients of average, or even high, risk.

For women with *BRCA1*, *BRCA2*, or MMR gene mutations, prophylactic bilateral salpingo-oophorectomy (BSO) is recommended after completion of childbearing. Prophylactic BSO is recommended by age 35 to 40 years for *BRCA1* carriers and by age 45 years for *BRCA2* carriers. For *BRCA1* or *BRCA2* carriers, prophylactic BSO decreases the risk of ovarian, fallopian tube, and primary peritoneal cancers by greater than 80% and decreases all-cause mortality to age 70 years by 77%. Recommendations for genetic testing for breast and ovarian cancer syndromes are discussed in Breast Cancer. In women with Lynch syndrome, BSO and hysterectomy are recommended because of the increased risk of endometrial cancer.

Oral contraceptives reduce the risk of ovarian cancer by 40% to 50%, with the greatest benefit seen after 15 years of use.

HVC

KEY POINTS

- Ovarian cancer screening is not recommended, even for women at high risk for ovarian cancer.
- Prophylactic bilateral salpingo-oophorectomy is recommended by age 35 to 40 years for *BRCA1* carriers and by age 45 years for *BRCA2* carriers.

Diagnosis

Ovarian cancer usually presents with advanced disease, either acutely with such symptoms as pleural effusions or bowel obstruction or subacutely with such symptoms as bloating, abdominal or pelvic pain, urinary frequency, or early satiety. An incidental ovarian mass may be found on routine examination. Initial studies for suspected ovarian cancer should include a pelvic examination, general physical examination, serum CA-125 level, complete blood count, liver chemistry tests, and transvaginal and transabdominal ultrasonography. Additional imaging with abdominal and pelvic CT or MRI and chest imaging with CT or chest radiography are added as clinically indicated. Patients with a high suspicion of ovarian cancer should be referred to a gynecologic oncologist.

For early ovarian cancer, surgical exploration is recommended for diagnosis because removing the ovarian cancer intact without rupture improves survival. For advanced ovarian cancers with peritoneal masses, ascites, or pleural effusions, fluid cytology or imaging-guided biopsy can be done, particularly in cases where the disease is not initially resectable and neoadjuvant chemotherapy may be used.

Staging and prognosis are shown in **Table 43**. Early stage, low grade, serous histology, extent of disease after surgical debulking, and young age are associated with improved survival. A recent analysis showed that 31% of patients diagnosed with ovarian cancer survived 10 years, with one third of these long-term survivors having stage III or IV cancer.

KEY POINTS

- Most women with ovarian cancer present with symptoms of advanced disease, either with acute symptoms such as pleural effusions or bowel obstruction, or with subacute symptoms such as bloating, abdominal or pelvic pain, urinary frequency, or early satiety.
- Diagnostic surgical exploration is most appropriate for early ovarian cancer because intact cancer removal improves survival, and fluid cytology or imaging-guided biopsy is more appropriate for advanced cancers, particularly those that are not initially resectable.

TABLE 43. International Federation of Gynecology and Obstetrics Ovarian Cancer Staging, Treatment, and Survival

Stage	Definition	Treatment	5-Year Survival
Stage I disease (favorable)[a]	Cancer in one or both ovaries, not high grade or clear cell, negative peritoneal washings, no rupture	Surgery alone	94% overall survival
Stage I disease (unfavorable); stage II disease	Unfavorable stage I disease: Confined to ovaries but with high-grade or clear cell histology, rupture, or positive peritoneal washings Stage II disease: spread beyond ovaries but confined to pelvis	Surgery followed by 3 to 6 cycles of chemotherapy (usually carboplatin and paclitaxel)	Stage I: 85% relative survival[b] Stage II: 70%-78% relative survival
Optimally debulked stage III disease	Spread to abdomen, with residual tumor masses <1 cm after debulking surgery	Surgery followed by IV or IV/IP chemotherapy	IV chemotherapy: 40% overall survival IV/IP chemotherapy: 50% overall survival (23% decreased risk of death with IP/IV versus IV chemotherapy)
Suboptimally debulked stage III disease or stage IV disease[c]	Stage III (suboptimal) disease: spread to abdomen with residual masses >1 cm after debulking surgery Stage IV disease: spread beyond abdomen	Surgery (usually done even for stage IV disease as it improves survival) and chemotherapy; preoperative (neoadjuvant) chemotherapy given for initially unresectable cancer	Stage III: 39% relative survival Stage IV: 17% relative survival

IP = intraperitoneal; IV = intravenous.

[a]Careful staging is critical: almost one third of patients with apparent early disease will have more advanced disease when thorough staging is completed.

[b]Relative survival is an estimate of the percentage of patients who would be expected to survive the effects of their cancer.

[c]According to recent guidelines by the American Society of Clinical Oncology (ASCO) and Society of Gynecologic Oncology (SGO), patients with stage IIIC or IV ovarian cancer who are at high perioperative risk or who have a low likelihood of optimal tumor debulking should receive neoadjuvant chemotherapy followed by reevaluation for cytoreductive surgery.

Treatment

Surgical staging includes total hysterectomy, BSO, peritoneal washings, omentectomy, and pelvic and para-aortic lymph node sampling. In advanced ovarian cancer, surgical debulking, including the resection of metastatic disease, improves prognosis. The volume of residual disease after surgery correlates inversely with survival. Neoadjuvant chemotherapy is usually recommended for patients with initially unresectable disease.

Patients with early-stage ovarian cancer who have favorable histology may be treated with surgical resection alone. All other patients should receive adjuvant chemotherapy. Patients with stage III disease have improved survival, albeit with increased toxicity, from intraperitoneal along with intravenous chemotherapy; nevertheless, intraperitoneal therapy remains underused. Platinum-taxane chemotherapy is generally used for all stages. According to recent guidelines by the American Society of Clinical Oncology (ASCO) and Society of Gynecologic Oncology (SGO), patients with stage IIIC or IV ovarian cancer who are at high perioperative risk or who have a low likelihood of optimal tumor debulking should receive neoadjuvant chemotherapy followed by reevaluation for cytoreductive surgery.

For patients who achieve a clinical remission after chemotherapy, maintenance therapy has not been shown to improve survival. Similarly, second-look laparotomy to determine if a patient is in a pathologic response has not been shown to be beneficial.

KEY POINTS

- Patients with early-stage ovarian cancer with favorable histology may be treated with surgery alone; all other patients should receive platinum-taxane chemotherapy.

- Intraperitoneal chemotherapy, when added to intravenous chemotherapy, leads to improved survival in patients with stage III ovarian cancer.

HVC
- Maintenance chemotherapy and second-look laparotomy do not improve survival in patients with ovarian cancer who achieve clinical remission.

Monitoring and Follow-up

Posttreatment surveillance consists of physical and pelvic examinations every 3 to 6 months for 5 years, then annually. The need to monitor serum CA-125 at each visit if initially elevated is controversial, as such monitoring does not improve survival. Other laboratory tests and imaging tests are recommended only as indicated for symptoms or findings suggesting recurrence.

Management of Recurrent Ovarian Cancer

Despite optimal treatment, 80% to 85% of women with stage III or IV ovarian cancer will relapse. Patients who relapse 6 months or more after initial chemotherapy are considered to have platinum-sensitive disease, have a better prognosis, and are usually treated with platinum-containing combination chemotherapy. Adding the angiogenesis inhibitor bevacizumab improves disease-free survival but not overall survival, and increases the risk of serious gastrointestinal toxicities including perforation. For patients with platinum-resistant disease, various single agents can be used palliatively, as can bevacizumab alone or with chemotherapy. For *BRCA1* or *BRCA2* carriers with recurrent ovarian cancer, the poly (ADP-ribose) polymerase (PARP) inhibitor olaparib can be given after progression on chemotherapy.

KEY POINT

- Patients who relapse more than 6 months after discontinuing platinum-based chemotherapy are considered to have platinum-sensitive disease and should be treated with platinum-based combination chemotherapy.

Cervical Cancer
Epidemiology and Risk Factors

In 2018, there will be an estimated 13,240 new patients diagnosed with invasive cervical cancer and 4170 deaths from cervical cancer in the United States. The mean age of diagnosis in the United States is 48 years. During the last 30 years, cervical cancer incidence and deaths in developed countries have decreased by more than 50%, primarily because of screening and preventive treatment. It remains the second most common cause of mortality from cancer in women worldwide, with more than 260,000 women dying each year of cervical cancer. More than 85% of deaths are in less developed countries.

Human papillomavirus (HPV) is the causative agent in most patients and can be detected in 99.7% of cervical cancers. Risk factors include sexual habits associated with a higher risk of acquiring HPV, such as earlier onset of sexual activity and several partners. Immunosuppression, including HIV infection, low socioeconomic status, and oral contraceptive use are additional risk factors. Cigarette smoking increases the risk of squamous cell carcinoma of the cervix. Squamous cell carcinoma is the histologic type in 69% of cervical cancers, with adenocarcinoma accounting for 25%. HPV vaccination decreases the incidence of cervical dysplasia and cervical cancer. Cervical cancer screening and HPV vaccination are covered in MKSAP 18 General Internal Medicine.

KEY POINT

- Human papillomavirus (HPV) is the causative agent in most patients with cervical cancer, and HPV vaccination significantly reduces the risk.

Diagnosis, Staging, and Treatment

Early cervical cancer is frequently asymptomatic. The most common symptoms are abnormal or heavy vaginal bleeding or vaginal discharge. Pelvic or back pain and bowel or bladder symptoms are presentations of advanced disease. Diagnosis is made by direct biopsy of a visible lesion, colposcopy, or cone biopsy (conization). Current guidelines for staging studies recommend a complete blood count, liver chemistry tests, kidney function studies, and imaging studies for moderate-risk and high-risk stage cancers. Chest radiography, CT or PET-CT scan, and MRI can be added as indicated. Cystoscopy and proctoscopy are optional. HIV testing should be considered. Cervical cancer staging and treatment are described in **Table 44**. For patients with tumors 2 cm in size or smaller that are confined to the cervix and with no lymph node involvement, fertility-sparing surgeries such as conization (only for stage IA) or radical trachelectomy are options. Vaginal radical trachelectomy involves removal of the cervix with conservation of the uterus. A permanent cerclage is placed in the uterine isthmus.

Patients with disease confined to the cervix who have tumors 2 cm or less in size and no node involvement can be treated by limited surgery that preserves fertility such as radical trachelectomy, which removes the cervix with conservation of the uterus. For high-risk disease, adding weekly cisplatin-based chemotherapy to radiation decreases the risk of recurrence by 34% and improves overall survival. Adding the anti–vascular endothelial growth factor monoclonal antibody bevacizumab to chemotherapy improves overall survival in patients with distant metastases.

KEY POINTS

- Early cervical cancer is frequently asymptomatic, but the most common symptoms are abnormal or heavy vaginal bleeding or vaginal discharge; advanced cervical cancer symptoms include pelvic or back pain and bowel or bladder symptoms.

- Select patients with cervical cancer confined to the cervix can be treated with surgery that preserves fertility.

- Patients with bulky or locally advanced cervical cancer are treated with cisplatin-based chemotherapy and radiation instead of surgery.

Prognosis and Surveillance

The 5-year relative survival for all stages of cervical cancer is 67.5%. The anatomic stage is the most important predictor of prognosis. Ninety percent of patients with localized disease survive 5 years. The 5-year survival rate drops to 58% for patients with regional disease and 17% for patients with disease extending outside of the true pelvis or involving the bladder or rectum.

Surveillance is recommended to monitor for recurrences that are potentially curable. Guidelines recommend doing a history and physical examination every 3 to 6 months for 2 years, every 6 to 12 months during years 3 to 5, and then annually based on the risk of recurrence. Annual vaginal cytology, cervical cytology, or both is recommended. Imaging and laboratory studies are recommended only if indicated based on symptoms or findings on examination that are suspicious for recurrence.

TABLE 44. International Federation of Gynecology and Obstetrics Cervical Cancer Staging and Treatment	
Stage	**Treatment**
I: Carcinoma is strictly confined to the cervix IA: Microscopic disease only, up to 5 mm in depth and up to 7 mm in horizontal spread IB: Clinically visible disease, or microscopic disease larger than IA criteria	IA and IB: Modified radical (for lesions <2 cm) or radical hysterectomy with pelvic lymph-node dissection is preferred; if poor functional status, radiation can be used instead. If treated with surgery, adjuvant radiation or chemoradiation is added if indicated based on final pathologic findings. Fertility preservation surgery is an option for cancers ≤2 cm with no lymph node metastases. IA: Simple hysterectomy, cone biopsy (conization), or removal of cervix (trachelectomy) are options.
IIA and IIB: Cervical carcinoma invades beyond the uterus, but not to the pelvic wall or lower third of the vagina. IIB has parametrial invasion.	IIA: Same as for stage I IIB: Same as for stage III
III: The tumor extends to the pelvic wall and/or involves the lower third of the vagina and/or causes hydronephrosis or nonfunctioning kidney	III: Radiation with concurrent platinum-based chemotherapy
IV: The carcinoma extends beyond the true pelvis or involves (biopsy proven) the mucosa of the bladder or rectum IVA: Spread to adjacent organs IVB: Distant metastases	IVA: Same as for stage III IVB: Palliative cisplatin-based chemotherapy, with radiation for local symptoms, such as bleeding or pain

KEY POINT

HVC
- Surveillance imaging and laboratory studies for cervical cancer survivors are recommended only if there are signs or symptoms suggestive of recurrence.

Gastroenterological Malignancies

Colorectal Cancer

Colorectal cancer (CRC) is the fourth most common cancer and the second leading cause of cancer death in North America, yet it is largely preventable through screening. CRC screening of average-risk patients is discussed in MKSAP 18 General Internal Medicine. Most colon cancers are adenocarcinomas that begin in the inner lining and progress to involve or spread beyond the full thickness of the bowel wall, then to regional lymph nodes, and subsequently to distant organ metastases. Epidemiology, pathophysiology, risk factors (and screening high-risk patients), and clinical manifestations will be discussed in MKSAP 18 Gastroenterology and Hepatology.

Recent evidence suggests tumors on the right side of the large intestine (cecum, ascending colon, and proximal two thirds of transverse colon) have a completely different biology, likely related to embryologic origin, and a substantially worse prognosis than tumors on the left side (distal one third of transverse colon, descending colon, sigmoid colon, and rectum). Symptoms may also differ based on tumor location, with left-side tumors more likely to cause a change in bowel habits. Cancer in the cecum, with a larger lumen and less formed stool, does not generally cause a change in bowel habits until the tumor is advanced in size, but may present with iron-deficiency anemia with occult, chronic blood loss. Colon cancer at any location may also present with hematochezia, pain, or acute clinical signs from perforation or obstruction.

Approximately 15% of CRCs lack one or more mismatch repair enzymes and are known as mismatch repair deficient (dMMR)–CRC. This manifests itself as increased microsatellite instability (MSI) in the cancer cell's DNA; the terms *dMMR* and *MSI* are essentially synonymous. Most guidelines now recommend that all CRCs should be screened for dMMR or MSI. Approximately 25% of patients with dMMR tumors will have Lynch syndrome, which is associated with a high lifetime risk of CRC as well as endometrial and other cancers. Patients and family members with Lynch syndrome require formal genetic counseling and more intense cancer surveillance. Mismatch repair status or the tumor can affect treatment choices in patients with stage II or stage IV cancer as discussed below.

KEY POINTS

- Recent evidence suggests tumors on the right side of the large intestine have a different biology and substantially worse prognosis than tumors on the left side.

(Continued)

KEY POINTS *(continued)*

- Tumors in all colorectal cancer patients should be screened for mismatch repair enzyme deficiency or microsatellite instability, which increases the risk of Lynch syndrome and other cancers.

Staging

Staging with the TNM cancer staging system is the first step in treatment planning (**Table 45**). Evaluation includes serum carcinoembryonic antigen (CEA) in addition to routine laboratory studies; a full colonoscopy (if possible); and contrast-enhanced CT scans of the chest, abdomen, and pelvis. Rectal cancers also require a rectal MRI or endorectal ultrasonography, both of which offer more precision in assessing tumor penetration and lymph node involvement. PET scans have not been demonstrated to provide greater accuracy in staging and should not be routinely used for preoperative staging or postoperative surveillance.

Treatment

Rectal Cancer

Rectal cancers without full thickness penetration of the bowel wall or enlarged lymph nodes are stage I and are treated with surgical resection. Small tumors may be resected by a transanal approach, decreasing postoperative morbidity. Unless more extensive disease is found at operation, no further treatment is warranted.

Full-thickness tumors (stage II) and involved lymph nodes (stage III) require radiation, chemotherapy, and surgery. The optimal sequencing and combining of the three treatment modalities is being studied. Attempts are made to preserve anal sphincter function, but distal rectal lesions may require an abdominal-perineal resection and permanent colostomy.

Intravenous 5-fluorouracil (5-FU) or oral capecitabine, a prodrug that is converted into 5-FU, is given concurrently with radiation therapy. The chemotherapy may be associated

TABLE 45.	**Staging of Colorectal Cancer**	
Stage	**Description**	**Approximate 5-Year Disease-Free Survival**
I	Tumor does not invade the full thickness of bowel wall (T1, T2); lymph nodes not involved (N0)	90%-95%
II	Tumor invades full thickness of the bowel and may invade into pericolonic or perirectal fat (T3, T4); lymph nodes not involved (N0)	70%-85%
III	One or more lymph nodes involved with cancer (N1, N2); any T stage	25%-70%
IV	Metastatic tumor spread to distant site (M1); any T stage; any N stage	0%-10%

with edema and erythema of the palms and soles that may progress to blistering and necrosis (hand-foot syndrome), mucositis, diarrhea, and neutropenia. Leucovorin, 5-FU, and oxaliplatin (FOLFOX) or capecitabine plus oxaliplatin (CAPOX) regimens are typically used for the chemotherapy-only portion of the treatment. Oxaliplatin often causes a peripheral neuropathy that does not resolve fully in some patients.

Following therapy, patients with rectal cancer should be evaluated at approximately 6-month intervals for up to 5 years with a history, physical examination, and serum CEA level assessment. Contrast-enhanced CT scans of the chest, abdomen, and pelvis are typically obtained annually for 5 years.

Colon Cancer

Nonmetastatic colon cancers are managed with initial surgery. Pathologic evaluation determines further treatment.

Patients with stage II cancer lacking high-risk features, such as poorly differentiated histology, T4 primary tumor, lymphovascular invasion, inadequate lymph node sampling, poorly differentiated histology, elevated postoperative CEA, or perforation or obstruction, are unlikely to benefit from adjuvant treatment. Patients with one or more of these risk factors may be considered for adjuvant 5-FU or capecitabine. All stage II colon tumors should be assessed for MSI or dMMR, because such tumors, when stage II, are at low risk for recurrence, do not benefit from adjuvant chemotherapy, and should not be treated regardless of the presence of other potential risk factors.

FOLFOX and CAPOX, given for approximately 6 months, are equally acceptable adjuvant chemotherapy regimens and reduce the risk of cancer recurrence and death in patients with stage III cancer.

As with rectal cancer, routine evaluation and serum CEA assessment should be done at approximately 6-month intervals, with annual CT scans for up to 5 years after therapy.

Postoperative surveillance following curative resection is used to identify oligometastatic disease in the liver or lung that may be resectable. Patients with metastatic foci confined to liver or lung should be referred for surgical evaluation. Complete resection of metastatic foci may lead to cure in 25% of these patients. Contrast-enhanced CT scans of the chest, abdomen, and pelvis are recommended annually for up to 5 years postoperatively. PET scanning should not be used for routine surveillance. Colonoscopy is recommended one year after resection (or 3 to 6 months after resection if a complete colonoscopy was not done preoperatively), and then in 3 years, followed by every 5 years, unless abnormalities are found. In 2016, the United States Multi-Society Task Force on Colorectal Cancer recommended that flexible sigmoidoscopy or endoscopic ultrasound be performed every 3 to 6 months for the first 2 to 3 years after surgery in patients with rectal cancer who are at increased risk for local recurrence.

KEY POINTS

- Pretreatment evaluation of rectal cancer requires a rectal MRI or endorectal ultrasonography.
- PET scans should not be used for preoperative staging or postoperative surveillance in colorectal cancer. **HVC**
- Standard treatment of stages II and III rectal cancer is either chemoradiotherapy (with 5-fluorouracil or capecitabine), followed by surgery and adjuvant chemotherapy, or neoadjuvant chemotherapy followed by chemoradiotherapy, followed by surgery.
- Patients with stage II colon cancer that lacks high-risk features are unlikely to benefit from adjuvant chemotherapy. **HVC**
- Posttreatment surveillance for patients with colon cancer includes periodic history; physical examination; serum carcinoembryonic antigen level testing; and CT of the chest, abdomen, and pelvis, as early detection and resection of isolated metastatic disease can still result in cure; repeat colonoscopy should be done at 1 year, then in 3 years, followed by every 5 years.

Metastatic Disease

All metastatic CRC requires molecular analysis for *KRAS*, *NRAS*, and *BRAF* gene mutation status as well as dMMR determination. This rarely affects the choice of first-line therapy but will define subsequent treatment options, discussed later. These tests can be done on either the primary tumor or a metastasis; rebiopsy of metastases for the purpose of these studies is rarely needed.

Patients with metastatic disease limited to the liver should be evaluated for surgical resection with curative intent. Unresectable metastatic CRC is treatable but not curable. Although chemotherapy may be palliative and even extend survival, patients who have a poor performance status may not benefit or may have unacceptable toxicity. A careful discussion should be undertaken with the patient to establish goals of care and expectations.

5-FU is at the center of most treatment regimens, with longer infusions preferable to bolus administration. Newer drugs have failed to replace 5-FU, but leucovorin is often combined with 5-FU, or capecitabine can be an alternative to 5-FU. Other cytotoxic agents used in metastatic CRC include irinotecan and oxaliplatin. The anti–vascular endothelial growth factor (VEGF) monoclonal antibody bevacizumab is often given concurrently with first-line cytotoxic chemotherapy regimens. This agent has essentially no antitumor activity in CRC on its own, but it does potentiate other chemotherapies, resulting in a modestly increased duration of progression-free survival, and in some studies, in increased duration of overall survival. Studies have shown that continuing an anti-VEGF agent with second-line chemotherapy also modestly improves overall survival. Bevacizumab commonly causes hypertension, sometimes requiring antihypertensive medication. It also interferes with wound healing and needs to be discontinued 6 to 8 weeks before elective surgery and withheld for at least a month after surgery. Very rare but potentially life-threatening side effects include arterial thrombotic events such as myocardial infarction, cerebrovascular accidents, and gastrointestinal perforations.

Panitumumab and cetuximab are monoclonal antibodies that bind to and block activation of the epidermal growth factor receptor (EGFR). They are potentially active only in tumors that are nonmutated (wild-type) *KRAS, NRAS,* and *BRAF* genes. In addition, more recent data suggest that these agents may only have activity in tumors derived from the left side of the large intestine. The major side effect of these agents is an acneiform rash, which can be painful, pruritic, and socially debilitating. There is a tight correlation between rash and anti-tumor activity, and patients who have only a mild skin rash are unlikely to benefit from these agents. Anti-EGFR agents should not be used concurrently with anti-VEGF agents; two large randomized trials found an unexpected detriment with concurrent use.

Thus far, immune checkpoint inhibitors have been inactive in metastatic CRC, with the exception of those rare tumors that are metastatic and dMMR. The programmed death 1 (PD-1) receptor inhibitors pembrolizumab and nivolumab have both shown activity in such patients; however, dMMR tumors make up only 1% or 2% of metastatic CRC.

Multigene sequencing may open some experimental options, but it does not yield actionable information in terms of standard management options at this time. Thus the expense is not warranted outside of a potential research setting.

KEY POINTS

- All metastatic colorectal cancers require molecular analysis for *KRAS, NRAS,* and *BRAF* gene mutation status as well as mismatch repair gene deficiency, which will determine treatment after first-line therapy.
- The anti–vascular endothelial growth factor antibody bevacizumab potentiates the efficacy of 5-fluorouracil combined with either leucovorin or capecitabine in treating metastatic colon cancer, but is associated with worsening hypertension, arterial thrombosis, poor wound healing, and gastrointestinal perforation and fistula formation.

Anal Cancer

Anal cancer is a human papillomavirus (HPV)–associated malignancy. Unlike rectal cancer, which is an adenocarcinoma, anal cancer is a squamous cell carcinoma. Anal cancer is often curable with combined radiation and chemotherapy; surgery is typically not indicated. Mitomycin plus 5-FU or capecitabine is the standard chemotherapy regimen. Although complete regression may be observed as soon as 8 weeks after radiation,

responding tumors may continue to regress for up to 6 months after radiation. If tumor growth is seen after radiation, then salvage surgery with a permanent colostomy is indicated. Distant metastases are rare. When they do develop, chemotherapy with oxaliplatin, cisplatin, or carboplatin is often active.

Although HPV vaccination would be expected to be as effective at cancer prevention as it is with other HPV-related malignancies, there is no evidence that HPV vaccination plays a role in treatment or post-treatment management of patients with anal cancer. See MKSAP 18 General Internal Medicine for further discussion of HPV vaccination.

KEY POINT

- Anal cancer, a squamous cell carcinoma linked to human papillomavirus, is often cured by combination radiation and chemotherapy, sparing the need for surgical resection and subsequent colostomy.

Pancreatic Cancer

There are approximately 53,000 patients diagnosed with exocrine pancreatic cancer per year in the United States. Mortality is high, with 42,000 deaths expected annually. Only patients who can undergo a complete resection have a chance of cure. When disease is unresectable because of invasion into critical vascular structures, median survival is approximately 1 year. For those with metastatic disease, median survival is typically less than half that.

Most pancreatic cancers lack a genetic predisposition, although 5% to 10% of patients have either a strong family history of pancreatic cancer, an identifiable mutation that confers increased risk, or both. Some rare familial pancreatic cancer syndromes have been recognized, including patients with *BRCA* gene mutations, but *BRCA* screening is not recommended for those without a strong family history. Chronic pancreatitis, obesity, type 2 diabetes mellitus, high red meat consumption, alcohol abuse, and tobacco use are implicated risk factors.

Painless jaundice, abdominal pain, weight loss, persistent fevers, or protracted nausea and vomiting may be presenting symptoms. Manifestations of hypercoagulability, including Trousseau syndrome (a migratory superficial thrombophlebitis of the lower extremities), chronic disseminated intravascular coagulation, deep venous thrombosis, or pulmonary embolism, may be the initial manifestations of underlying pancreatic cancer. **H**

A contrast-enhanced CT of the chest and abdomen (or noncontrast chest CT and abdominal MRI) are appropriate for staging and treatment planning. PET scans have not been shown to add value in pancreatic cancer and are not part of standard management. For patients whose disease is confined to the pancreas with or without involved local regional lymph nodes, resectability is the most important question. Endoscopic ultrasonography may help in staging and is used to more precisely guide diagnostic needle biopsy. Some patients with clinical features that strongly suggest malignancy may not require such preoperative biopsy, as false-negative results would not obviate the need for surgical resection. Magnetic resonance cholangiopancreatography may also be useful in delineating resectability in borderline patients. Conversion therapy—using radiation or chemotherapy to convert locally unresectable disease to resectable—has garnered interest, but evidence defining how successful this approach actually is remains limited and preliminary.

Patients without evidence of metastatic disease who appear to have technically resectable disease should undergo resection.

Patients who are medically well enough to receive chemotherapy after resection should do so. A trial that compared single-agent gemcitabine to observation showed improved survival for patients who received gemcitabine, and a more recent trial comparing single-agent gemcitabine to gemcitabine plus capecitabine showed improved survival for the combination arm. The data for use of adjuvant radiation therapy are controversial.

Patients experience considerable morbidity following resection of pancreatic cancer, with most requiring pancreatic enzyme replacement therapy and those with the most extensive pancreatic resection needing lifelong insulin therapy.

For metastatic disease, the combination regimen of oxaliplatin, irinotecan, 5-FU, and leucovorin (FOLFIRINOX) or the combination of nab-paclitaxel and gemcitabine has each shown better antitumor activity and modest survival benefits over single-agent gemcitabine in randomized trials, but the combination regimens have higher toxicity. In second-line therapy, liposome-encapsulated irinotecan added to 5-FU has shown activity. Clinical trials are needed to define second-line therapy for metastatic pancreatic cancer.

KEY POINTS

- Patients without metastatic disease who have clinical staging suggesting resectable or borderline resectable pancreatic cancer should undergo resection as it is the only option for cure.
- PET scans have not been shown to add value in the staging of pancreatic cancer and are not part of standard management.
- The use of adjuvant chemotherapy with gemcitabine and capecitabine following successful pancreatic resection will prolong survival.

Gastroesophageal Cancer

Epidemiology, risk factors, and clinical manifestations of esophageal and gastric cancer are discussed in MKSAP 18 Gastroenterology and Hepatology.

Upper gastrointestinal tract cancers are a major cause of cancer deaths worldwide, particularly in Asia and Africa. The incidence has been increasing significantly in the United States and Western countries, albeit with changing pathology. With the dramatic rise in the incidence of adenocarcinoma of the distal esophagus and proximal stomach, gastroesophageal cancer is now considered a single entity.

Smoking and alcohol use remain the major risk factors for the traditional squamous cell carcinoma of the esophagus. Risk factors for adenocarcinoma also include smoking along with gastroesophageal reflux disease (GERD) and obesity. The development of Barrett esophagus as a result of GERD, especially with dysplastic features, is a further risk for developing adenocarcinoma of the esophagus, and regular surveillance is indicated. See MKSAP 18 Gastroenterology and Hepatology for more detailed information on Barrett esophagus and GERD.

Pain or difficulty on swallowing, weight loss, nausea, vomiting, or persistent dyspepsia may be presenting symptoms. Upper endoscopy and biopsy establishes the diagnosis. Endoscopic ultrasonography is routinely used to assess the depth of tumor penetration and presence of involved lymph nodes. In contrast to the evaluation of other gastrointestinal tumors, PET-CT is widely used as part of standard preoperative staging.

Surgery is the primary treatment of locoregional disease, found in approximately one third of patients. Data have shown a survival benefit for preoperative therapy with either neoadjuvant chemotherapy or the combination of neoadjuvant chemotherapy and radiation therapy. For those patients with cancer who undergo surgery first and whose cancer is more advanced than stage I, adjuvant chemotherapy is warranted. A recently reported trial of adjuvant chemotherapy with or without adjuvant radiation therapy showed no difference in outcome, raising questions as to the utility of radiation in this setting. Unfortunately, recurrence rates following surgical resection remain high, even with the use of adjuvant therapy.

Treatment of recurrent or metastatic disease is only modestly effective and is not curative.

Approximately 25% of gastroesophageal cancers overexpress the human epidermal growth factor receptor 2 (*HER2*), and it is now standard practice to evaluate gastroesophageal tumors for *HER2* overexpression. For these patients only, the addition of the anti-*HER2* monoclonal antibody trastuzumab to chemotherapy provides a modest but statistically significant survival benefit. More recently, the anti-VEGF receptor monoclonal antibody ramucirumab has shown modest activity as a non–first-line treatment, either alone or in combination with a taxane.

KEY POINTS

- Smoking, obesity, and gastroesophageal reflux disease, especially with the development of Barrett esophagus, are risk factors for adenocarcinoma of the esophagus, gastroesophageal junction, and proximal stomach.
- In contrast to other gastrointestinal tumors, PET-CT is widely used as part of standard preoperative staging of gastroesophageal cancer.
- Upper gastrointestinal tumors should be evaluated for human epidermal growth factor 2 (*HER2*) overexpression; adding trastuzumab to chemotherapy regimens for patients with *HER2* overexpression provides a modest survival benefit.

Gastric Lymphoma

The stomach may be the primary site for extranodal lymphoma, a heterogeneous group of B-cell and T-cell neoplasms, generally treated with combination chemotherapy. A specific variant, mucosa-associated lymphoid tissue (MALT) lymphomas, are indolent tumors that often present with localized disease and concomitant *Helicobacter pylori* infection. In that setting, standard treatment to eradicate the *H. pylori* infection results in sustained complete remission in the majority of patients without the need for additional chemotherapy or radiation therapy. MALT is discussed further in Lymphoid Malignancies.

Neuroendocrine Tumors

Gastrointestinal neuroendocrine tumors (NETs) (formerly called carcinoid tumors) arise from the endocrine cells of the digestive tract. Pancreatic NETs arise from the islets of Langerhans cells and were previously called islet cell tumors. Although histologically similar, gastrointestinal and pancreatic NETs behave differently, with several drugs showing activity against pancreatic NETs but not gastrointestinal NETs. The clinical features of pancreatic NETs are discussed in MKSAP 18 Gastroenterology & Hepatology. NETs are rare in incidence but are typically indolent, and patients frequently survive many years, resulting in a high prevalence relative to the incidence.

Well-differentiated NETs exhibit indolent growth. These range from low grade (low proliferative index) to intermediate grade (somewhat higher proliferative index). As would be expected, intermediate-grade tumors are generally, but not always, more aggressive than low-grade tumors. Poorly differentiated, high-grade NETs are highly aggressive tumors that are treated with etoposide plus cisplatin regimens used for small cell lung cancer.

Most NETs do not produce hormones and are termed "nonfunctional," but approximately 25% do produce a hormone, in which case the hormone-related symptoms are often both the source of presentation and morbidity. Gastrointestinal NETs can produce serotonin, which can cause the classic carcinoid syndrome of diarrhea and facial flushing.

Nonfunctional NETs are often discovered incidentally. The liver is the most common site of metastases, and metastatic disease may be present asymptomatically for years before it is identified.

Given the indolent nature of NETs, observation and serial imaging are appropriate initially; asymptomatic patients may do well, with minimal growth and no symptoms for years, even with metastatic disease. Follow-up examination and imaging at approximately 3 months is appropriate. In patients whose disease appears stable at the 3-month CT scan, further monitoring with serial imaging at 3-month to 6-month intervals is appropriate.

In tumors with somatostatin receptors, the somatostatin analogs octreotide or lanreotide may be used for hormonal control or for stabilization of progressing disease. Hepatic arterial embolization, radiofrequency ablation, or surgical debulking are sometimes used to decrease hormone production or to relieve symptoms of tumor bulk.

When treatment is needed, pancreatic NETs can be treated with temozolamide plus capecitabine, or sunitinib (an anti-VEGF tyrosine kinase inhibitor), or everolimus (a mammalian target of rapamycin [mTOR] inhibitor). Everolimus has more modest activity in gastrointestinal NETs, but the other agents used for pancreatic NETs are inactive in gastrointestinal NETs.

KEY POINTS

- Gastrointestinal neuroendocrine tumors (NETs) arise from the endocrine cells of the digestive tract, whereas pancreatic NETs arise from the islets of Langerhans cells; although histologically similar, gastrointestinal and pancreatic NETs behave differently, with several drugs showing activity against pancreatic NETs but not gastrointestinal NETs.

- Gastrointestinal neuroendocrine tumors can produce serotonin, which can cause the carcinoid syndrome characterized by diarrhea and facial flushing.

- Well-differentiated neuroendocrine tumors are indolent and only require observation and serial imaging.

HVC

Gastrointestinal Stromal Tumors

Gastrointestinal stromal tumors (GISTs), derived from the precursors of the interstitial cells of Cajal, are sarcomas characterized by an activating mutation in the c-*kit* proto-oncogene, which leads to constitutive activation of the receptor tyrosine kinase. Histologically, GISTs are identified by overexpression of the *KIT* gene, the immunohistochemical marker for KIT protein. Although these tumors may be asymptomatic or discovered during an endoscopic or imaging procedure done for another purpose, most are associated with nonspecific gastrointestinal symptoms, and some may cause overt bleeding, pain, or signs of obstruction. They are most commonly located in the stomach, which confers a better prognosis, and in the proximal intestine. Other prognostic factors include tumor size and mitotic rate.

For patients undergoing a potentially curative resection of a localized GIST, low-risk tumors do not benefit from further treatment. Higher-risk tumors are treated with adjuvant tyrosine kinase inhibitor imatinib; 3 years of imatinib yields outcomes superior to 1 year of treatment. Imatinib is also used to treat patients who present with unresectable or metastatic disease.

KEY POINT

- High-risk gastrointestinal stromal tumors should be treated with surgery and 3 years of adjuvant imatinib.

Lung Cancer

This section will focus on treatment and follow-up of patients with lung cancer. See MKSAP 18 Pulmonary and Critical Care Medicine for discussion of epidemiology, screening, clinical manifestations, diagnosis, and staging of patients with lung cancer. Initial biopsy can distinguish tumors as either non–small cell lung cancer (NSCLC) or small cell lung cancer (SCLC). NSCLC can be divided into pathologic subtypes, including large cell, adenocarcinoma, and squamous cell cancer. Although these subtypes have characteristic clinical features, the diagnosis, staging, and therapy for all forms of NSCLC are similar. The staging criteria and treatment of SCLC differ from NSCLC.

Non-Small Cell Lung Cancer

Treatment of NSCLC, like that of most other solid malignancies, is based largely on disease stage. For the purposes of this discussion, it is best to divide NSCLC into early stage, locally advanced, and metastatic categories.

Early-Stage Disease

Early-stage disease refers to lung cancer that is amenable to surgical resection at the time of diagnosis. This typically encompasses stage I and II cancers, though some patients with stage II cancer are not amenable to resection based on location or extent of the primary tumor. Stages I and II are differentiated by hilar nodal metastatic disease (present in some patients with stage II cancer, but not present in stage I) and also by the size and invasiveness of the primary tumor into adjacent structures. As in many other cancers, multidisciplinary evaluation is of vital importance to these patients in order to make the most accurate determination regarding optimal treatment.

Patients deemed potential surgical candidates based on imaging need to have a rigorous functional evaluation to help predict their anticipated pulmonary reserve after surgery. The initial evaluation consists of FEV_1 and D_{LCO} measurement. If both test variables are favorable, then no further evaluation is needed. However, if one or the other variable falls in a range suggesting impaired lung function, then calculation of the predicted postoperative FEV_1 and D_{LCO} should be performed, which is determined by baseline values and assessment of the fractional contribution of the lung to be resected. If the predictive postoperative lung function values indicate mild to moderate impairment, then exercise testing is often used. Based on the results of these assessments, a decision can be made regarding suitability for resection. Patients with pathologic stage I cancer who are undergoing surgical resection have a 60% to 70% survival rate at 5 years and patients with stage II cancer have approximately a 40% survival rate.

For patients who are not surgical candidates, other options are available, including stereotactic body radiation and other ablative treatments that can be used to treat the primary tumor. Such treatments have been shown to have excellent rates of local control, but they are only suitable for patients with relatively small tumors. For larger tumors, conventional radiation is used. There are no data supporting the use of chemotherapy combined with radiation in patients with stage I or II disease. Despite the adverse effect of their comorbid lung disease, patients with localized tumors treated with radiation have a mean survival of greater than 3 years.

Lobectomy is the preferred surgical procedure in early-stage disease. Proximal tumors may be less amenable to lobectomy. In those patients, sleeve resection (resection of the involved lobe and a portion of the main stem bronchus) has fewer postoperative complications and is preferable to pneumonectomy. Sublobar resection is not recommended but can be considered in selected patient populations (such as elderly patients and those with stage I cancer).

Patients treated surgically for stage I or II disease who have positive margins benefit from postoperative radiation therapy and show an improvement in overall survival. This is not the case for patients with negative surgical margins.

Cisplatin-based adjuvant chemotherapy has been shown to improve survival after resection in patients with resected stage II or III lung cancer. The LACE meta-analysis, which used patient data from five different cisplatin-based adjuvant chemotherapy trials, found a 5.4% decrease in the risk of death at 5 years in patients with resected stage II or III disease. Another meta-analysis identified a 4% improvement in survival at 5 years in patients treated with cisplatin-based chemotherapy after surgery and radiation. Approximately 50% of patients who had surgically resected stage I, II, or IIIA cancer survived 5 years. Chemotherapy consists of cisplatin with a second agent and is typically given for four cycles. The most commonly used chemotherapy partners are vinorelbine, pemetrexed, gemcitabine, and docetaxel.

After completion of treatment, patients with early-stage disease remain at risk for both distant and local recurrence. Many patients with smoking histories are also at risk for developing a second primary lung cancer and cancers of the head, neck, and other sites. Current accepted recommendations for surveillance include history, physical examination, and chest CT at least every 6 months for the first 2 years and then annually. Smoking cessation decreases the risk of new primary lung cancers, although the magnitude of benefit is uncertain, ranging from 20% to 90%; the risk steadily declines beginning 5 years after quitting, but it never quite reaches the incidence found in nonsmokers.

KEY POINTS

- Lobectomy is the preferred surgical procedure in early-stage disease.
- Potential surgical candidates with early-stage lung cancer must have FEV_1 and D_{LCO} measurement to predict their anticipated postoperative pulmonary reserve and suitability for resection.

(Continued)

- Patients with early-stage lung cancer who are not surgical candidates can be treated with radiation therapy; stereotactic body radiation is appropriate for small tumors, but conventional radiation is used for large tumors.

- Postoperative radiation therapy is used to treat patients with resected localized lung cancer and positive tumor margins; cisplatin-based adjuvant chemotherapy is standard treatment of all resected stage II and III lung cancer.

Locally Advanced Disease

Locally advanced lung cancer is most commonly defined by the presence of clinically detectable lymphadenopathy in the mediastinum or by a primary tumor that invades into local structures, such as the mediastinum, heart, trachea, esophagus, or great vessels.

Safer, more refined surgical technique, along with more precise preoperative staging that more accurately defines the primary tumor, has expanded the number of patients eligible for surgical resection, although it is unclear whether this has resulted in improved survival outcomes. For example, some patients with T4 tumors showing invasion into adjacent vital structures, with no evidence of mediastinal node involvement, can have surgical resection and their disease treated as stage III disease. Patients with satellite nodules in the same lobe (T3) or in another ipsilateral lobe (T4) were previously considered to have metastatic disease, but can be resected with curative intent. Even patients with an isolated tumor nodule in the contralateral lung, traditionally considered incurable metastatic disease, can now undergo resection to remove all sites of cancer under the assumption that the nodule could represent a second localized primary lung cancer. Finally, patients with limited ipsilateral mediastinal node involvement, a single node station, and nonbulky disease can undergo surgical resection. These patients will all generally receive neoadjuvant or adjuvant chemotherapy or radiation treatment.

Patients who present with bulky or multistation (widespread mediastinal or hilar lymph node involvement) mediastinal lymphadenopathy are treated with combined platinum-based chemotherapy and radiation, which has been found to be superior to sequential treatment. Unfortunately, the risk of recurrence, both locoregional and distant, is very high after chemoradiation treatment (approaching 70% to 90%).

- Surgical techniques have improved substantially and, along with better preoperative staging, allow surgical therapy with curative intent for various patients who were traditionally considered to have unresectable disease.

Metastatic Disease

Metastatic lung cancer is defined as the spread of disease to distant sites such as liver, bone, or brain. The presence of one or more tumor nodules in the contralateral lung also qualifies as metastatic disease, but as the prognosis for that pattern of metastatic disease is notably better than that of patients with distant disease, it has been reclassified as M1a, with other distant sites given the designation of M1b.

In the past, all patients with metastatic NSCLC were treated with the same chemotherapy regimens. With the recent development of precision medicine, specific molecular and genetic targets have been discovered, resulting in more tailored treatments. Furthermore, it is now understood that patients with different histologic types of lung cancer respond differently to various chemotherapy agents. Immunotherapy has now been shown to have an impact on the treatment of advanced lung cancer. Despite these advances, however, metastatic NSCLC remains incurable. Level 1 evidence supports early palliative care interventions in this patient population. Their quality of life will be improved even as they continue to receive aggressive chemotherapy.

Before deciding the optimal treatment for any given patient, it is essential to define histology, assess for molecular alterations, and determine performance status. For patients with non-squamous histology (particularly adenocarcinoma), testing for molecular alterations is mandatory. At present, it is considered standard care to test for mutation in the epidermal growth factor receptor (*EGFR*) gene and for translocations involving *ALK* or *ROS1*. If an *EGFR* mutation is identified, initial treatment with erlotinib is recommended. If an *ALK* or *ROS1* translocation is identified, initial treatment with crizotinib is recommended. Erlotinib and crizotinib are both small molecule tyrosine kinase inhibitors that are specific for those genetic alterations. Although many other molecular and genetic alterations have been identified in patients with NSCLC, further investigation is required before changes in treatment become evidence-based care.

If a patient has negative findings for the alterations noted above, treatment with chemotherapy is indicated only if the patient has a good performance status. Patients with poor performance status do not benefit from chemotherapy treatment. Front-line chemotherapy is given with a platinum-based doublet regimen. Either cisplatin or carboplatin can be used; cisplatin is slightly more active, but carboplatin is more commonly used because of its more favorable side-effect profile. Histologic assessment can help guide choice of the second agent, as patients with adenocarcinoma have been shown to respond well to pemetrexed, whereas those with squamous cell carcinoma respond better to gemcitabine, based on the results of a phase III clinical trial comparing these two agents. Other commonly used second agents in this setting include paclitaxel, docetaxel, and vinorelbine. Chemotherapy is administered for four to six cycles and can be given in combination with bevacizumab. Bevacizumab is a monoclonal antibody directed against vascular endothelial growth factor and when given in combination with platinum-based chemotherapy for patients with non–squamous cell forms of NSCLC in the first-line setting, it has been shown to improve both progression-free survival and overall survival, though the degree of benefit is modest. In addition, bevacizumab carries the risk of thrombosis, stroke, myocardial infarction, and hemoptysis in some patients. For patients who respond to front-line chemotherapy, maintenance treatment with docetaxel, pemetrexed, or gemcitabine has been shown to improve progression-free survival, and pemetrexed has also been shown to improve overall survival.

Immunotherapy with agents that act on the programmed cell death ligand 1 (PD-L1) have shown impressive activity in metastatic NSCLC. Pembrolizumab is superior to chemotherapy in the first-line treatment of patients with NSCLC who have PD-L1 expression greater than 50% with a higher response rate, progression-free survival, and overall survival when compared to standard chemotherapy. Pembrolizumab and nivolumab are also both more active than chemotherapy in the second-line setting.

KEY POINTS

- Metastatic non–small cell lung cancer that demonstrates an epidermal growth factor receptor gene mutation should be treated initially with erlotinib; if an *ALK* or *ROS1* translocation is identified, initial treatment should be with crizotinib.

- If metastatic non–small cell lung cancer is negative for gene mutations or translocations, platinum-based doublet chemotherapy in combination with bevacizumab is appropriate for patients with good performance status.

Small Cell Lung Cancer

SCLC, a neuroendocrine neoplasm, has been decreasing in incidence during the past several years, and currently it accounts for approximately 10% of lung cancer cases. SCLC is almost exclusively caused by smoking. In unfortunate contrast to the advances made in the treatment of NSCLC, little has changed in the prognosis or treatment of SCLC patients. Most patients initially present with distant metastatic disease. SCLC is known to be associated with paraneoplastic syndromes, most prominently syndrome of inappropriate antidiuretic hormone secretion and Eaton-Lambert myasthenia. The staging of SCLC is straightforward and defines patients with "limited disease" that can be encompassed by a hemithoracic radiation portal; all others, including those with distant metastases, have "extensive disease." Patients should undergo routine CT scan of the thorax, abdomen, and pelvis, but even those who have no bone or central nervous system symptoms should undergo whole body bone scintigraphy and an MRI of the brain.

Typically, primary SCLC presents with proximal and often large tumors, but occasionally it presents as a solitary pulmonary nodule (see Lung Tumors: Pulmonary Nodule Evaluation)

and is often not diagnosed until after surgical resection. After resection, these rare patients can be treated with adjuvant chemotherapy, but radiation therapy can be avoided if surgical margins are negative. Surgery can also be performed for small primary tumors without lymph node spread, although preoperative evaluation in those patients should include endobronchial ultrasonography or, if that procedure is not available, mediastinoscopy to rule out occult nodal involvement. Those patients should also receive adjuvant chemotherapy.

Most patients with SCLC will not meet the criteria for primary surgery. Treatment of limited disease consists of combined cisplatin-based chemotherapy, typically cisplatin plus etoposide, and radiation. Chemotherapy is continued after radiation for up to six cycles; prophylactic cranial irradiation should be used in patients with responsive disease because this treatment decreases the rate of subsequent brain metastases and improves overall survival.

For patients who present with extensive disease, treatment consists of platinum-based chemotherapy without radiation, again for up to six cycles. Patients with limited disease that is responsive to treatment and no evidence of brain metastases should be treated with prophylactic cranial irradiation. Patients with extensive disease who have a favorable response to chemotherapy but persistent involvement in the lung can be treated with additional radiation therapy.

Despite treatment response, recurrences are very common, even in patients with limited disease at the time of diagnosis. For patients who had a disease-free interval of more than 3 months, treatment with the initial platinum-based doublet regimen can be used because the likelihood of response is good. However, for patients who relapsed earlier, treatment options and outcomes are generally poor. As in NSCLC, addressing goals of care and aggressive symptom management are of significant importance in this setting.

KEY POINTS

- Routine staging of patients with small cell lung cancer includes whole body bone scintigraphy and MRI of the brain, even if they have no bone or central nervous system symptoms, along with routine CT scan of the thorax, abdomen, and pelvis.

- Although patients with SCLC typically present at an advanced stage, those with early-stage disease can be considered for resection and adjuvant chemotherapy without radiation if surgical margins are negative.

- Treatment of limited-disease SCLC consists of combined cisplatin-based chemotherapy and radiation to the area of lung involvement; treatment of extensive disease consists of analogous chemotherapy, but additional radiation treatment is not indicated.

- Patients with both limited- and extensive-stage SCLC who respond to chemotherapy should receive prophylactic radiation to the central nervous system.

Head and Neck Cancer

Head and neck cancers include primary tumors of the oral cavity, oropharynx, nasopharynx, hypopharynx, larynx, paranasal sinuses, thyroid, and salivary glands. Squamous cell carcinoma is the most common form of head and neck cancer and is therefore the focus of this chapter. Thyroid cancer is discussed in MKSAP 18 Endocrinology and Metabolism.

Risk Factors

The most important risk factor for head and neck cancer is tobacco use, which includes smoked and smokeless tobacco. Alcohol use is also a known risk factor, and the combination of alcohol and tobacco has been found to synergistically increase risk.

Human papillomavirus (HPV), more likely to be found in men and women with behavioral risk for other sexually transmitted diseases, is a recently recognized and increasingly important cause of head and neck cancer, with most HPV-associated cancers arising in the oropharynx (tonsil and base of tongue most commonly). The prognosis of HPV-associated cancer is significantly better than that for non-HPV-related cancer, but smoking can mitigate this improvement. Treatment of head and neck cancer is not altered based on HPV status, although several ongoing studies are addressing this issue.

KEY POINTS

- Tobacco and alcohol use are important risk factors for head and neck cancer, and their combined use synergistically increases risk.
- Human papillomavirus infection is an important cause of oropharyngeal cancer; it does not affect therapy, but the prognosis is better than that for non-HPV-related cancer.

Clinical Manifestations

Presenting symptoms vary with the location of the cancer, but concerning signs and symptoms that generally should raise suspicion of head and neck cancer include persistent or progressive lymph node enlargement or other neck mass, unilateral hearing loss, unilateral ear pain, nasal obstruction, oral pain, nonhealing oral ulcers, dysphagia, odynophagia, and hoarseness.

Evaluation and Staging

Initial evaluation of patients suspected of having head and neck cancer includes history, physical examination, and direct laryngoscopy. Fine-needle aspiration of suspicious lesions will generally establish the diagnosis. Assessment of HPV status using tumor staining for p16, which is overexpressed in HPV-positive cancers, is standard. Although HPV positivity significantly improves prognosis, this finding is not currently used to make treatment decisions.

Once a diagnosis has been established, imaging studies are indicated for accurate assessment of the extent of local disease and evaluation of nodal and distant metastatic disease. MRI is generally superior to CT for anatomic assessment of the primary tumor. PET-CT is useful to identify primary tumors and for evaluating regional lymph nodes, tumor invasion, and distant metastatic disease, although it is not accurate in nodes 5 mm or smaller.

The staging of head and neck cancers is complex, as each subsite uses a different staging system. In general, however, staging of primary tumors is based on both size and extent of invasion into adjacent structures, with higher-stage tumors exhibiting greater degrees of invasiveness. Nodal staging is predicated on the number of nodes involved, size, and presence or absence of bilateral lymphadenopathy. The stage of head and neck cancer, as with many other malignancies, is the single-most important determinant of prognosis. Patients with localized disease have 70% to 90% long-term survival. Given the complexity of head and neck cancer treatment, multimodality tumor board discussion is valuable for determining the proper course of treatment.

KEY POINT

- In patients suspected of having head and neck cancer, fine-needle aspiration should be performed to establish the diagnosis.

Treatment

Approximately one third of patients present with localized or early-stage head and neck cancer, generally small tumors that have no lymph node metastases. Although surgery is preferred for early-stage oral cancer and radiation for early laryngeal disease, early-stage head and neck cancer can be effectively treated with either surgery or radiation therapy. Treatment decisions weigh the accessibility of the lesion and complications expected with surgical resection, including quality-of-life issues such as appearance and preservation of speech, with the expected morbidity of radiation therapy, including acute mucositis and fatigue, along with more long-lasting alterations in taste, xerostomia, dental disease, and an increased risk of second malignancies. The need for and extent of additional dissection of lymph nodes in the neck is determined by the site and stage of the primary tumor, anatomy of lymphatic drainage, presence or absence of enlarged nodes, and the results of diagnostic imaging.

The need for adjuvant radiation for patients with primary surgical resection is based on tumor pathology and is recommended for patients with one or more high-risk features (**Table 46**). Combined chemotherapy and radiation can be used for patients felt to be at very high risk for recurrence, most commonly in the setting of extracapsular extension or positive or close margins. Adjuvant chemoradiation is typically given with single-agent cisplatin and concomitant radiation.

TABLE 46. High-Risk Pathologic Features in Head and Neck Cancer

T3 or T4 tumor
Positive or close resection margins
Lymph node extracapsular extension
≥2 positive lymph nodes (N2 or N3)
Perineural invasion
Lymphovascular invasion

Data from Adelstein D, Gillison ML, Pfister DG, Spencer S, Adkins D, Brizel DM, et al. NCCN guidelines insights: head and neck cancers, version 2.2017. J Natl Compr Canc Netw. 2017;15:761-770. [PMID: 28596256] doi:10.6004/jnccn.2017.0101

For patients with more advanced disease at the time of diagnosis, based on either having an unresectable primary tumor or extensive nodal disease, initial treatment with combined chemotherapy and radiation is recommended. Surgery is reserved for treatment of persistent disease or in the setting of inadequate response to treatment. In patients treated with definitive chemoradiotherapy, systemic therapy can be given with cisplatin, a platinum agent, or with cetuximab, a monoclonal antibody directed against the epidermal growth factor receptor.

Treatment of nasopharyngeal carcinoma differs somewhat from that of other sites. Nasopharyngeal carcinoma is rarely resectable at the time of diagnosis, and therefore surgery plays little role in the treatment of this disease. For very early-stage disease, radiation alone can be used with excellent control rates. However, for all other patients, initial treatment with chemoradiotherapy is used. The role of additional adjuvant chemotherapy in more advanced disease is uncertain.

KEY POINTS

- Early-stage oral head and neck cancers are generally treated with surgery, although radiation therapy is preferred for localized tumors of the larynx.

- Adjuvant therapy for locally advanced head and neck cancer includes radiation alone or in combination with single-agent cisplatin chemotherapy.

- Advanced head and neck cancer includes patients with unresectable tumors or extensive nodal disease and should be treated with combined chemotherapy (cisplatin or cetuximab) and radiation; surgery is reserved for treatment of persistent disease or inadequate response to treatment.

Posttreatment Surveillance

After treatment of localized disease, a history and physical examination, including direct laryngoscopy, nasopharyngoscopy, or both, to evaluate for local recurrence and second primary cancers should be conducted every 1 to 3 months

for the first year after primary treatment, decreasing in frequency thereafter, with annual evaluation at 5 years. Patients treated with radiotherapy that includes the thyroid bed are at risk for hypothyroidism and thyroid carcinoma. Periodic assessment of thyroid function and a physical examination of the thyroid are indicated, although thyroid ultrasonography should not be performed. Similarly, PET-CT or other imaging surveillance following a negative posttreatment scan is not indicated. Imaging should be performed as needed based on signs and symptoms suggestive of recurrent disease. Patients should be offered lung cancer screening if they meet high-risk criteria.

KEY POINTS

- Posttreatment surveillance for head and neck cancer consisting of history and physical examinations should be performed every 1 to 3 months for the first year, decreasing in frequency through year 5, and then annually.

- Routine imaging for head and neck cancer after a negative posttreatment scan is not indicated unless there are signs and symptoms suggestive of recurrent disease. **HVC**

Management of Recurrent Head and Neck Cancer

For patients with recurrent head and neck cancer, it is important to decide whether potentially curative therapy is still possible or if treatment instead should be palliative. Cure is most likely in patients whose recurrence is with small localized disease, who have a longer time to recurrence (also termed longer disease-free survival), and who have a site of recurrence in the larynx or nasopharynx. Patients with limited recurrence are treated with surgery and adjuvant therapy as needed. For patients with unresectable local recurrence, treatment with radiation or chemoradiation is appropriate. Reirradiation can be associated with long-term survival, but it is also associated with a potentially significant risk of toxicity including pain, tissue necrosis, infection, and fatal bleeding.

For patients with distant metastatic disease or unresectable persistent local disease not amenable to surgery or radiation, systemic chemotherapy is the mainstay of treatment. The current standard front-line treatment of patients with good performance status is the combination of a platinum agent (cisplatin or carboplatin) with 5-fluorouracil and cetuximab. If progression occurs after front-line therapy, single-agent therapy is indicated, using drugs not previously used. The programmed cell death 1 (PD-1) inhibitors pembrolizumab and nivolumab are FDA approved for treatment following progression after platinum-containing chemotherapy. Patients with distant metastases and unresectable local disease have a poor prognosis, especially if their performance status is declining; treatment decisions should include options for palliative and hospice care.

- Favorable factors of recurrent head and neck cancer include small, localized disease; longer time to recurrence; and site of recurrence in the larynx or nasopharynx.
- Patients with good performance status and advanced disease not amenable to surgery or radiation should first receive a combination of a platinum agent (cisplatin or carboplatin) with 5-fluorouracil and cetuximab.

Genitourinary Cancer

Prostate Cancer

Epidemiology and Risk Factors

Adenocarcinoma of the prostate remains one of the most commonly diagnosed types of cancer among men in the United States, with an estimated lifetime risk of one in seven. Age is a very important risk factor; prostate cancer is rarely diagnosed before age 40 years, but after that point, the incidence increases significantly. Ethnicity is also an important risk factor, with the incidence significantly greater for black men than for white or Hispanic men. Further, black men are more likely to be diagnosed at a younger age with higher-risk disease. Genetics and family history also play an important role in risk. Men with a first-degree relative diagnosed with prostate cancer are twice as likely to be diagnosed. Prostate cancer is also linked with germline mutations in different genes, such as *BRCA2*, *HOXB13*, and the Lynch syndrome genes.

Diagnosis and Staging

Prostate cancer is most commonly diagnosed after identification of an elevated serum prostate-specific antigen (PSA) level during screening and in the absence of symptoms. See MKSAP 18 General Internal Medicine for a discussion of current issues relating to prostate cancer screening.

Although urinary symptoms might be present in patients with prostate cancer, they are usually related to benign prostatic hyperplasia and not to the cancer. In some men diagnosed with metastatic disease at the time of initial presentation, bone pain or back pain can be the presenting symptom. If the diagnosis is suspected on the basis of an elevated serum PSA level, the elevation should first be confirmed by a second measurement at least 1 month later. Persistent serum PSA elevation should prompt urology referral, as should a palpable abnormal finding in the prostate on digital rectal examination.

Prostate biopsy is performed using transrectal ultrasonography for guidance, and several cores should be taken from different regions of the gland. Studies have found that increasing the number of cores improves diagnostic accuracy without causing a significant increase in complications. Most commonly, at least five to seven cores are taken per side to provide a sufficient diagnostic yield. Atypical small acinar proliferation and multifocal high-grade prostatic intraepithelial neoplasia are both associated with a high risk of underlying cancer and should prompt rebiopsy.

Risk stratification using serum PSA, Gleason score, and TNM cancer staging based on biopsy results and digital rectal examination is essential for determining prognosis and treatment options (**Table 47**). Imaging studies need not be done in patients whose risk is very low or low but should be obtained in others to evaluate regional lymph node involvement and metastatic disease.

- Prostate cancer is most commonly diagnosed after identification of an elevated serum prostate-specific antigen level during screening and in the absence of symptoms.

Treatment

Treatment options for men with newly diagnosed localized prostate cancer include active surveillance, radiation, and radical prostatectomy. For men with limited life expectancy or significant medical comorbidities, observation is most appropriate.

Active surveillance is deferral of curative-intent therapy in lieu of regular monitoring for evidence of disease progression. It is an option for men with very-low-risk or low-risk prostate cancer who have a life expectancy of at least 10 years. Active surveillance should consist of digital rectal examination (not more than every 12 months), serial measurement of

TABLE 47. Prostate Cancer Risk Stratification

Risk Category	Definition[a]
Very low	Stage T1c, serum PSA <10 ng/mL (10 µg/L), Gleason score ≤6, fewer than 3 biopsy cores positive, ≤50% cancer in each core, PSA density <0.15 ng/mL/g
Low	T1-T2a, Gleason score ≤6, PSA <10 ng/mL (10 µg/L)
Intermediate	T2b-T2c OR Gleason score 7 OR PSA 10-20 ng/mL (10-20 µg/L)
High	T3a OR Gleason score 8-10 OR PSA >20 ng/mL (20 µg/L)
Very high	T3b-T4, primary Gleason pattern 5, >4 cores with Gleason score 8-10

PSA = prostate-specific antigen.

[a]T1 = tumors that are not palpable or seen on imaging; T1a (<5% of specimen) and T1b (>5% of specimen) are discovered incidentally in a pathologic specimen resected for benign disease; T1c discovered in prostate biopsy for elevated serum PSA.

T2 = palpable tumors; T2a involves <50% of one lobe; T2b involves >50% of one lobe; T2c are in both lobes of the prostate.

T3a extends through the prostate capsule; T3b involves the seminal vesicles.

T4 tumors are fixed to adjacent structures.

Data from NCCN Clinical Guidelines in Oncology. Prostate Cancer. Version 2.2017. NCCN.org. https://www.nccn.org/professionals/physician_gls/pdf/prostate.pdf. Accessed February 17, 2018.

serum PSA (assessing level changes and calculating PSA doubling time), and repeat biopsy. A PSA doubling time of less than 3 years is considered an indication for treatment. Repeat biopsy is typically done at 1 year, and if no high-grade disease is identified, it can be done less often after that. Fifteen-year metastasis-free survival is as high as 97% in appropriately selected patients.

Active treatment of low-risk localized prostate cancer is typically a choice between external beam radiation and radical prostatectomy. Brachytherapy, in which radioactive implants are inserted into the prostate, is also an option for men with low-risk cancer or selected men with low-volume intermediate-risk cancer.

Radiation is associated with short-term risks of enteritis (approximately 20% of men) and cystitis (approximately 50% of men). These conditions become long-term complications in a very small percentage of men. Erectile dysfunction typically increases over time after radiation, such that by 2 years, approximately 60% to 70% of men have at least moderate erectile dysfunction.

With radical prostatectomy, the main risks are urinary incontinence and erectile dysfunction. Urinary incontinence is relatively common immediately after surgery. The rate of chronic moderate to severe incontinence is approximately 5% to 10%. Erectile dysfunction is relatively common after surgery and can persist for several years. Approximately 40% of men reported erectile dysfunction 2 years after surgery.

A recent study showed no difference in survival after 10 years for patients with localized prostate cancer detected through serum PSA screening who were randomized to receive active surveillance, surgery, or radiation therapy. There was a trend toward improved survival for patients older than 65 years of age who received either of the active interventions. Patients receiving surgery or radiation had decreased disease progression and decreased metastatic disease.

For men with intermediate-risk or higher-risk localized disease who are treated with radiation therapy, the addition of a gonadotropin-releasing hormone (GnRH) agonist will delay disease progression. It has also been shown to improve overall survival in men with high-risk and very-high-risk prostate cancer. For those men with high-risk or very-high-risk localized prostate cancer, six cycles of adjuvant docetaxel given after radiation therapy in addition to androgen deprivation therapy improves disease-free survival and overall survival.

After definitive local treatment, men are monitored for evidence of recurrence with serial serum PSA measurements every 3 to 4 months and digital rectal examination yearly unless PSA is undetectable. After radical prostatectomy, the PSA should rapidly become undetectable, but after radiation treatment, the PSA will fall gradually, will reach a nadir, and will not necessarily become undetectable. PSA recurrence after surgery is defined as a detectable PSA level that increases on at least two measurements; after radiation, PSA recurrence is defined as an increase in the PSA level by at least 2 ng/mL (2 µg/L) above the nadir PSA.

For men with PSA-only recurrence, an evaluation to look for evidence of clinical local or metastatic disease with imaging studies is indicated. If men were treated with initial surgery and metastatic disease has not been identified, salvage radiation with or without androgen deprivation therapy (ADT) can be offered. Likewise, if men were treated initially with radiation, salvage surgery can be offered, but it is only indicated if a transrectal ultrasound–guided biopsy specimen is positive and no metastatic disease is identified; if the specimen is negative, then ADT can be considered.

It is important to note that for men with PSA-only recurrence, with or without clinical metastatic disease, observation is a reasonable consideration depending on patient and disease-specific factors, such as symptoms and PSA doubling time. This is especially true for men with PSA-only recurrence, as it can take several years for clinical metastatic disease to develop in that setting.

KEY POINTS

- Active surveillance, including serial serum prostate-specific antigen (PSA) and repeat biopsy, is appropriate for men with very-low-risk or low-risk prostate cancer.

- Treatment of localized low-risk prostate cancer is typically either external beam radiation or radical prostatectomy, in which both have equal efficacy; brachytherapy is also an option.

- Gonadotropin deprivation is typically administered after radiation therapy for localized intermediate-risk or high-risk prostate cancer.

- Patients with PSA-only recurrence may be treated with androgen deprivation therapy, although observation is a reasonable choice because it may take several years for overt metastatic disease to develop.

HVC

Metastatic Prostate Cancer

Once distant metastatic disease is diagnosed, the mainstay of therapy is ADT. Options for providing ADT include orchiectomy, GnRH-agonist therapy (with or without antiandrogen) and GnRH-antagonist therapy (**Table 48**). Psychological aversion to orchiectomy by both patients and physicians has limited its use in the United States, although it is a rapidly acting and cost-effective way to achieve androgen depletion and remains the mainstay of ADT in other parts of the world.

At present, there is no clear advantage to combined androgen blockade using a GnRH agonist or antagonist plus an antiandrogen. In patients who have clinical metastatic disease, antiandrogen therapy should precede or be started at the same time as a GnRH agonist, and the combination should be continued for at least 7 days because of the risk of a transient worsening of disease-related symptoms, termed a flare reaction. Continuation is not necessary if a GnRH antagonist is used. Intermittent ADT is not typically recommended in men with clinical metastatic disease, although it can be offered to

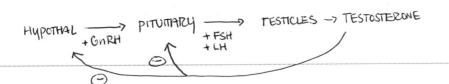

TABLE 48.	Treatments for Metastatic Prostate Cancer		
Class	**Agents**	**Mechanism of Action**	**Indications**
GnRH agonist	Leuprolide, goserelin, triptorelin, buserelin, histrelin	Binds to GnRH receptor, causes initial release of FSH/LH (and also testosterone) followed by suppression	Metastatic prostate cancer; neoadjuvant/adjuvant ADT in combination with radiation
GnRH antagonist	Degarelix	Binds to GnRH receptor and suppresses activity without initial increase in activity seen with GnRH agonists	Metastatic prostate cancer; neoadjuvant/adjuvant ADT in combination with radiation
Antiandrogen	Bicalutamide, flutamide	Binds to androgen receptor with competitive inhibition of testosterone binding	Metastatic castrate-sensitive prostate cancer (not indicated as monotherapy, only in combination with GnRH agonist or antagonist)
CYP17 inhibitor	Abiraterone plus prednisone	Blocks androgen synthesis in tumor tissue, testes, and adrenal glands	Metastatic castrate-resistant prostate cancer; used in combination with prednisone as it can cause adrenal insufficiency
Androgen receptor blockade	Enzalutamide	Binds to the androgen binding site of the androgen receptor in a non-competitive fashion	Metastatic castrate-resistant prostate cancer
Tumor vaccine	Sipuleucel-T	Autologous dendritic cell therapeutic vaccine Aims to increase T cell response to prostatic acid phosphatase	Asymptomatic or minimally symptomatic metastatic castrate-resistant prostate cancer with no visceral metastatic disease Not indicated for PSA-only relapse; does not result in PSA response
Bone-seeking isotope	Radium-223	Alpha particle–emitting isotope that concentrates in bone	Metastatic castrate-resistant prostate cancer with symptomatic bone metastases and no known visceral metastatic disease
Chemotherapeutic	Docetaxel plus prednisone	Antimicrotubule agent	Metastatic castrate-resistant prostate cancer with clinical metastatic disease Metastatic castrate-sensitive prostate cancer in combination with ADT in men with clinical metastatic disease Adjuvant therapy after radiation in men with high-risk or very-high–risk prostate cancer, in combination with ADT
Chemotherapeutic	Cabazitaxel plus prednisone	Antimicrotubule agent	Metastatic castrate-resistant prostate cancer following disease progression after docetaxel treatment

ADT = androgen-deprivation therapy; CYP17 = 17α-hydroxy/17,20-lyase; FSH = follicle-stimulating hormone; GnRH = gonadotropin-releasing hormone; LH = luteinizing hormone; PSA = prostate-specific antigen.

mitigate side effects. Response can be assessed most easily by serial serum PSA measurement, but imaging also plays a role. The serum testosterone level should be less than 50 ng/dL (1.7 nmol/L) in men treated with ADT.

Men with clinical metastatic disease who respond to ADT are considered to have castrate-sensitive prostate cancer. In this population, evidence from two recently reported phase III randomized clinical trials indicates that treatment with docetaxel for six cycles with ADT results in improved disease-free survival and overall survival.

ADT results in many short-term and long-term side effects. Short-term effects include loss of lean body mass, fatigue, gynecomastia, hair loss, decreased libido, erectile dysfunction, and vasomotor symptoms. Long-term risks include a possible increase in cardiovascular disease, increased risk of venous thromboembolism, and reduction in bone density. Osteoporosis is a prevalent and underappreciated complication of ADT. All men being treated with ADT should take supplemental calcium and vitamin D, and baseline fracture risk should be assessed using a dual-energy x-ray absorptiometry (or "DEXA") scan. Osteoclast inhibitors will reduce bone pain and lower fracture risk in men with ADT-resistant, metastatic prostate cancer.

After identification of progressive disease in men being treated with ADT (castrate-resistant prostate cancer), many treatment options exist (see Table 48). There is no optimal sequence of therapies. Initial treatment options for castrate-resistant prostate cancer include docetaxel with prednisone, abiraterone with prednisone, enzalutamide, radium-223 (for symptomatic bone metastases), and secondary hormone therapy. Secondary hormone therapies are older treatments that are generally not as effective as newer treatments. Secondary hormone therapies include the addition of an antiandrogen in men not previously exposed to one, addition of ketoconazole (with or without hydrocortisone), antiandrogen withdrawal and use of diethylstilbestrol, or another form of estrogen. For patients who develop progressive disease after treatment with docetaxel, cabazitaxel with prednisone can be used.

KEY POINTS

- Continuous androgen deprivation therapy (ADT), including orchiectomy, gonadotropin-releasing hormone–agonist therapy, and gonadotropin-releasing hormone–antagonist therapy is most appropriate for metastatic prostate cancer.

- Men who respond to ADT and then receive docetaxel chemotherapy will have prolonged survival without disease progression and prolonged overall survival.

- All men who are treated with ADT should take supplemental calcium and vitamin D and have measurement of baseline bone mineral density because osteoporosis is a prevalent and underappreciated complication of ADT.

Testicular Cancer

Testicular cancer is the most common solid tumor diagnosed in men aged 15 to 35 years, although it accounts for only about 1% of all cancers diagnosed in the United States. It is also one of the most curable forms of cancer, due in large part to its sensitivity to chemotherapy. It most commonly presents as a unilateral testicular swelling or mass. However, other presentations are also possible in men with more advanced disease at diagnosis.

Patients with localized symptoms should have a scrotal ultrasound to rule out benign cystic or infectious causes of scrotal enlargement and baseline tumor markers, including α-fetoprotein and β-human chorionic gonadotropin. Diagnosis is made most commonly through inguinal orchiectomy. Needle biopsy of a testicular mass is contraindicated because of concern regarding tumor seeding to the scrotum and inguinal nodes. When the diagnosis is confirmed, evaluation with chest radiography, CT of the abdomen and pelvis, and tumor marker levels after orchiectomy are used for staging. It is important to realize that marker levels fall at predictable rates after surgery, with serum α-fetoprotein the slowest to fall because of its longer serum half-life. Therefore, sufficient time is needed before concluding that markers remain elevated after orchiectomy.

The most common site of spread is to retroperitoneal nodes. Histologically, testicular cancers are either pure seminomas or nonseminomatous germ cell tumors. Management depends on histology, the results of staging studies, and the presence or absence of serum tumor marker elevation after orchiectomy. It is essential to discuss and offer cryopreservation of sperm before initiating additional treatment.

For pure seminoma, active surveillance can be offered after surgery for early-stage disease; adjuvant radiation or chemotherapy with one to two cycles of carboplatin is also appropriate options. Stage II seminoma is defined by retroperitoneal lymph node metastases. For patients with low-volume lymph node metastatic disease, either adjuvant radiation or cisplatin-based combination chemotherapy can be used. In general, as the size of the largest lymph node metastasis increases to more than 2 cm, chemotherapy is preferred over radiation. For stage III seminoma disease, which signifies distant metastatic disease, cisplatin-based chemotherapy is used. PET-CT can be used to determine whether residual masses after chemotherapy require resection. Residual masses that show negative results on PET scan may be benign and can be followed, with resection based on any further increase in size. Residual masses that show positive results on PET scan should be promptly resected, as cure remains possible.

Patients with early-stage nonseminomatous germ cell tumors can be managed with active surveillance (in selected patients), retroperitoneal lymph node dissection (RPLND), or limited chemotherapy. Adjuvant chemotherapy can be considered in patients with positive findings on RPLND. Persistence of tumor marker elevation after orchiectomy without abnormal imaging findings is an indication for chemotherapy. Patients with clinically metastatic retroperitoneal nodes can be managed with RPLND or primary chemotherapy if markers are negative and nodal metastases are limited and small. For patients with several positive nodes, large nodes (>5 cm), or elevated markers, chemotherapy is recommended. Any residual masses after chemotherapy should be resected.

For the first year after treatment, patients should be seen for interview and examination every 2 to 3 months and should have tumor marker measurement and imaging studies periodically, with specific intervals determined by histology, stage, and previous treatment. After the first year, evaluations can be performed less often.

Patients with recurrent disease are treated with combination chemotherapy and can also be treated with high-dose chemotherapy and autologous hematopoietic stem cell transplantation.

Men treated with chemotherapy for testicular cancer are at risk for many different long-term complications, including cardiovascular disease, metabolic syndrome, pulmonary toxicity, hypogonadism, infertility, chronic kidney disease, and neurotoxicity. Further, there is a well-described risk of a second malignancy among men treated for testicular cancer. The risk of a second solid tumor is approximately twofold higher than in men without a history of testicular cancer.

- Measurement of serum tumor markers (α-fetoprotein, lactate dehydrogenase, β–human chorionic gonadotropin) are important before and after inguinal orchiectomy for staging and prognosis of testicular cancer.

- Patients with stage II seminoma, defined by retroperitoneal lymph node metastasis, can be treated with adjuvant radiation or cisplatin-based chemotherapy, although chemotherapy is preferred if the largest metastasis increases above 2 cm.

- Patients with seminoma and residual masses after chemotherapy should receive PET-CT; masses with negative findings on PET-CT can be observed with follow-up imaging to assess progression, and masses with positive findings should be resected.

- Patients with nonseminoma and clinically metastatic nodes can be treated with retroperitoneal lymph node dissection or primary chemotherapy; chemotherapy is preferred if there are several positive nodes, large nodes (>5 cm), or elevated serum tumor markers.

Renal Cell Carcinoma

Renal cancers typically arise in the cortex of the kidney. The most common histology is clear cell carcinoma, which is also the most responsive to medical treatment. In the past, the most common presenting symptoms of renal cell carcinoma were hematuria, abdominal mass, and weight loss, but most patients are currently diagnosed incidentally based on imaging studies done for other reasons. Ultrasonography can be used to differentiate benign cysts from complex cysts or solid masses. If a lesion is not clearly a benign cyst, CT is indicated for further evaluation. Biopsy is only indicated if CT does not clearly indicate renal cell carcinoma.

Many different paraneoplastic syndromes can be seen in patients with renal cell carcinoma, including anemia, hepatic dysfunction in the absence of liver metastases (known as Stauffer syndrome), fever, hypercalcemia, erythrocytosis, AA amyloidosis, thrombocytosis, and polymyalgia rheumatica. Many of these conditions can improve with resection of the primary tumor, metastatic sites, or both.

For localized disease, surgery is indicated. This consists of either radical nephrectomy or partial nephrectomy, depending on the size and location of the primary tumor. In most patients no adjuvant therapy is indicated. Sunitinib has recently been approved by the US Food and Drug Administration (FDA) for use as adjuvant treatment in patients with high risk clear cell carcinoma of the kidney following definitive surgery. In a phase III trial it improved disease free survival by 1.2 years compared with no treatment. Postoperative surveillance to identify recurrent disease is indicated, with the frequency of interventions depending on the extent of local disease. This typically consists of a history and physical examination, basic laboratory studies, and imaging of the chest and abdomen.

Cryoablation, radiofrequency ablation, or even active surveillance may be indicated for managing small tumors in frail patients who have a high risk of postoperative complications.

Resection of the primary renal cell cancer improves survival for select patients with metastatic disease. Debulking nephrectomy can be considered because there is evidence indicating that this procedure is associated with improved survival. Surgery also has a possible role in the treatment of isolated or several easily resected areas of metastatic disease.

No specific front-line therapy has been shown superior for patients who present with metastatic clear cell or non-clear cell histology. Various novel agents, including the programmed death 1 (PD-1) receptor antibody nivolumab and the vascular endothelial growth factor (VEGF) inhibitors lenvatinib and axitinib, have shown activity for patients with disease recurrence.

- Many different paraneoplastic syndromes can be seen in patients with renal cell carcinoma, including anemia, hepatic dysfunction in the absence of liver metastases, fever, hypercalcemia, erythrocytosis, AA amyloidosis, thrombocytosis, and polymyalgia rheumatica. Resecting a primary renal cell cancer may improve the response to chemotherapy in patients with metastatic disease.

Bladder Cancer

Bladder cancer is the most common cancer of the genitourinary tract. Most patients have transitional cell carcinoma, which is the focus of this section. The most common presenting symptom is hematuria, which is often gross hematuria and may be intermittent. It is typically painless, although irritative urinary symptoms can be present with or without hematuria. It is important to assess for gross hematuria in review of systems questioning for all patients and confirm with a urinalysis if a patient does note hematuria. Any patient with gross hematuria should be referred for urologic evaluation, as should any patient confirmed to have persistent microscopic hematuria after evaluating benign causes, such as urinary tract infection, nephrolithiasis, or underlying kidney disease with a glomerular source of erythrocytes. Notably, use of anticoagulants does not alter these recommendations.

The primary modality of initial evaluation is cystoscopy combined with urine cytology, with biopsy of any visible tumor or mucosal abnormality. Random biopsy is performed if no abnormality is seen. If cancer is confirmed, then transurethral resection of the bladder tumor (TURBT) and examination under anesthesia is performed to determine histology and also depth of invasion.

Most patients are found to have non–muscle invasive disease. This can include exophytic lesion (Ta, which can be low grade or high grade), carcinoma in situ (Tis, always high grade), or early-stage invasive cancer (T1). Small low-grade Ta tumors are treated with TURBT followed by a single dose of intravesical chemotherapy. All other noninvasive disease (including recurrent low-grade Ta disease) is treated with TURBT followed by six treatments of intravesical chemotherapy, most commonly bacillus Calmette-Guérin or mitomycin, although other compounds are used. After primary treatment, cystoscopic surveillance is indicated because of the risk for recurrent disease. There is a higher risk for muscle invasive recurrence for patients with larger tumors, less differentiated tumors, tumors that invade into the lamina propria, and tumors with multifocal or noninvasive recurrence. Most patients require cystoscopy 3 months after initial therapy, with subsequent cystoscopy at 3-month to 1-year intervals based on risk of recurrence. Cystectomy can be considered for patients at high risk for developing muscle-invasive disease.

If muscle-invasive disease is diagnosed, cystectomy is indicated, with or without neoadjuvant cisplatin-based chemotherapy. Partial cystectomy can be considered in very carefully selected patients. If bladder preservation is desired, maximal TURBT can be combined with concurrent chemoradiotherapy. Adjuvant chemotherapy after surgical resection is appropriate to consider in patients with poor-risk features, such as positive nodes and extension beyond the bladder.

Treatment of metastatic disease requires systemic therapy, and treatment outcomes remain poor. Cisplatin-based combination chemotherapy remains the evidence-based choice in patients eligible to receive cisplatin. After further progression, single-agent therapy is recommended. Immunotherapy plays a role here with the recent FDA approval of atezolizumab, a monoclonal antibody directed against the programmed death ligand 1 (PD-L1) receptor.

KEY POINTS

- Any patient with gross hematuria should be referred for urologic evaluation, as should any patient confirmed to have microscopic hematuria in the absence of an apparent benign cause; use of anticoagulants does not alter these recommendations.

- Bladder cancer typically does not invade the muscle, and treatment includes transurethral resection of the bladder tumor (TURBT) plus intravesical chemotherapy, usually bacillus Calmette-Guérin or mitomycin.

- Muscle-invasive bladder cancer is treated with cystectomy with or without neoadjuvant cisplatin-based chemotherapy; partial cystectomy with bladder preservation through maximal TURBT and concurrent chemoradiotherapy can be performed in select patients.

Lymphoid Malignancies
Epidemiology and Risk Factors

The American Cancer Society estimates that in 2018 83,180 new cases of lymphoma will be diagnosed in the United States. The lifetime risk of developing non-Hodgkin lymphoma is 2.1%, whereas the lifetime risk of developing Hodgkin lymphoma is considerably less. Although incidence has only slightly declined recently, death rates have decreased significantly owing to improvements in treatment. The incidence of non-Hodgkin lymphoma rises with increased age, whereas the incidence of Hodgkin lymphoma shows a bimodal age distribution, with an early peak in the second and third decades of life, then a decline, followed by a sustained increase with older age.

Although most of these cases seem sporadic, familial clustering can be seen, with an increased relative risk in first-degree relatives. Patients with both congenital and acquired immunosuppression (such as HIV infection, organ transplantation, or an inherited immunodeficiency) are at greater risk.

Various viral infections are also associated with increased risk. Epstein-Barr virus is associated with Burkitt lymphoma, seen in African pediatric patients, as well as some cases of Hodgkin lymphoma. Human T-cell lymphotropic virus type 1 (HTLV-1) is associated with T-cell leukemias and lymphomas, endemic in Japan, West Africa, Central America, the southeastern United States, and the Caribbean. Hepatitis C virus is associated with an increased risk of lymphoma, particularly splenic marginal zone lymphoma. HIV infection is associated with an increased risk of principally B-cell lymphomas, typically with aggressive histology, more advanced stage, more B symptoms, and a higher risk of extranodal and central nervous system involvement. Kaposi sarcoma herpesvirus (human herpesvirus 8) is associated not only with Kaposi sarcoma but also with primary effusion lymphoma.

Patients with autoimmune rheumatic disorders, such as Sjögren syndrome, systemic lupus erythematosus, and rheumatoid arthritis, have an increased risk of non-Hodgkin lymphoma. The strongest association is with Sjögren syndrome and extranodal marginal zone lymphomas.

Evaluation and Diagnosis

Enlarged lymph nodes are the most common sign of lymphoma. There are many causes of lymphadenopathy, and in most patients, it is of benign origin (infectious or inflammatory). Palpable small and modest-sized cervical and inguinal lymph nodes may be noted in otherwise healthy adults and need not be evaluated further. This finding in young adults and of brief (less than 3 to 4 weeks) duration is likely to be benign. CT scan of the chest, abdomen, and pelvis can assess palpable lymph nodes not amenable to physical examination but generally should not be done in asymptomatic patients. When the size, distribution, or persistence of enlarged lymph nodes or systemic symptoms raises concern for lymphoma, a diagnosis is generally established based on lymph node biopsy. An excisional biopsy is often preferable to a core needle biopsy as it may better determine nodal architecture. Fine-needle aspiration cytology is generally inadequate to make a specific diagnosis, but it may show features suspicious for lymphoma, requiring a more definitive excisional biopsy or, conversely, may reveal findings consistent with inflammation that make lymphoma less likely. Flow cytometry on cytology can demonstrate B-cell or T-cell markers, as well as features consistent with monoclonality.

Although most patients with lymphoma present with lymph node involvement, presentation in extranodal sites is not uncommon.

KEY POINTS

- Lymphadenopathy is the most common sign of lymphoma; increase in size, distribution, and persistence, along with systemic symptoms, raises the concern for lymphoma.
- Diagnosis of lymphoma is generally established by excision or core needle biopsy.

Classifications, Staging, and Prognosis of Malignant Lymphoma

Malignant lymphoma represents a spectrum of disorders. Diagnosis and classification are established not just on standard histopathologic staining looking at cell type and nodal architecture but also on flow cytometry, various immunohistochemical stains, and cytogenetic and molecular genetic features. The classification systems are complex and have continued to evolve during the past decades. The most commonly recognized system is the World Health Organization update on the Revised European-American Lymphoma classification. Experienced hematopathologists are essential to obtaining proper classification. However, there can be significant discordance among experts and some overlap among tumor types.

Staging the anatomical extent of spread can be simplified through the Ann Arbor staging criteria (**Figure 21**).

Lymphomas are staged I to IV based on the number of sites of disease and the presence of extranodal involvement. Staging involves physical examination, CT scans, and PET scans in most patients. However, PET scans tend not to be sensitive for some very indolent lymphomas (such as small lymphocytic lymphoma and marginal zone lymphomas). Bone marrow aspiration and biopsy have typically been part of staging for many lymphomas, but the use of PET scans may obviate the need for bone marrow biopsies in many patients with Hodgkin lymphoma and large cell lymphoma as marrow involvement is rarely found if it is not suggested by PET.

Lymphoma stages are also designated A or B; A indicates no systemic symptoms are present, and B indicates the presence of one or more of the following: fever, drenching night sweats, or unexplained weight loss.

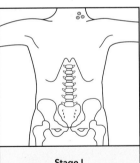

Stage I

- Involvement of single lymph node region; or
- Involvement of single extralymphatic site (stage IE)

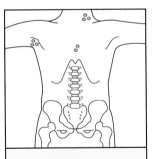

Stage II

- Involvement of ≥2 lymph node regions on same side of diaphragm
- May include localized extralymphatic involvement on same side of diaphragm (stage IIE)

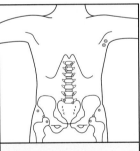

Stage III

- Involvement of lymph node regions on both sides of diaphragm
- May include involvement of spleen (stage IIIS) or localized extranodal disease (stage IIIE) or both (IIIE+S)

For Hodgkin lymphoma:

III1

- Disease limited to upper abdomen—spleen, splenic hilar, celiac, or portahepatic nodes

III2

- Disease limited to lower abdomen—periaortic, pelvic or inguinal nodes

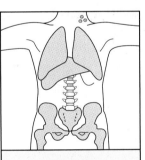

Stage IV

- Disseminated (multifocal) extralymphatic disease involving one or more organs (e.g., liver, bone, marrow, lung, skin), +/– associated lymph node involvement; or
- Isolated extralymphatic disease with distant (nonregional) lymph node involvement

FIGURE 21. Ann Arbor Staging System for Hodgkin and non-Hodgkin lymphoma. Reprinted with permission from Skarkin, A. The Atlas of Diagnostic Oncology, 3rd Edition. Philadelphia, PA: Mosby. Copyright Elsevier, 2002.

The prognosis of the lymphoma varies greatly depending on the subtype, stage, and comorbidities. Immunophenotypic, cytogenetic, and molecular genetic classifications also commonly inform the prognosis. Prognostic indices have been reported and validated for most common types, including the International Prognostic Index for large cell lymphoma, the Follicular Lymphoma International Prognostic Index, and the Mantle cell lymphoma Prognostic Index.

KEY POINTS

- Staging of lymphoma involves physical examination, CT scans, and PET scans in most patients.

HVC
- A negative PET scan may obviate the need for bone marrow biopsies in many patients with Hodgkin and large cell lymphoma, but PET scans are not sensitive to very indolent lymphomas.

Non-Hodgkin Lymphomas

Approximately 85% of non-Hodgkin lymphomas are B-cell derived and express surface immunoglobulin and B-cell markers, whereas 15% are T-cell derived.

Indolent B-Cell Lymphomas

The indolent lymphomas may be present for many years without symptoms and typically have a favorable response to various sequential therapies when needed, but all have a tendency for continued relapse.

Follicular Lymphoma

Follicular lymphomas demonstrate lymph node architecture with a follicular morphology. They arise from the germinal center B cells of the lymph node and are characterized by the presence of a t(14;18) translocation that causes an overexpression of the *BCL2* oncogene. Follicular lymphomas are classified based on their dominant cell type: predominantly smaller cells (grade 1), a mixture of smaller and larger cells (grade 2), and predominantly large cells (grade 3). Grades 1 and 2 are commonly combined as the distinction between them is somewhat subjective. Grade 3 follicular lymphoma can be divided into 3A and 3B, with the latter composed of sheets of more uniform poorly differentiated cells. Grade 3A follicular lymphoma is more akin in behavior and treatment to grades 1 and 2, whereas 3B is treated more like diffuse large B-cell lymphoma, although this is somewhat controversial.

Follicular lymphoma is the most common indolent B-cell lymphoma and accounts for approximately 30% of non-Hodgkin lymphomas. Many patients are not symptomatic at diagnosis and in some cases do not require therapy for many years. There is no clear evidence that early treatment leads to improved outcomes, so asymptomatic patients without bulky disease are usually observed. Some patients may undergo spontaneous, although generally transient, regression of disease.

Most patients with follicular lymphoma will present with stage III or IV disease. Single-agent rituximab is associated with high response rates and durable remissions. Combining rituximab with chemotherapy (such as the alkylating agent bendamustine) leads to remission in more than 90% of patients. The use of maintenance rituximab after induction of an initial remission is associated with prolonged duration of remission or relapse-free survival, but no clear improvement in overall survival. Patients with relapsing or refractory cases can be treated with various other approaches, including alternate chemotherapy regimens (such as rituximab plus cyclophosphamide, doxorubicin, vincristine, and prednisone [R-CHOP]), the anti-CD20 antibody obinutuzumab, the phosphoinositide 3-kinase inhibitor idelalisib, radioimmunotherapy with ibritumomab tiuxetan, as well as autologous or allogeneic hematopoietic stem cell transplantation (HSCT).

A minority of patients present with localized disease and can be approached with radiation therapy with curative intent rather than with systemic therapy. Whether systemic therapy, such as rituximab, with or without chemotherapy should be used in addition to or as an alternative to radiotherapy in patients with localized follicular (and other low-grade) lymphomas is controversial.

Histologic transformation, most typically to a diffuse large B-cell lymphoma, occurs in approximately 30% of patients with follicular lymphomas and is associated with an aggressive course and poor prognosis. Transformation may be suggested by a change in the clinical pattern of disease with new systemic symptoms or rapid progression of a localized area of disease, a rise in serum lactate dehydrogenase, or markedly higher areas of standardized uptake values on PET scans. A new biopsy is required to establish that transformation has occurred.

KEY POINTS

- Many patients with follicular lymphoma are not symptomatic at diagnosis and may not require therapy for many years. HVC

- In advanced-stage follicular lymphoma, rituximab plus chemotherapy leads to remission in more than 90% of patients, although the disease will recur in most patients.

- Histologic transformation of follicular lymphoma to a diffuse large B-cell lymphoma, which should be confirmed by obtaining another lymph node biopsy, occurs in approximately 30% of patients and is associated with a poor prognosis.

Mucosa-associated Lymphoid Tissue Lymphoma

Mucosa-associated lymphoid tissue (MALT) lymphoma is an extranodal marginal zone lymphoma. Gastric MALT lymphoma may be the best known, particularly given its common association with *Helicobacter pylori* infection. However, MALT lymphomas can arise in other sites such as the gastrointestinal tract, thyroid, orbits, skin, and lung and generally demonstrate indolent behavior and a low propensity for transformation. Repetitive immune stimulation, from underlying chronic infection or an autoimmune process, is likely to play a role in the pathogenesis of this tumor.

H. pylori–associated gastric MALT lymphoma should be treated with antibiotics and proton pump inhibitors initially. Other localized MALT lymphomas may be treated with radiation, to which they are quite sensitive. When systemic therapy is required, rituximab alone or in combination with chemotherapy is associated with high response rates.

KEY POINT

- *Helicobacter pylori*–associated gastric MALT lymphoma should be treated with antibiotics and proton pump inhibitors initially; other localized MALT lymphomas may be treated with radiation.

Chronic Lymphocytic Leukemia

Chronic lymphocytic leukemia (CLL) is generally easy to diagnose because it manifests as an increase in absolute lymphocytes on complete blood count. The lymphocytes are predominantly small and mature appearing, although they may be fragile and form "smudge cells" on the peripheral smear. Flow cytometry using peripheral blood is essential in establishing the diagnosis and will reveal B-cell antigens (CD19, 20, and 23), coexpression of CD5 (normally a T-cell marker), and low levels of a monoclonal surface immunoglobulin. Bone marrow aspiration and biopsy are no longer necessary to diagnose and stage most patients with CLL.

Although less common, other lymphomas may present similarly to CLL in peripheral blood smears and must be distinguished by morphology, flow cytometry, and genetic studies. These other disorders include hairy cell leukemia, marginal and mantle zone lymphomas, T-cell lymphoma, and prolymphocytic leukemia.

CLL and small lymphocytic lymphoma represent the same disease, with the designation as leukemia or lymphoma based on the dominant clinical manifestation in either peripheral blood and marrow or nodal involvement, respectively. Both CLL and small lymphocytic lymphoma are treated the same. CLL is now grouped more with the lymphomas than with the leukemias in treatment centers.

CLL is typically an indolent disease, and many patients require no therapy for many years and sometimes decades. Prognosis can relate to clinical staging (Rai and Binet staging systems are based on the extent of cytopenias, organomegaly, and degree of nodal involvement) but also on cytogenetic and molecular genetic characteristics. The specific nature of the mutation can help indicate the prognosis.

The past decade has seen a rapid advance in the number and efficacy of active agents for CLL. Although these therapies are not curative, most patients can now achieve durable remissions once treatment is required. Treatment options available include alkylating agents (chlorambucil, cyclophosphamide,

bendamustine), purine nucleoside analogues (fludarabine, cladribine, pentostatin), monoclonal antibodies (rituximab, alemtuzumab, ofatumumab, obinutuzumab), and the phosphoinositide-3 kinase inhibitor idelalisib. There has been an increase in use of the Bruton kinase inhibitor ibrutinib, which is now approved for first-line therapy and active in a broad spectrum of patients, including those with 17p deletion. Venetoclax, a *BCL2* inhibitor, is active in refractory cases, induces brisk apoptosis, and occasionally induces tumor lysis syndrome. Lenalidomide, an immune modulator approved for myeloma and myelodysplasia, is also active. Allogeneic HSCT is rarely performed in CLL but has been used in refractory cases in appropriate patients. Anti-CD19 chimeric antigen receptor (CAR) T-cell therapy has also been shown to be active in refractory cases. Older chemoimmunotherapy regimens, although quite active, may increasingly give way to targeted therapies.

Patients with CLL are prone to infection, in part related to commonly associated hypogammaglobulinemia. In patients with repeated infections and hypogammaglobulinemia, regular treatment with intravenous gamma globulin reduces infectious events. The infection risk increases in more advanced disease, a result of both impaired T-cell–mediated and B-cell–mediated immune response along with treatment-induced immunosuppression. Patients with CLL and small lymphocytic lymphoma may also develop autoimmune cytopenias such as immune thrombocytopenic purpura and autoimmune hemolytic anemias. Transformation to a large cell lymphoma (known as Richter transformation) occurs in about 5% of patients with CLL and small lymphocytic lymphoma and is generally associated with a poor prognosis and refractory disease.

[handwritten margin note: AUTOIMMUNE CYTOPENIAS]

KEY POINTS

- Chronic lymphocytic leukemia and small lymphocytic lymphoma are the same disease, but the former predominates in peripheral blood and bone marrow, whereas the latter predominates in lymph nodes.

- The diagnosis of chronic lymphocytic leukemia manifests as an increase in absolute lymphocytes on complete blood count; the lymphocytes are predominantly small and mature appearing and may form "smudge cells" on the peripheral smear.

- Patients with low-stage, asymptomatic chronic lymphocytic leukemia can be observed without therapy for decades.

Hairy Cell Leukemia   *[handwritten: BRAF MUTATION]*

Like CLL, hairy cell leukemia is a low-grade B-cell disorder but with characteristic clinical, pathologic, immunophenotypic, and genetic changes. Patients typically present with cytopenias and splenomegaly; lymphadenopathy is typically absent. Circulating "hairy cells," characterized by cytoplasmic projections, are often identified in the peripheral blood smear (**Figure 22**); when seen

R: RITUXIMAB / RITUXAN
C: CYCLOPHOSPHAMIDE / CYTOXAN
H: HYDROXY - DOXORUBICIN
O: ONCOVIN / VINCRISTINE
P: PREDNISONE

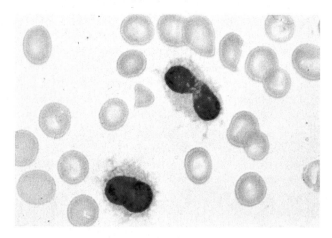

FIGURE 22. Hairy cell leukemia depicted by a peripheral blood smear showing atypical lymphocytes with thread-like cytoplasmic projections from the cell surface.

on bone marrow biopsy, these cells have a lacunar appearance. Classically, the bone marrow aspirate is a dry tap due to some degree of marrow fibrosis. Flow cytometry shows hairy cells positive for characteristic surface markers. In addition, the presence of a *BRAF* V600E mutation has been associated with hairy cell leukemia in most patients and represents not only a diagnostic marker but also a therapeutic target.

As with CLL and other low-grade lymphomas, some patients with hairy cell leukemia do not require immediate treatment if not symptomatic. However, the front-line therapy remains purine nucleoside agents, typically pentostatin or cladribine. These agents are highly active, and almost all patients respond, many with durable responses, with only one course of treatment. Relapses can be treated with the alternate purine nucleoside agent. Rituximab is also active in relapse. The selective *BRAF* inhibitor vemurafenib has also shown activity in relapsed patients.

Hairy cell leukemia variant is a distinct entity that typically presents with a high circulating leukocyte count, as opposed to the leukopenia seen in the classic form. These patients respond less well to cladribine and have shorter durations of response.

KEY POINTS

- Patients with hairy cell leukemia typically present with circulating "hairy cells," cytopenias, and splenomegaly but no lymphadenopathy.

- Durable remissions of hairy cell leukemia can often be achieved with one course of a purine nucleoside agent such as pentostatin or cladribine.

Aggressive B-Cell Lymphomas

The more aggressive lymphomas, such as diffuse large B-cell and Burkitt lymphoma, are more likely to present with systemic symptoms or signs of rapid tumor progression. Diagnosis

should be promptly pursued because these patients have a greater potential for cure with therapy.

Diffuse Large B-Cell Lymphoma

CD 20+
CD 19+

Diffuse large B-cell lymphoma represents approximately 30% of non-Hodgkin lymphomas. Although diffuse large B-cell lymphoma can be subdivided based on gene expression profiling (activated B-cell versus germinal center type), and although this subtyping may be associated with prognostic differences, there is no clear indication yet that the initial treatment approach should be altered based on the subtype. These patients often present with symptomatic enlarging lymphadenopathy in the neck or abdomen. Approximately 40% may have symptoms or signs of extranodal disease, and one third have systemic symptoms. Biopsy specimens show diffuse effacement of normal nodal architecture by large, atypical lymphoid cells with prominent nucleoli and basophilic cytoplasm. Flow cytometry reveals B-cell antigens, and most patients have monoclonal surface immunoglobulin. The B-cell lymphoma 6 (*BCL6*) gene shows rearrangement or other mutations that lead to overexpression in most patients.

Sixty percent of patients have advanced (stage III or IV) disease at diagnosis, and standard therapy is R-CHOP. Consolidative radiation therapy may be given to sites of bulky disease. Residual masses, which are often benign, may remain after treatment. PET may help determine if these represent active disease or just scarring.

Patients with poor prognostic features, such as elevated serum lactate dehydrogenase level, extensive tumor burden, and poor performance status, may receive more aggressive initial therapy. Those patients who present with localized disease can be treated with a shorter course of chemotherapy with consolidative radiation therapy. In addition to further standard chemotherapy, autologous HSCT and anti-CD19 chimeric antigen receptor (CAR) T-cell therapy may be used as salvage therapy in patients who relapse.

Primary mediastinal large cell lymphoma is a distinct clinical, morphologic, and genetic lymphoma, often presenting in younger patients. It putatively arises from thymic B cells. It has a female predilection, a tendency to present with bulky but localized disease, and a relatively high cure rate. It may have significant overlap histologically and genetically with nodular sclerosing Hodgkin lymphoma, and some cases may be difficult to classify as one or the other; these are called mediastinal gray-zone lymphomas.

KEY POINTS

- Aggressive B-cell lymphomas, such as diffuse large B-cell and Burkitt lymphoma, progress more quickly than indolent lymphomas but have a greater potential for cure.

- Standard therapy for most patients with advanced-stage diffuse large B-cell lymphoma is rituximab plus cyclophosphamide, doxorubicin, vincristine, and prednisone.

Mantle Cell Lymphoma

Mantle cell lymphomas represent approximately 3% to 6% of non-Hodgkin lymphomas. Median age at diagnosis is 68 years, and there is a 3-to-1 male predominance. It is defined and presumably initiated by a t(11;14) translocation, which leads to constitutive overexpression of cyclin D1, a cell-cycle gene regulator. Patients can present with nodal or extranodal disease, and the disease is usually widely disseminated at diagnosis. Gastrointestinal involvement with several polyps (lymphomatoid polyposis) is well described, as is involvement of the peripheral blood and bone marrow.

Although mantle cell lymphoma is responsive to various conventional chemotherapy regimens and newer agents, it is associated with a predilection for continued relapse. There is no clear consensus on the optimal therapeutic approach, with treatments spanning a spectrum of least aggressive (lenalidomide or bendamustine plus rituximab) to more aggressive (R-CHOP with or without HSCT). A subset of patients with indolent disease may not require therapy for many years.

Burkitt Lymphoma

DOUBLING TIME 24-48 hr

A relatively rare lymphoma, Burkitt lymphoma, is remarkable for its extremely rapid growth. The endemic form occurs primarily in Africa, is a common cause of childhood cancer, and is associated with Epstein-Barr virus infection. Patients may present with a large jaw mass (**Figure 23**). The sporadic form is more typically seen in the United States, occurs at a somewhat later age, and is more likely to present with abdominal or pelvic involvement. A third variety of Burkitt lymphoma is the immunodeficiency-associated form and occurs in HIV-infected patients. *MYC* gene activation is characteristic of this lymphoma. The serum lactate dehydrogenase level is typically high.   Ki-67, CD20+, CD10+, CD5-   t(8,14)

Early signs of the tumor lysis syndrome are often present in patients with Burkitt lymphoma even before treatment is initiated and should be anticipated because the tumor is quite chemosensitive. Various aggressive multiagent chemotherapy regimens with rituximab have been associated with high cure rates. These regimens are more intensive than standard lymphoma therapy and are associated with some risk of treatment-related mortality (for a more complete discussion, see Oncologic Emergencies and Urgencies). Treatment of occult central nervous system involvement is included in initial treatment regimens because of the risk for leptomeningeal involvement. 🄷

KEY POINT

- Prophylaxis to manage tumor lysis syndrome should be instituted before initiation of chemotherapy for patients with Burkitt lymphoma.

T-Cell Lymphomas

T-cell lymphomas represent approximately 10% to 15% of lymphomas in Western countries but are more common in Asia. They include various subtypes and are a heterogeneous group

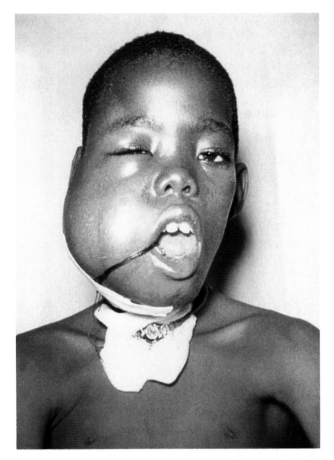

FIGURE 23. A large jaw mass associated with Burkitt lymphoma.

of disorders characterized by distinct presentations and morphology. Diagnosis can be made on routine pathology and supplemented by flow cytometry and immunohistochemistry. Monoclonality can be confirmed by findings of clonal rearrangements of the T-cell receptor genes detected by polymerase chain reaction. In general, T-cell lymphomas are more refractory to therapy than B-cell lymphomas. Although various new agents are available for treatment, studies are small and many responses are transient.

Cutaneous T-Cell Lymphoma

Mycosis fungoides and Sézary syndrome are the two major subtypes of cutaneous T-cell lymphoma. The skin findings in mycosis fungoides are quite heterogeneous, ranging from non-specific macular-papular eruptions or plaques, to more defined skin tumors with ulceration, to diffuse erythroderma. There is often a preceding prodromal illness, or "premycotic" period, with milder skin disease that waxes and wanes or that may progress for months or even years without a definitive diagnosis; skin biopsies done during that interval are nonspecific. Pruritus is common and can be debilitating. Ultimately, as skin involvement becomes more extensive, the disease progresses to involve extracutaneous sites, including lymph nodes and organs, such as the lung, liver, and gastrointestinal tract. Infections are more common as a function of underlying immunodeficiency and disruption of the protective barrier provided by healthy skin. The Sézary syndrome is a more aggressive form of cutaneous T-cell lymphoma in which diffuse erythroderma characterizes the skin involvement and malignant T cells circulate in the blood.

The staging of cutaneous T-cell lymphoma is dependent on the extent of skin disease and involvement of lymph nodes and extranodal sites. Early stages of cutaneous T-cell lymphoma are confined to the skin and managed with topical therapy, such as glucocorticoids, retinoids, or ultraviolet light therapy, that may be combined with interferon. Survival is greater than 10 years. More advanced disease is associated with a survival of less than 4 years and requires more aggressive skin treatment with electron beam radiation along with systemic chemotherapy. Patients with Sézary syndrome require systemic chemotherapy. Extracorporeal photopheresis uses psoralens, compounds that enter cells and sensitize them to injury after activation with ultraviolet light; this technique is also used in Sézary syndrome.

Peripheral T-Cell Lymphoma, Not Otherwise Specified

Peripheral T-cell lymphoma, not otherwise specified, is the most commonly diagnosed subtype of peripheral T-cell lymphoma. It typically presents in older adults at an advanced stage, has a male predominance, and has a generally poor clinical outcome compared to B-cell lymphomas.

Various combination chemotherapy regimens have been used. The addition of etoposide to standard combination chemotherapy may provide some benefit as part of initial therapy. The use of chemotherapy designed for acute lymphoblastic leukemia or management with HSCT, both autologous and allogeneic, may benefit some patients, although there is controversy as to when and in whom these are best used. As with other T-cell lymphomas, newer chemotherapy agents such as pralatrexate and romidepsin yield responses in some patients with relapsed disease.

Anaplastic Large Cell Lymphoma

Anaplastic large cell lymphoma can present with nodal as well as extranodal disease, including skin, bone marrow, and bone. Patients commonly have B symptoms. Tumor cells are typically CD30 positive. An important prognostic and potentially therapeutic distinction is the presence or absence of a t(2;5) or variant *ALK* gene translocation and protein expression.

CD 30+

ALK-positive patients are younger (mean age at diagnosis is approximately 35 years) and have a much more favorable prognosis with conventional chemotherapy and may also respond to treatment with crizotinib, an oral targeted agent also active in lung cancer with *ALK* gene translocations.

Angioimmunoblastic T-Cell Lymphoma

Angioimmunoblastic T-cell lymphoma, initially termed angio-immunoblastic lymphadenopathy, was thought to be a disease of impaired immune regulation rather than a true malignancy; however, patients with this disease are now recognized to have clonal rearrangement of T-cell receptors consistent with a T-cell neoplasm. Patients with angioimmunoblastic T-cell lymphoma often present with systemic B symptoms, generalized lymphadenopathy, hepatosplenomegaly, and a skin rash. They commonly show polyclonal hypergammaglobulinemia and elevated erythrocyte sedimentation rate and C-reactive protein level. Autoimmune manifestations (such as a Coombs-positive autoimmune hemolytic anemia) may be present. Although the lymphoma in some patients is responsive to glucocorticoids and conventional chemotherapy, it typically has a moderately aggressive clinical course and median survival of less than 2 years.

KEY POINTS

- The skin findings in mycosis fungoides, a subtype of cutaneous T-cell lymphoma, range from nonspecific macular-papular eruptions or plaques, to more defined skin tumors with ulceration, to diffuse erythroderma.

- The Sézary syndrome is a more aggressive subtype of cutaneous T-cell lymphoma in which diffuse erythroderma characterizes the skin involvement and malignant T cells circulate in the blood.

- Peripheral T-cell lymphoma, not otherwise specified, is treated with combination chemotherapy.

Lymphoblastic Lymphoma

Lymphoblastic lymphoma is an aggressive lymphoma that can be of T- or B-cell origin. It is akin to and treated with protocols for acute lymphoblastic leukemia. Presentation with a mediastinal mass, blood or bone marrow, and central nervous system involvement is typical.

Hodgkin Lymphoma

Hodgkin lymphoma represents approximately 10% of lymphomas and is curable in most, but not all, patients. It has a bimodal incidence, although it most commonly presents in young adults. Presentation with mediastinal, cervical, and supraclavicular involvement is particularly common for the nodular sclerosing subtype (**Figure 24**). Patients may also present with B symptoms, although that is more commonly seen in elderly patients with more advanced disease. Pruritus may also be a presenting symptom.

The diagnosis is established with a lymph node biopsy specimen showing Reed-Sternberg cells (**Figure 25**), malignant cells that originate from germinal center B cells and are seen in an inflammatory infiltrate. The number of Reed-Sternberg cells and variability in the composition of the infiltrate lead to pathologic subtypes, including nodular sclerosis, mixed cellularity, lymphocyte predominant, and lymphocyte depleted. Patients are staged by physical examination and PET-CT scan. Staging laparotomies, including diagnostic splenectomy, are no longer done. Routine bone marrow biopsy, in the absence of unexplained blood abnormalities, is not indicated.

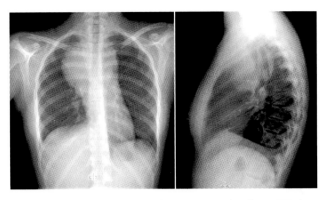

FIGURE 24. Hodgkin lymphoma is the most common lymphoma to involve the mediastinum, shown in this chest radiograph (left) as a mass that originates from the mediastinum, given the convex angles resulting from the mass impinging on the pleura. The lateral film (right) localizes the mass to the anterior mediastinum. Hodgkin lymphoma is the most common cause of anterior mediastinal masses in patients aged 20 to 30 years.

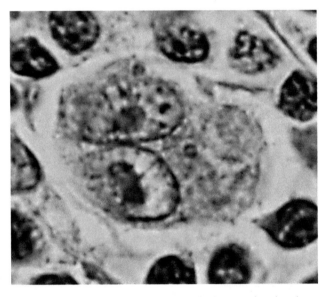

FIGURE 25. Reed-Sternberg cells are large and either are multinucleated or have a bilobed nucleus ("owls eye" appearance) with prominent eosinophilic inclusion-like nucleoli. They can be seen with light microscopy in biopsies from individuals with Hodgkin lymphoma. They are usually derived from B lymphocytes. When seen against a sea of B cells, they give the tissue a "starry sky" or "moth-eaten" appearance. The absence of Reed-Sternberg cells has very high negative predictive value for Hodgkin disease.

More than 90% of patients present with "classic" Hodgkin lymphoma pathology and, even with early-stage disease, receive chemotherapy because this has been shown to result in higher cure rates. The doxorubicin, bleomycin, vinblastine, and dacarbazine (ABVD) regimen is most commonly used in the United States. ABVD has replaced alkylating agent–based regimens such as mechlorethamine, vincristine, procarbazine, and prednisone, in part because of higher rates of fertility preservation and a lower risk of secondary acute leukemia. For patients with early-stage, favorable disease, treatment can consist of short-course chemotherapy (as short as two cycles of ABVD) and involved

field radiation. Chemotherapy alone (ABVD for four to six cycles) in patients with good response is also an option. For more advanced disease, chemotherapy alone is used. Although the regimen is usually well tolerated, up to 25% of patients may develop bleomycin-induced lung injury during treatment or within 6 months of its conclusion. A portion of those patients will have sustained exertional dyspnea associated with a decline in pulmonary function.

Complete response indicated by PET scan after two to three cycles of chemotherapy is a reliable prognostic indicator. Early repeat PET scan is an appropriate response-adapted strategy in Hodgkin lymphoma and may allow some patients with early-stage disease to forgo radiation therapy and thereby reduce the risks of late radiation side effects.

For patients with relapsed or refractory disease, salvage chemotherapy and autologous or allogeneic HSCT may provide curative options. Brentuximab vedotin (an anti-CD30 monoclonal antibody conjugated with a peptide link to monomethyl auristatin E [MMAE]) is active in refractory disease and has also been used for consolidation after autologous HSCT. The programmed death 1 (PD-1) antibodies (pembrolizumab and nivolumab) are highly active in relapsed or refractory disease. The incorporation of these drugs in earlier treatment regimens is being studied.

Nodular lymphocyte–predominant Hodgkin lymphoma is distinct clinically and pathologically from classic Hodgkin lymphoma (nodular sclerosis, mixed cellularity, and lymphocyte depleted). It represents approximately 10% of Hodgkin lymphomas and is more likely to present with localized disease but is associated with a high rate of late relapse. Early-stage disease may be treated with radiation therapy alone. Single-agent rituximab or combined with chemotherapy may be used for more advanced or relapsed disease.

KEY POINTS

- All patients with classic Hodgkin lymphoma, regardless of stage, receive chemotherapy. Patients with early-stage nodular lymphocyte–predominant Hodgkin lymphoma may be treated with radiation alone, but in the more advanced stages, they should be treated with rituximab with or without chemotherapy.

- Complete response indicated by PET scan after two to three cycles of chemotherapy can allow some patients with early-stage classical Hodgkin lymphoma to forgo radiation therapy.

Cancer of Unknown Primary Site

Introduction

Despite steady improvements in diagnostic and imaging techniques during the past decades, a reasonable evaluation will not identify the source of cancer in a small number (less than 5%) of all patients presenting with metastatic cancer. This heterogeneous group of patients is classified as having cancer of unknown primary (CUP). As diagnostic imaging continues to improve, the frequency of CUP diagnoses is decreasing.

Diagnosis and Evaluation

On identification of metastatic cancer, a full medical history and physical examination should be obtained, as well as contrast-enhanced CT of the chest, abdomen, and pelvis. Histologic evaluation of the most accessible tumor mass should include a limited number of immunohistochemical stains to assess the nature of the tumor and to identify or exclude treatable histologies (such as lymphoma or germ cell tumor). Patterns of clinical presentation, or subgroups (discussed later), that also suggest a potential for better outcome should be sought. In addition, specific symptom or presentation-related evaluations may be pursued, such as upper endoscopy and colonoscopy in patients with symptoms or evidence of gastrointestinal bleeding. Patients with regional lymphadenopathy require focused evaluation, such as pan-endoscopic evaluation of the head and neck for patients with isolated or dominant cervical lymphadenopathy or anoscopy for those with isolated inguinal lymphadenopathy. In female patients, breast examination and mammography should be done to search for a breast primary cancer, and a gynecologic evaluation should be performed to look for an ovarian primary. Male patients require a testicular examination and, in those with bone metastases, a prostate examination and serum prostate-specific antigen to evaluate for prostate cancer. Nonspecific tumor markers, such as serum carcinoembryonic antigen, CA-19-9, CA-15-3, or CA-125, are not definitive for identifying a specific site of origin and are not routinely recommended. PET may in some patients suggest the possible primary location, but false-positive results are significant and PET scan findings are not apt to change the treatment plan. The use of gene expression arrays has been commercially promoted, but the clinical utility of these tests to identify more effective therapy is unknown. As these add expense without clear benefit, their routine use in the evaluation of CUP is not recommended.

Ultimately, CUP is a diagnosis of exclusion after evaluation has failed to identify the primary tumor, which either may be too small to be detected or may have been destroyed immunologically and is no longer present. Both patients and clinicians tend to overemphasize the importance of identifying the primary site. Such efforts often deflect focus from the major issue, which is the presence of metastatic cancer. Once the more treatable possibilities have been excluded, specific identification of the site of origin is very unlikely to improve treatment options or clinical outcome. At that point, it should be determined if the metastatic cancer has a favorable or unfavorable prognosis and if there is a specific, efficacious therapy for that patient.

- In patients with a metastatic cancer of unknown primary site, CT scans and histologic, endoscopic, and gender-specific cancer evaluations are reasonable; however, nonspecific tumor markers, PET scans, and gene expression arrays are not definitive and have not been shown to be beneficial and should not be done.

- After reasonable attempts to identify primary cancer have failed, management should shift focus, treating the metastasis based on histology and prognostic factors as finding the primary site is unlikely to improve treatment options or clinical outcome.

HVC

Favorable Prognostic Subgroups of Cancer of Unknown Primary Site

For patients with CUP, the identification of a favorable prognostic subgroup allows selection of specific surgical, radiation, or chemotherapy to which patients are more likely to respond and on occasion achieves long-term remission and cure.

Poorly Differentiated Cancer of Unknown Primary Site

Poorly differentiated cancers are usually more aggressive than well-differentiated cancers, and metastatic poorly differentiated adenocarcinoma has a poor prognosis; however, some patients with poorly differentiated CUP that is not definitively an adenocarcinoma may have specific treatment options as a result of their histology. In particular, young men with poorly differentiated carcinoma that is predominantly in the midline, such as those with large retroperitoneal or mediastinal lymphadenopathy, or both, should be carefully evaluated for the possibility of a germ cell tumor. Serum α-fetoprotein and β-human chorionic gonadotropin levels should be measured, and a testicular examination and ultrasonography should be performed. Even if these evaluations have negative findings, an unrecognized germ cell tumor may still exist, and these patients should be treated for this possibility with a platinum-based chemotherapy regimen.

Patients with poorly differentiated neuroendocrine tumors also warrant careful consideration. These tumors frequently both metastasize like small cell lung cancers and respond similarly to platinum-based chemotherapy.

Isolated Regional Lymphadenopathy

A group of patients with CUP who may have a more favorable prognosis is women found to have adenocarcinoma in isolated axillary lymphadenopathy. These patients should be presumptively considered to have locoregional breast cancer. If mammography is unrevealing, a breast MRI should be performed. If the MRI scan is negative, the patient is still assumed to have a presumptive stage II breast cancer. Given the inability to identify the primary, a mastectomy or whole breast radiation therapy is recommended. These patients should all receive adjuvant treatment consistent with a stage II breast cancer diagnosis. Patients with isolated or dominant cervical lymphadenopathy should undergo full endoscopic examination of the upper aero-digestive tract to evaluate for a head and neck primary. Even if a primary is not identified, treatment along a head and neck paradigm with chemotherapy and radiation therapy is often appropriate. In particular, patients with high cervical lymphadenopathy with squamous cell cancer occasionally achieve cure. Supraclavicular lymphadenopathy or adenocarcinoma makes a head and neck primary far less likely, and therapy is less efficacious.

Isolated inguinal lymphadenopathy should prompt a careful examination of the anal, perineal, and genital regions that includes anoscopy. Even in the absence of a defined primary tumor, definitive resection or radiation to inguinal or other isolated solitary or regional lymph nodes may provide long-term tumor control and cures in rare circumstances.

Peritoneal Carcinomatosis in Women

Women who have adenocarcinoma with abdominal carcinomatosis and ascites should be presumptively treated for ovarian cancer. Ovarian cancer paradigms, including initial cytoreductive surgery and ovarian cancer chemotherapy regimens, should be used.

KEY POINTS

- Patients with cancer of unknown primary who have poorly differentiated carcinoma predominantly in the midline, such as those with large retroperitoneal or mediastinal lymphadenopathy, are likely to have a germ cell tumor and should be treated for that possibility with platinum-based chemotherapy.

- Women with a cancer of unknown primary who have axillary lymphadenopathy and a negative breast MRI scan should be treated for presumptive stage II breast cancer.

- Women with adenocarcinoma with abdominal carcinomatosis and ascites should be treated for presumptive ovarian cancer.

- Patients with isolated or dominant cervical lymphadenopathy and cancer of unknown primary should be treated along a head and neck cancer paradigm with chemotherapy and radiation therapy.

Nonfavorable Subgroups of Cancer of Unknown Primary Site

Therapy for CUP that does not fall into one of the favorable subgroups is empirically directed with chemotherapy and radiation therapy based on the pattern of presentation. CUP presenting above the diaphragm should be evaluated and managed as metastatic lung cancer. CUP that is predominantly below the diaphragm should be managed as gastrointestinal cancer.

Chronic medical comorbidities and performance status of the patient greatly influences the range of treatment options.

As with other solid tumors, patients with several comorbidities and poor performance status are far less likely to benefit from aggressive chemotherapy and are far more likely to experience serious or life-threatening toxicity. Palliative and hospice care should be considered in such patients. Clinical trials that may demonstrate tumor response are typically restricted to patients with normal organ function and good performance status. The results of those trials are unlikely to be informative regarding the response to therapy or prognosis for patients who are not well enough to have qualified for entry into those trials.

KEY POINTS

- Therapy for cancer of unknown primary that does not fall into one of the favorable subgroups should be managed based on pattern of presentation; cancer presenting above the diaphragm should be treated as metastatic lung cancer and cancer presenting below the diaphragm should be treated as gastrointestinal cancer.

- Palliative or hospice care is appropriate for patients with an unfavorable subtype of cancer of unknown primary site who have comorbidities and poor performance status. **HVC**

Melanoma

Melanoma has been steadily increasing in incidence worldwide, with risk related to sun exposure. Most melanomas begin in and present with cutaneous disease, but they can also begin in mucosal sites. About half arise in preexisting nevi, but many begin in apparently normal skin. Melanoma can also present in nodal or visceral sites without a known cutaneous or mucosal primary. About 10% of patients with melanoma have a familial history, and mutations in certain genes, such as *CDKN2A*, have been identified in some families. Ocular melanoma is the most common cancer of the eye, and uveal melanomas have a distinct biology and behavior. Epidemiology, diagnosis, and staging of melanoma are discussed in MKSAP 18 Dermatology.

Advances in systemic therapy during the past decade have resulted in significant improvements in survival for metastatic melanoma patients. These advances include the use of molecular therapy targeted at specific gene mutations and immunotherapy, including the use of immune checkpoint inhibitors.

Treatment of Melanoma

Melanoma has the potential to behave quite aggressively, but it is a highly curable disease when detected and treated early with simple excision. For localized melanomas, prognosis is related to the depth of invasion, either by Clark level (I to V) or by Breslow's depth. A high mitotic rate, lymphovascular invasion, and the presence of bleeding or ulceration are poor prognostic signs. Surgical resection margins for melanomas do not have to be excessive: 1-cm margins are acceptable for lesions that are less than 1 mm in thickness. Patients with melanomas between 1 mm and 2 mm in thickness should be resected with a 2-cm margin provided that a skin graft is not required for closure. Patients with lesions that are greater than 2 mm in thickness should be resected with 2-cm margins. Early-stage patients can be assessed clinically and do not need radiographic staging (for example, CT and PET) and surveillance.

As the depth of invasion increases, the risk of nodal and ultimately distant metastasis increases. Nodal metastases are uncommon and need not be assessed if the patient has thin lesions with a Breslow depth of less than 1 mm. Assessing for lymph node metastasis with lymphatic mapping and sentinel lymph node biopsy is often recommended for intermediate and thicker melanomas. If the sentinel node is positive, a lymph node dissection commonly yields other positive nodes. Although prophylactic lymphadenectomies or completion node dissections for those with positive sentinel nodes have not definitively shown an overall survival benefit, node dissections can be curative in 20% to 50% of patients who present with or who develop regional nodal disease. The use of interferon as adjuvant therapy for resected high-risk disease has been extensively studied and is FDA approved. Although there is some demonstrated improvement in disease-free survival, the overall survival benefit is uncertain, and this therapy is associated with considerable side effects. Adjuvant ipilimumab (see below) also has shown modest benefit in disease-free survival, but as of yet, no overall survival benefit has been shown. Adjuvant nivolumab has been recently shown to be more effective than ipilimumab in node-positive disease.

For distant metastatic disease, surgery may still play a significant role. Melanoma can present with solitary or oligometastatic disease amenable to resection that is curable in some patients. Standard cytotoxic chemotherapy is associated with low response rates and no longer plays a large role in the treatment of metastatic melanoma. The biologic agents interferon-alfa and interleukin-2 can induce responses in some patients, but they cause considerable toxicity and are generally used only in specialized referral centers. The current focus is on targeted therapy for patients with specific gene mutations and on the use of checkpoint inhibitors of programmed cell death transmembrane proteins.

Approximately one half of melanomas harbor a *BRAF* gene mutation (most commonly V600E), and another 20% have a *MEK* or *NRAS* mutation; all of these mutations activate the mitogen-activated protein kinase pathway. Melanomas with these mutations may respond to oral therapy with the *BRAF* inhibitors vemurafenib and dabrafenib. Combining *BRAF* inhibitors with MEK inhibitors trametinib and cobimetinib improves the rate and duration of response. These are available as combined oral agents.

In addition to the efficacy of *BRAF* inhibitors, the use of immune checkpoint inhibitors has revolutionized the therapy and prognosis of patients with metastatic melanoma. Cellular immunity is based on T cells recognizing peptide fragments expressed on the surface of antigen-presenting cells when bound to histocompatibility complex molecules. Cytotoxic T-lymphocyte associated protein 4 (*CTLA4*) is a potent down-regulator of this process. *CTLA4* is stimulated by T-cell activation and various cytokines, serving as an inhibitory factor or braking "checkpoint" on immune activation. The antibody against *CTLA4*, ipilimumab, can result in dramatic tumor response, albeit in a small percentage of patients. Tumor response is independent of *BRAF* status.

The programmed cell death-1 (PD-1) receptor is another transmembrane protein that acts as an inhibitory molecule when bound to the PD-ligand 1 and stops tumor cell apoptosis while down-regulating other aspects of T-cell immune response. Nivolumab and pembrolizumab are both anti-PD-1 antibodies that can result in significant melanoma response rates with sometimes durable response and dramatic survival improvement. Ipilimumab alone has a relatively low response rate and is associated with considerable toxicity, with various immune-related adverse events that can include colitis, hepatitis, pneumonitis, and endocrine insufficiency syndromes. Similar side effects can occur with nivolumab and pembrolizumab but are less frequent, and these antibodies are associated with a higher response rate (30% to 40%). Combining ipilimumab with nivolumab improves results compared with ipilimumab or nivolumab alone. The best dosage, schedule, and sequence for these newer agents continue to be explored.

KEY POINTS

- Surgical resection can be curative in many patients with melanoma, including those with solitary or oligometastatic disease.

- Nodal metastases are uncommon and need not be assessed in patients with thin melanoma lesions (Breslow depth less than 1 mm). **HVC**

- More than one half of patients have melanoma that harbors a V600E *BRAF* or *MEK* gene mutation, which may respond to the *BRAF* inhibitors vemurafenib and dabrafenib combined with MEK inhibitors trametinib and cobimetinib.

- The combination of ipilimumab, a checkpoint inhibitor targeting cytotoxic T-lymphocyte associated protein 4 (*CTLA4*), and nivolumab, an antibody against programmed cell death-1 receptor, has shown significant improvements in survival for patients with metastatic melanoma.

Follow-up

All patients should be encouraged to perform skin self-examinations as well as receive annual skin evaluations by a dermatologist for life. Patients with early-stage melanoma need not undergo routine blood testing or imaging studies in the absence of signs or symptoms.

H Oncologic Urgencies and Emergencies

Structural Urgencies and Emergencies

Superior Vena Cava Syndrome

Obstruction of the superior vena cava (SVC), or SVC syndrome, occurs in approximately 15,000 persons in the United States each year. Most cases are caused by malignancies with large mediastinal masses. Patients typically present with edema of the head, neck, and arms, often with cyanosis, plethora, and distended cutaneous collateral vessels. They may have headache, cough, dyspnea, hoarseness, or syncope. The severity of symptoms depends on the degree of narrowing of the SVC and the speed of onset, with slower development allowing venous collaterals to develop. Most patients do not require emergency intervention, and deaths due to SVC syndrome are rare, although tumors in that region may cause other emergencies, such as bronchial obstruction or cardiac tamponade. A chest CT scan with intravenous contrast usually confirms the diagnosis (**Figure 26**). Lung cancer accounts for almost 75% of cases of SVC syndrome, with lymphoma and metastatic disease each causing approximately 10%; rarer tumors, such as germ cell tumor, thymoma, or mesothelioma, account for the remainder.

Management is based on the severity of symptoms and the underlying malignancy. In patients requiring immediate treatment of respiratory distress, an SVC stent can be placed without tissue diagnosis and results in prompt improvement

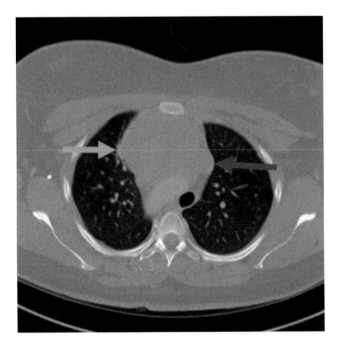

FIGURE 26. Superior vena cava (SVC) syndrome often presents on chest CT scan with bronchial obstruction due to mediastinal mass (*blue arrow*) and SVC compression (*red arrow*).

in symptoms. For most patients, a tissue diagnosis is obtained, with treatment directed by the type of cancer. Options for obtaining diagnostic tissue include mediastinoscopy, bronchoscopy, thoracentesis (if a pleural effusion is present), or biopsy of a peripheral area of lymphadenopathy. Complication rates are usually low.

Types of cancer that are highly responsive to chemotherapy, such as small cell lung cancer, lymphoma, and germ cell cancers, are treated with initial chemotherapy. Non–small cell lung cancer may be treated with initial chemotherapy, radiation therapy, or both. Initial surgery may be required in thymoma and mesothelioma. Although glucocorticoids and loop diuretics are often used, there is no clear evidence of their effectiveness. If thrombosis is present, anticoagulation should be added unless contraindicated.

Treatment of curable malignancies should not be compromised by the presence of SVC syndrome. The survival is the same as in patients with the same malignancies without this presentation. H

KEY POINTS

- Most patients with superior vena cava syndrome do not require emergency intervention; a tissue diagnosis should be obtained first with treatment directed by the type of cancer.
- Presentation with superior vena cava syndrome does not worsen prognosis in patients who present with otherwise curable malignancies.

Central Nervous System Emergencies

Increased Intracranial Pressure

Elevated intracranial pressure can result from primary brain malignancies or from brain metastases, which occur in 10% to 20% of adults cancer patients. The most common types of primary cancer that cause brain metastases are lung cancer, breast cancer, and melanoma. Median survival after diagnosis of brain metastases varies from less than 3 months to more than 25 months.

Symptoms of increased intracranial pressure include headache, depressed global consciousness, vomiting, and even signs and symptoms of herniation. Emergent CT or MRI imaging will confirm the diagnosis. Glucocorticoids relieve symptoms in 75% of patients by decreasing tumor-related vasogenic edema. Patients with severe symptoms are treated with a loading dose of dexamethasone of 10 to 20 mg followed by 4 to 6 mg every 6 hours. The most critically ill patients may require other measures, including osmotic diuresis with mannitol, head elevation, hyperventilation, and possibly decompressive surgery. Antiepileptic drugs should be used in the 25% of patients who present with seizures. See MKSAP 18 Neurology for further discussion of antiepileptic drugs. Anticoagulation can be safely used when indicated. Lumbar puncture is contraindicated in patients with an increased intracranial pressure because of the risk of herniation.

Spinal Cord Compression

CONT.

Neoplastic epidural spinal cord compression (ESCC) develops in approximately 2.5% of patients with metastatic cancer. The most common types of cancer that cause ESCC in adults are lung, breast, and prostate cancer; myeloma; and lymphoma. Approximately 85% of ESCC cases are due to epidural extension from vertebral body metastases. Lymphomas are more likely to involve a paraspinal mass that extends through the neural foramina to cause cord compression. Pain, often worse with recumbency, is present in more than 80% of patients and usually precedes neurologic symptoms by several weeks. The absence of neurologic signs should not delay evaluation of such pain. At times, ESCC may be the first sign of cancer, although patients with such a presentation often have other systemic signs, such as anorexia and weight loss. Pain can be radicular. Weakness is present in more than 60% of patients at presentation. If a sensory level is present, it is typically one to five levels below the actual level of cord compression. Bowel and bladder dysfunction is a late finding that is present in up to half of patients. MRI of the entire thecal sac is the preferred imaging test when ESCC is suspected.

The patient's neurologic status at diagnosis is the most important predictor of outcome. Of patients who are able to walk when starting treatment, 80% remain ambulatory; however, less than 20% of nonambulatory patients regain the ability to walk. Patients are initially treated with glucocorticoids at either a moderate or high dose if paraparesis or paraplegia is present. Definitive treatment with surgery, radiation, or both depends on whether the patient has a known cancer diagnosis, as well as the stability of the spine, the sensitivity of the cancer to radiation, and the patient's overall prognosis. For patients who are acceptable surgical candidates with an expected survival of at least 3 months, initial decompressive surgery followed by radiation increases the likelihood of ambulation compared with radiation alone. See MKSAP 18 Neurology for further discussion of spinal cord compression.

KEY POINTS

- Neoplastic spinal cord compression is initially treated with glucocorticoids; definitive treatment with surgery, radiation, or both depends on the whether the patient has a known cancer diagnosis, stability of the spine, the sensitivity of the cancer to radiation, and the patient's overall prognosis.

- Neurologic status is the most important predictor of outcome for patients with neoplastic spinal cord compression; ambulatory patients tend to remain ambulatory with treatment, but nonambulatory patients typically do not regain the ability to walk.

Malignant Pleural and Pericardial Effusions

Types of cancer that most commonly cause malignant pleural effusions include lymphomas; mesotheliomas; and carcinomas of the breast, lung, gastrointestinal tract, and ovaries.

Patients present with progressive dyspnea and may or may not have concomitant chest pain. See MKSAP 18 Pulmonary and Critical Care Medicine for further discussion of pleural effusions. Chest radiography is the initial diagnostic study, often followed by CT imaging, which provides more precise anatomic detail. Therapeutic thoracentesis is used as the initial treatment of symptomatic effusions. Further management depends on the rate of reaccumulation, the severity of symptoms, and the patient's prognosis. Recurrent effusion is common, unless the tumor is responsive to systemic therapy. Repeat thoracentesis is appropriate for slowly recurring effusions. For effusions with more rapid reaccumulation, the best options for management are placement of an indwelling pleural catheter with intermittent outpatient drainage or pleurodesis, with similar palliation obtained by either method. Less frequently, pleurectomy can be done to control malignant pleural effusions.

Malignancy accounts for 13% to 23% of pericardial effusions and may be the first presentation of the disease. Lung, breast, and esophageal cancers; melanoma; lymphoma; and leukemia are the most common malignancies that cause pericardial effusions. Cardiac tamponade results when the pericardial fluid pressure impairs filling of one or both ventricles, leading to decreased cardiac output. Patients present with dyspnea, chest discomfort, or fatigue. They usually have elevated jugular venous distention and may have hypotension and peripheral edema. Pulsus paradoxus, a greater than 10-mm decrease in systolic pressure with inspiration, is also typically present. Echocardiography usually establishes the diagnosis. Symptoms from progressive cardiac tamponade may be inappropriately attributed to nonspecific systemic signs of cancer or heart failure until cardiac filling and cardiac output is emergently compromised. See MKSAP 18 Cardiovascular Medicine for further discussion of cardiac tamponade.

Treatment of symptomatic pericardial effusion involves percutaneous pericardiocentesis or drainage during surgical placement of a pericardial window. The most common treatments to prevent recurrence are prolonged catheter drainage or surgical decompression with a pericardial window.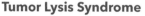

KEY POINT

- For slowly recurring malignant pleural effusions, repeat thoracentesis is appropriate; for more rapidly recurring pleural effusions, either an indwelling pleural catheter with intermittent outpatient drainage or pleurodesis is used.

Metabolic Urgencies and Emergencies

Tumor Lysis Syndrome

Tumor lysis syndrome (TLS) is caused when tumor cells release their contents into the bloodstream, either spontaneously or as a result of treatment, leading to hyperuricemia, hyperkalemia,

CONT.

hyperphosphatemia, and hypocalcemia. These electrolyte abnormalities can lead to acute kidney injury, cardiac arrhythmias, seizures, and death. TLS is seen most often in highly proliferative hematologic malignancies such as acute leukemia and high-grade lymphomas, but can develop in many other cancers.

The risk of TLS can be categorized based on the volume of cancer mass present; the cell-lysis potential of the cancer; and patient characteristics of preexisting kidney failure, dehydration, acidosis, hypotension, or nephrotoxin exposure. Patients at intermediate risk for TLS can be managed with monitoring of laboratory values, hydration, and allopurinol, and those at high risk should receive intravenous hydration and rasburicase, a urate oxidase enzyme that metabolizes uric acid, before receiving chemotherapy. There is no clear benefit of alkalinization to increase uric acid excretion, particularly given the availability of rasburicase. Alkalinization increases the risk of hyperphosphatemia.

Patients who develop TLS require continuous cardiac monitoring; serum measurement of electrolytes, creatinine, and uric acid every 4 to 6 hours; and correction of electrolyte abnormalities. Rasburicase should be given and patients should receive aggressive hydration if kidney function allows, with the use of a loop diuretic if needed to improve urinary output. Patients may require renal replacement therapy for severe oliguria or anuria, persistent hyperkalemia, symptomatic hypocalcemia, or a calcium–phosphate product greater than or equal to 70 mg²/dL².

KEY POINT

- Tumor lysis syndrome should be treated with rasburicase and aggressive hydration if kidney function allows; patients require continuous cardiac monitoring and measurement of electrolyte, creatinine, and uric acid levels every 4 to 6 hours.

Hypercalcemia of Malignancy

Hypercalcemia of malignancy (HCM) occurs in 20% to 30% of patients with advanced cancer. It is most frequent in patients with myeloma and cancer of the lung, breast, kidney, and head and neck. Osteolytic bone metastases are usually the cause of HCM in breast cancer and myeloma, although the incidence of hypercalcemia in these patients may be decreasing with the prophylactic use of bisphosphonates. Paraneoplastic production of parathyroid hormone–related protein may occur in localized tumors without widespread bone metastases. Lymphomas can cause hypercalcemia by overproduction of 1,25-dihydroxyvitamin D. Malignancies such as ovarian cancer can produce ectopic parathyroid hormone.

Patients may present with nausea, vomiting, constipation, fatigue, polyuria, polydipsia, altered mental status, or muscle weakness. Symptoms depend on both the serum calcium level and the rate of rise. Rapidly rising levels and levels greater than 14 mg/dL (3.5 mmol/L) are most likely to cause severe symptoms. Hypercalcemia can result in dehydration, nephrogenic diabetes insipidus, and acute kidney injury.

Patients with severe or symptomatic hypercalcemia should receive isotonic saline volume expansion. Loop diuretics are not recommended unless kidney failure or heart failure is present, in which case volume expansion should precede the administration of loop diuretics to avoid hypotension and further kidney injury. Calcitonin increases kidney excretion of calcium and decreases bone resorption; it can decrease calcium within several hours in responsive patients. The most effective agents are bisphosphonates, such as zoledronic acid, which inhibit bone resorption and can lower calcium levels to normal in 50% of patients in 4 days and in 88% of patients in 10 days. The receptor activator of nuclear factor κB ligand denosumab can be considered for patients who do not respond to zoledronic acid. It can be safely used in patients with kidney failure where bisphosphonates may be contraindicated. Effective treatment of the underlying malignancy remains the most appropriate means of controlling hypercalcemia.

KEY POINT

- Patients with severe or symptomatic hypercalcemia should receive isotonic saline volume expansion, calcitonin, and bisphosphonates; loop diuretics are not recommended unless kidney failure or heart failure is present.

Effects of Cancer Therapy and Survivorship

Effects of Cancer Therapy

Hematologic Toxicity

The major toxicity of many traditional chemotherapeutic agents remains myelosuppression, leading to anemia, neutropenia, and thrombocytopenia.

Neutropenia and Fever

The risk of infection increases with the magnitude and the duration of neutropenia, which typically occurs 5 to 15 days after chemotherapy administration. Serious infectious complications are more likely when the absolute neutrophil count is below 500/μL (0.5×10^9/L) and the expected duration is more than 7 days. Fever in a patient with neutropenia is an emergency, as patients can become septic quickly. Prompt evaluation, including blood count and other appropriate cultures, and administration of empiric, broad-spectrum antibiotics, typically a third-generation cephalosporin alone or in combination (even in the absence of a documented or suspected site of infection), is critical. Selected patients without significant comorbidities who are medically stable and adherent, and in whom a short duration of neutropenia is anticipated, can be treated on an outpatient basis with intravenous or oral antibiotics.

The prophylactic use of granulocyte colony-stimulating factor or granulocyte-macrophage colony-stimulating factor reduces the risk of febrile neutropenia. These medications may be given to patients receiving regimens associated with a high risk of this complication or as secondary prophylaxis in patients with a previous episode of neutropenic fever. Growth factors are not used in the treatment of patients with neutropenic fever unless the patient has either persistent fever despite antibiotic treatment or severe neutropenia (absolute neutrophil count less than 100/μL [0.1 × 10⁹/L]) expected to last more than 7 days.

> **KEY POINT**
>
> HVC
> - Growth factors are not used in the treatment of patients with neutropenic fever unless the patient has either persistent fever despite antibiotic treatment or severe neutropenia (absolute neutrophil count less than 100/μL [0.1 × 10⁹/L]) expected to last more than 7 days.

Anemia and Thrombocytopenia

Anemia in patients with cancer may be multifactorial, related to chronic inflammation, bone marrow suppression, blood loss, and chemotherapy. Anemia contributes significantly but not solely to the fatigue patients with cancer endure. Erythrocyte transfusions and erythropoietin administration are sometimes required. The enthusiasm for erythropoietin has been tempered by studies suggesting that symptom improvement is achieved at a cost of more rapid cancer progression and increased risk of venous thromboembolism. This concern has prompted increased regulation and a significant decrease in the use of erythropoietin therapy in patients with cancer, particularly for those receiving curative or adjuvant treatments.

Thrombocytopenia is generally managed with platelet transfusions, when needed, and appropriate dose reductions and delays.

Nausea and Vomiting

Although nausea and vomiting are still common side effects of chemotherapy, their incidence and severity have been markedly reduced by antiemetic medications. Delayed nausea (more than 1 day after treatment), especially with cisplatin regimens, has not been as effectively prevented. Chemotherapy agents can be separated into mild, moderate, and severe emetogenic effect categories. For patients receiving moderate to severely emetogenic drugs, administration of serotonin receptor antagonists (such as ondansetron or the longer-acting palonosetron) in combination with high-dose glucocorticoid therapy is standard. Improvement in both acute and delayed nausea and vomiting is seen with the addition of neurokinin 1 receptor blockers (such as aprepitant and netupitant). Further benefit has been reported with the antipsychotic agent olanzapine.

Dermatologic Effects

Cutaneous toxicities vary in frequency, severity, and type. Alopecia is the most common but does not occur with all chemotherapy agents. Almost all drugs have the potential to cause allergic reactions; examples of severe reactions include toxic epidermal necrolysis and Stevens-Johnson syndrome.

Fluoropyrimidines (5-fluorouracil and capecitabine) are associated with palmar-plantar erythrodysesthesia ("hand-foot syndrome"), described as redness, peeling, and tenderness of the palms and soles. Small-molecule epidermal growth factor receptor (EGFR) inhibitors, such as erlotinib and gefitinib, used to treat *EGFR*-mutated lung cancer, are associated with pustular acneiform eruptions and other skin changes, including dryness. Monoclonal antibodies against EGFR (cetuximab and panitumumab) are associated with a similar and often more severe acneiform eruption. See MKSAP 18 Dermatology for further discussion of dermatologic chemotherapy reactions.

Disorders of Pulmonary Function

A wide variety of chemotherapy agents can be associated with pulmonary injury, likely from various mechanisms. Bleomycin, nitrosoureas, and gemcitabine may have the strongest associations with pulmonary toxicity, but many others have toxicity potential. In addition, various monoclonal antibodies and targeted therapies can be associated with pulmonary toxicities, including rituximab, trastuzumab, cetuximab, and erlotinib.

Radiation therapy can be associated with a pneumonitis, typically occurring within 1 to 3 months of treatment, and may lead to the development of radiation fibrosis. See MKSAP 18 Pulmonary and Critical Care Medicine for further discussion of disorders of pulmonary function related to chemotherapy.

Disorders of Genitourinary and Kidney Function

Several chemotherapy agents can affect kidney function. Cisplatin is the most common agent and is associated with acute tubular necrosis. The risk is reduced with the use of aggressive hydration. Ifosfamide can be associated with kidney disease and significant tubular toxicity, with long-term potassium, magnesium, and bicarbonate wasting. Both ifosfamide and cyclophosphamide, in high doses, may cause a hemorrhagic cystitis. Hemolytic uremic syndrome is associated with various chemotherapy agents, most commonly with mitomycin and gemcitabine. Kidney failure can occur with tumor lysis syndrome.

Neurologic Toxicity

Peripheral neuropathy is a common toxicity of several chemotherapy agents, most commonly occurring with platinums, taxanes, and vinca alkaloids, as well as with newer agents, such as bortezomib. Oxaliplatin causes a transient hypersensitivity to cold—patients must avoid eating, drinking, or even touching cold items for several days after infusions—as well as a non–temperature-dependent persistent peripheral neuropathy that may be more problematic in the long term. Therapies are sometimes continued with appropriate dose reductions if there are only mild sensory symptoms. However, when patients develop significant symptoms with dysfunction, pain, and motor weakness, therapies are discontinued. Although symptoms may alleviate over time, some patients are left with significant deficits. Medications such as gabapentin and duloxetine may help alleviate discomfort but no definitive neuroprotective agents or strategies have proved to reliably prevent or resolve these symptoms.

Rituximab, along with other immunosuppressive agents, rarely has been associated with progressive multifocal leukoencephalopathy. 5-Fluorouracil and high-dose cytosine arabinoside are associated with cerebellar toxicity. The reversible posterior encephalopathy syndrome, consisting of headache, visual disturbances, delirium, and seizures associated with characteristic white matter edema in the posterior brain, has been linked to chemotherapy that targets vascular endothelial growth factor, such as bevacizumab or sunitinib.

Whole brain radiation can cause impairment of cognitive function. In some situations, this toxicity can be reduced by the use of focused high-dose radiation (gamma knife or stereotactic radiosurgery) to identified lesions. See MKSAP 18 Neurology for further discussion of disorders of peripheral neuropathy related to chemotherapy.

Toxicities Related to Immune Dysregulation

With the increasing use of checkpoint inhibitors for various tumors, patients with cancer are at risk for toxicities associated with the induction of autoimmunity. Antibodies such as ipilimumab (anti–cytotoxic T-lymphocyte associated protein 4 [CTLA4]), pembrolizumab and nivolumab (anti–programmed death receptor-1 [PD-1]), and atezolizumab (anti–programmed death ligand-1 [PDL1]), are associated with immune-related toxicities, including colitis, pneumonitis, hepatitis, dermatitis, hypophysitis, thyroiditis, and adrenalitis. These toxicities occur in a small but significant minority of patients and require prompt recognition and often glucocorticoid therapy as well as hormone replacement, if indicated. H

KEY POINTS

- Fever in a neutropenic patient with cancer is an emergency requiring prompt evaluation and administration of empiric broad-spectrum antibiotics.
- **HVC** Patients with febrile neutropenia expected to be of short duration, who lack significant comorbidity and who have reliable home care and follow-up, can be treated with oral antibiotics on an outpatient basis.
- Standard antiemetic treatment of patients taking moderate to severe emetogenic chemotherapy drugs is a serotonin receptor antagonist (ondansetron or palonosetron) and a high-dose glucocorticoid.

Survivorship Issues

As patients with cancer live longer, being either cured or surviving for more extended periods, survivorship issues have assumed greater importance. Survivorship embodies the care that follows patients on completion of their treatments, including screening for recurrence and secondary malignancies; monitoring for late organ dysfunction; and helping patients cope with the psychological, sexual, vocational, and other effects of treatment. An initial treatment plan for cancer may be based not only on providing the highest probability of cure but also on a strategy to reduce the risk of long-term complications.

Late Effects of Cancer Therapy
Effects on Bone Health

Bone loss occurs at an increased rate in female cancer survivors who have taken long-term glucocorticoids; those who have undergone surgical, radiation, or chemotherapy-induced premature menopause; and those taking aromatase inhibitors for breast cancer. Men treated for prostate cancer with androgen deprivation therapy may also develop osteoporosis. Multiple myeloma, in addition to causing lytic bone disease, can be associated with generalized bone loss. Assessment of bone density and treatment or prophylaxis should be considered to reduce the risk of fracture. Treatment commonly includes routine supplements of vitamin D and calcium (while monitoring serum calcium levels) and bisphosphonates or denosumab (a receptor activator of nuclear factor κB ligand monoclonal antibody). Vigilance for complications with these agents, which can include osteonecrosis of the jaw and atypical subtrochanteric spiral fractures of the femur, is required for patients on these agents.

Disorders of Cardiac Function

Radiation therapy to the heart can lead to valvular disease, myocardial and pericardial disease, and coronary disease. These risks have been reduced owing to advances in dosing, treatment planning, and modern radiation techniques. Doxorubicin and other anthracyclines can cause irreversible cardiomyopathy; the risk for this increases with cumulative dosing. Trastuzumab can also induce non-dose-dependent cardiomyopathy; the risk increases when trastuzumab is combined with anthracyclines. Fluoropyrimidines (5-fluorouracil and capecitabine) have been associated with a risk of coronary spasm and ischemia during administration.

Newer-generation tyrosine kinase inhibitors for treatment of chronic myeloid leukemia have been associated with cardiovascular morbidity, nilotinib and ponatinib are associated with coronary insufficiency, and dasatinib is associated with pulmonary hypertension. The anti–vascular endothelial growth factor antibody bevacizumab is associated with an increased risk of coronary and other vascular events, both arterial and venous.

Monitoring for and management of cardiac complications in cancer survivors is discussed in MKSAP 18 Cardiovascular Medicine.

Sexual Function and Fertility

Surgery, radiation, and chemotherapy all have the potential to affect sexual function and fertility of both men and women. Altered body image after breast surgery or other radical resection and the generalized fatigue associated with most radiation or chemotherapy may reduce libido. Anxiety and depression further diminish interest in sex. Individual counseling and support groups may be helpful.

In women, premature menopause and infertility can result from both pelvic radiotherapy and chemotherapy, particularly with alkylating agents. Risk factors for infertility relate to the dose and duration of chemotherapy as well as patient age, with older women being at greater risk for premature menopause. Consultation with experts in fertility should be considered in younger women who desire future childbearing; egg and embryo harvests may be options. Fertility evaluations can often be done on an emergency basis so delay in the initiation of definitive cancer treatment is minimized. Men may be offered the option of semen cryopreservation.

Hormonal therapy for women with breast cancer, including tamoxifen, aromatase inhibitors, and ovarian suppression, may cause menopausal symptoms, decreased libido, and vaginal dryness. Men with prostate cancer commonly suffer from erectile dysfunction after surgery, radiation, and androgen suppression therapy.

Cognitive Decline

Short-term and long-term declines in cognitive function are now recognized as a complication after cancer therapy. It remains unclear whether cancer and its treatment unmasks preexisting cognitive impairment that was not yet manifest, whether the decline represents a sign of more rapid aging, or whether there is a more specific neurotoxic effect. Symptoms may include impairment of multitasking and executive function, memory, and verbal ability. Behavioral therapy may be beneficial. Patients with cancer who complain of a decline in cognitive function should have their experience acknowledged and validated, and behavioral therapy should be offered.

KEY POINTS

- Fertility preservation options before cancer treatment include egg and embryo harvests for women and semen cryopreservation for men.

- Patients with cancer who complain of a decline in cognitive function should have their experience acknowledged and validated, and behavioral therapy should be offered.

Survivorship Care Plan

Patients with cancer go through distinct phases of management, beginning with the initial therapy and any maintenance or adjuvant treatment needed to achieve and prolong remission. Once in remission, these patients go through a phase of surveillance for disease recurrence. Whereas the duration of the surveillance phase and the extent of active assessment through physician examination and diagnostic imaging differs based on the underlying cancer, patients eventually reach the "survivor" phase, wherein disease recurrence becomes unlikely.

Providing patients with a prescription for survivorship is an important responsibility of oncologists. Patients are given a formal document summarizing their diagnosis, stage, and treatment details, along with recommended follow-up by the oncologist as they return to their internist. Recommendations can include surveillance for cancer recurrence; lifestyle modifications, such as diet, exercise, and avoiding tobacco and alcohol to reduce the risk of a second malignancy; and a discussion of the late effects of cancer treatment that may occur and any strategies for preventing or reducing them.

Cancer survivors should, at a minimum, have age- and gender-appropriate cancer screening. Secondary malignancies may develop in cancer survivors owing to a preexisting genetic predisposition, a "field" effect from previous carcinogen exposure, or late effects of previous cancer treatments. Patients with *BRCA* gene mutations have an increased risk of breast and ovarian cancer. Patients with smoking-related head and neck cancer are prone to second head and neck cancers, as well as lung and esophageal cancers. Patients exposed to chemotherapy with alkylating agents have an increased risk of myelodysplastic syndromes and acute leukemia. Radiation to the neck can be associated with the development not just of hypothyroidism but also of thyroid cancer years later. Women receiving radiation to the mediastinum for Hodgkin lymphoma and other cancers have a marked increase of breast cancer, particularly if they were treated in adolescence and early adulthood, with the increased risk beginning within 8 years of treatment. Screening MRI, mammography, or a combination of both modalities is recommended for these patients beginning at age 25 years or 8 years after completion of radiation therapy, whichever occurs last.

KEY POINTS

- A "prescription for survivorship" provides the patient with recommendations regarding surveillance for cancer recurrence, lifestyle modifications to reduce the risk of a second malignancy, and strategies to prevent or reduce the late effects of cancer treatment.

- Various factors, including genetic predisposition, "field" effect, and the carcinogenic effects of cancer therapies, all increase the risk of secondary malignancies in patients in remission after therapy for their primary cancer.

- Mediastinal radiation is associated with a marked increase of breast cancer beginning within 8 years of treatment; screening MRI, mammography, or a combination of both modalities is recommended for women beginning at age 25 years or 8 years after completion of radiation therapy, whichever occurs last.

Bibliography

Hematopoietic Stem Cells and Their Disorders

Al Ustwani O, Gupta N, Bakhribah H, Griffiths E, Wang E, Wetzler M. Clinical updates in adult acute lymphoblastic leukemia. Crit Rev Oncol Hematol. 2016;99:189-99. [PMID: 26777876] doi:10.1016/j.critrevonc.2015.12.007

Diller L. Clinical practice. Adult primary care after childhood acute lymphoblastic leukemia. N Engl J Med. 2011;365:1417-24. [PMID: 21995389] doi:10.1056/NEJMcp1103645

Döhner H, Weisdorf DJ, Bloomfield CD. Acute myeloid leukemia. N Engl J Med. 2015;373:1136-52. [PMID: 26376137] doi:10.1056/NEJMra1406184

Fenaux P, Haase D, Sanz GF, Santini V, Buske C; ESMO Guidelines Working Group. Myelodysplastic syndromes: ESMO Clinical Practice Guidelines for diagnosis, treatment and follow-up. Ann Oncol. 2014;25 Suppl 3:iii57-69. [PMID: 25185242] doi:10.1093/annonc/mdu180

Greenberg PL, Stone RM, Bejar R, Bennett JM, Bloomfield CD, Borate U, et al; National comprehensive cancer network. Myelodysplastic syndromes, version 2.2015. J Natl Compr Canc Netw. 2015;13:261-72. [PMID: 25736003]

Killick SB, Bown N, Cavenagh J, Dokal I, Foukaneli T, Hill A, et al; British Society for Standards in Haematology. Guidelines for the diagnosis and management of adult aplastic anaemia. Br J Haematol. 2016;172:187-207. [PMID: 26568159] doi:10.1111/bjh.13853

Smith TJ, Bohlke K, Lyman GH, Carson KR, Crawford J, Cross SJ, et al; American Society of Clinical Oncology. recommendations for the use of WBC growth factors: American Society of Clinical Oncology Clinical Practice Guideline Update. J Clin Oncol. 2015;33:3199-212. [PMID: 26169616] doi:10.1200/JCO.2015.62.3488

Spivak JL. Myeloproliferative neoplasms. N Engl J Med. 2017;376:2168-2181. [PMID: 28564565] doi:10.1056/NEJMra1406186

Vannucchi AM, Barbui T, Cervantes F, Harrison C, Kiladjian JJ, Kröger N, et al; ESMO Guidelines Committee. Philadelphia chromosome-negative chronic myeloproliferative neoplasms: ESMO Clinical Practice Guidelines for diagnosis, treatment and follow-up. Ann Oncol. 2015;26 Suppl 5:v85-99. [PMID: 26242182] doi:10.1093/annonc/mdv203

Vannucchi AM, Kiladjian JJ, Griesshammer M, Masszi T, Durrant S, Passamonti F, et al. Ruxolitinib versus standard therapy for the treatment of polycythemia vera. N Engl J Med. 2015;372:426-35. [PMID: 25629741] doi:10.1056/NEJMoa1409002

Multiple Myeloma and Related Disorders

Chng WJ, Dispenzieri A, Chim CS, Fonseca R, Goldschmidt H, Lentzsch S, et al; International Myeloma Working Group. IMWG consensus on risk stratification in multiple myeloma. Leukemia. 2014;28:269-77. [PMID: 23974982] doi:10.1038/leu.2013.247

Gillmore JD, Wechalekar A, Bird J, Cavenagh J, Hawkins S, Kazmi M, et al; BCSH Committee. Guidelines on the diagnosis and investigation of AL amyloidosis. Br J Haematol. 2015;168:207-18. [PMID: 25312307] doi:10.1111/bjh.13156

Kumar S, Dispenzieri A, Lacy MQ, Hayman SR, Buadi FK, Colby C, et al. Revised prognostic staging system for light chain amyloidosis incorporating cardiac biomarkers and serum free light chain measurements. J Clin Oncol. 2012;30:989-95. [PMID: 22331953] doi:10.1200/JCO.2011.38.5724

Leblond V, Kastritis E, Advani R, Ansell SM, Buske C, Castillo JJ, et al. Treatment recommendations from the Eighth International Workshop on Waldenström's Macroglobulinemia. Blood. 2016;128:1321-8. [PMID: 27432877] doi:10.1182/blood-2016-04-711234

Lokhorst HM, Plesner T, Laubach JP, Nahi H, Gimsing P, Hansson M, et al. Targeting CD38 with daratumumab monotherapy in multiple myeloma. N Engl J Med. 2015;373:1207-19. [PMID: 26308596] doi:10.1056/NEJMoa1506348

Palumbo A, Rajkumar SV, San Miguel JF, Larocca A, Niesvizky R, Morgan G, et al. International Myeloma Working Group consensus statement for the management, treatment, and supportive care of patients with myeloma not eligible for standard autologous stem-cell transplantation. J Clin Oncol. 2014;32:587-600. [PMID: 24419113] doi:10.1200/JCO.2013.48.7934

Rajkumar SV, Dimopoulos MA, Palumbo A, Blade J, Merlini G, Mateos MV, et al. International Myeloma Working Group updated criteria for the diagnosis of multiple myeloma. Lancet Oncol. 2014;15:e538-48. [PMID: 25439696] doi:10.1016/S1470-2045(14)70442-5

van de Donk NW, Palumbo A, Johnsen HE, Engelhardt M, Gay F, Gregersen H, et al; European Myeloma Network. The clinical relevance and management of monoclonal gammopathy of undetermined significance and related disorders: recommendations from the European Myeloma Network. Haematologica. 2014;99:984-96. [PMID: 24658815] doi:10.3324/haematol.2013.100552

Erythrocyte Disorders

Barcellini W. Immune hemolysis: diagnosis and treatment recommendations. Semin Hematol. 2015;52:304-12. [PMID: 26404442] doi:10.1053/j.seminhematol.2015.05.001

Brodsky RA. Complement in hemolytic anemia. Blood. 2015;126:2459-65. [PMID: 26582375] doi:10.1182/blood-2015-06-640995

Da Costa L, Galimand J, Fenneteau O, Mohandas N. Hereditary spherocytosis, elliptocytosis, and other red cell membrane disorders. Blood Rev. 2013;27:167-78. [PMID: 23664421] doi:10.1016/j.blre.2013.04.003

Finberg KE. Regulation of systemic iron homeostasis. Curr Opin Hematol. 2013;20:208-14. [PMID: 23426198] doi:10.1097/MOH.0b013e32835f5a47

Chapter 1: Diagnosis and evaluation of anemia in CKD. Kidney Int Suppl (2011). 2012;2:288-291. [PMID: 25018948]

Lopez A, Cacoub P, Macdougall IC, Peyrin-Biroulet L. Iron deficiency anaemia. Lancet. 2016;387:907-16. [PMID: 26314490] doi:10.1016/S0140-6736(15)60865-0

Luzzatto L, Nannelli C, Notaro R. Glucose-6-phosphate dehydrogenase deficiency. Hematol Oncol Clin North Am. 2016;30:373-93. [PMID: 27040960] doi:10.1016/j.hoc.2015.11.006

Moretti D, Goede JS, Zeder C, Jiskra M, Chatzinakou V, Tjalsma H, et al. Oral iron supplements increase hepcidin and decrease iron absorption from daily or twice-daily doses in iron-depleted young women. Blood. 2015;126:1981-9. [PMID: 26289639] doi:10.1182/blood-2015-05-642223

Piel FB, Steinberg MH, Rees DC. Sickle cell disease. N Engl J Med. 2017;376:1561-1573. [PMID: 28423290] doi:10.1056/NEJMra1510865

Rund D. Thalassemia 2016: Modern medicine battles an ancient disease. Am J Hematol. 2016;91:15-21. [PMID: 26537527] doi:10.1002/ajh.24231

Shipton MJ, Thachil J. Vitamin B12 deficiency - a 21st century perspective . Clin Med (Lond). 2015;15:145-50. [PMID: 25824066] doi:10.7861/clinmedicine.15-2-145

Vichinsky E. Non-transfusion-dependent thalassemia and thalassemia intermedia: epidemiology, complications, and management. Curr Med Res Opin. 2016;32:191-204. [PMID: 26479125] doi:10.1185/03007995.2015.1110128

Iron Overload Syndromes

Bacon BR, Adams PC, Kowdley KV, Powell LW, Tavill AS; American Association for the Study of Liver Diseases. Diagnosis and management of hemochromatosis: 2011 practice guideline by the American Association for the Study of Liver Diseases. Hepatology. 2011;54:328-43. [PMID: 21452290] doi:10.1002/hep.24330

Brittenham GM. Iron-chelating therapy for transfusional iron overload. N Engl J Med. 2011;364:146-56. [PMID: 21226580] doi:10.1056/NEJMct1004810

Platelet Disorders

Fakhouri F, Zuber J, Frémeaux-Bacchi V, Loirat C. Haemolytic uraemic syndrome. Lancet. 2017;390:681-696. [PMID: 28242109] doi:10.1016/S0140-6736(17)30062-4

George JN. Measuring ADAMTS13 activity in patients with suspected thrombotic thrombocytopenic purpura: when, how, and why? [Editorial]. Transfusion. 2015;55:11-3. [PMID: 25582234] doi:10.1111/trf.12885

Greinacher A. CLINICAL PRACTICE. Heparin-induced thrombocytopenia. N Engl J Med. 2015;373:252-61. [PMID: 26176382] doi:10.1056/NEJMcp1411910

McGowan KE, Makari J, Diamantouros A, Bucci C, Rempel P, Selby R, et al. Reducing the hospital burden of heparin-induced thrombocytopenia: impact of an avoid-heparin program. Blood. 2016;127:1954-9. [PMID: 26817956] doi:10.1182/blood-2015-07-660001

Neunert C, Noroozi N, Norman G, Buchanan GR, Goy J, Nazi I, et al. Severe bleeding events in adults and children with primary immune thrombocytopenia: a systematic review. J Thromb Haemost. 2015;13:457-64. [PMID: 25495497] doi:10.1111/jth.12813

Paniccia R, Priora R, Liotta AA, Abbate R. Platelet function tests: a comparative review. Vasc Health Risk Manag. 2015;11:133-48. [PMID: 25733843] doi:10.2147/VHRM.S44469

Tarantino MD, Fogarty PF, Shah P, Brainsky A. Dental procedures in 24 patients with chronic immune thrombocytopenia in prospective clinical studies of eltrombopag. Platelets. 2015;26:93-6. [PMID: 24433306] doi:10.3109/09537104.2013.870333

Warkentin TE, Pai M, Linkins LA. Direct oral anticoagulants for treatment of HIT: update of Hamilton experience and literature review. Blood. 2017;130:1104-1113. [PMID: 28646118] doi:10.1182/blood-2017-04-778993

Wei Y, Ji XB, Wang YW, Wang JX, Yang EQ, Wang ZC, et al. High-dose dexamethasone vs prednisone for treatment of adult immune thrombocytopenia: a prospective multicenter randomized trial. Blood. 2016;127:296-302; quiz 370. [PMID: 26480931] doi:10.1182/blood-2015-07-659656

Bleeding Disorders

Blackshear JL, Wysokinska EM, Safford RE, Thomas CS, Shapiro BP, Ung S, et al. Shear stress-associated acquired von Willebrand syndrome in patients with mitral regurgitation. J Thromb Haemost. 2014;12:1966-74. [PMID: 25251907] doi:10.1111/jth.12734

Donohoe K, Levine R. Acquired factor V inhibitor after exposure to topical human thrombin related to an otorhinolaryngological procedure. J Thromb Haemost. 2015;13:1787-9. [PMID: 26270511] doi:10.1111/jth.13114

Ferraris VA, Boral LI, Cohen AJ, Smyth SS, White GC 2nd. Consensus review of the treatment of cardiovascular disease in people with hemophilia A and B. Cardiol Rev. 2015;23:53-68. [PMID: 25436468] doi:10.1097/CRD.0000000000000045

Franchini M, Mannucci PM. Acquired haemophilia A: a 2013 update. Thromb Haemost. 2013;110:1114-20. [PMID: 24008306] doi:10.1160/TH13-05-0363

Marks PW. Hematologic manifestations of liver disease. Semin Hematol. 2013;50:216-21. [PMID: 23953338] doi:10.1053/j.seminhematol.2013.06.003

Ng C, Motto DG, Di Paola J. Diagnostic approach to von Willebrand disease. Blood. 2015;125:2029-37. [PMID: 25712990] doi:10.1182/blood-2014-08-528398

Roberts JC, Morateck PA, Christopherson PA, Yan K, Hoffmann RG, Gill JC, et al; Zimmerman Program Investigators. Rapid discrimination of the phenotypic variants of von Willebrand disease. Blood. 2016;127:2472-80. [PMID: 26917779] doi:10.1182/blood-2015-11-664680

Yates SG, Gavva C, Agrawal D, Sarode R. How do we transfuse blood components in cirrhotic patients undergoing gastrointestinal procedures? Transfusion. 2016;56:791-8. [PMID: 26876945] doi:10.1111/trf.13495

Transfusion Medicine

Carson JL, Grossman BJ, Kleinman S, Tinmouth AT, Marques MB, Fung MK, et al; Clinical Transfusion Medicine Committee of the AABB. Red blood cell transfusion: a clinical practice guideline from the AABB*. Ann Intern Med. 2012;157:49-58. [PMID: 22751760]

Delaney M, Wendel S, Bercovitz RS, Cid J, Cohn C, Dunbar NM, et al; Biomedical Excellence for Safer Transfusion (BEST) Collaborative. Transfusion reactions: prevention, diagnosis, and treatment. Lancet. 2016;388:2825-2836. [PMID: 27083327] doi:10.1016/S0140-6736(15)01313-6

Goldstein JN, Refaai MA, Milling TJ Jr, Lewis B, Goldberg-Alberts R, Hug BA, et al. Four-factor prothrombin complex concentrate versus plasma for rapid vitamin K antagonist reversal in patients needing urgent surgical or invasive interventions: a phase 3b, open-label, non-inferiority, randomised trial. Lancet. 2015;385:2077-87. [PMID: 25728933] doi:10.1016/S0140-6736(14)61685-8

Goodnough LT, Levy JH, Murphy MF. Concepts of blood transfusion in adults. Lancet. 2013;381:1845-54. [PMID: 23706801] doi:10.1016/S0140-6736(13)60650-9

Murphy GJ, Pike K, Rogers CA, Wordsworth S, Stokes EA, Angelini GD, et al; TITRe2 Investigators. Liberal or restrictive transfusion after cardiac surgery. N Engl J Med. 2015;372:997-1008. [PMID: 25760354] doi:10.1056/NEJMoa1403612

Schwartz J, Winters JL, Padmanabhan A, Balogun RA, Delaney M, Linenberger ML, et al. Guidelines on the use of therapeutic apheresis in clinical practice-evidence-based approach from the Writing Committee of the American Society for Apheresis: the sixth special issue. J Clin Apher. 2013;28:145-284. [PMID: 23868759] doi:10.1002/jca.21276

Villanueva C, Colomo A, Bosch A, Concepción M, Hernandez-Gea V, Aracil C, et al. Transfusion strategies for acute upper gastrointestinal bleeding. N Engl J Med. 2013;368:11-21. [PMID: 23281973] doi:10.1056/NEJMoa1211801

Thrombotic Disorders

Kearon C, Akl EA, Ornelas J, Blaivas A, Jimenez D, Bounameaux H, et al. Antithrombotic therapy for VTE disease: CHEST Guideline and Expert Panel Report. Chest. 2016;149:315-52. [PMID: 26867832] doi:10.1016/j.chest.2015.11.026

Pollack CV Jr, Reilly PA, Eikelboom J, Glund S, Verhamme P, Bernstein RA, et al. Idarucizumab for dabigatran reversal. N Engl J Med. 2015;373:511-20. [PMID: 26095746] doi:10.1056/NEJMoa1502000

Raja AS, Greenberg JO, Qaseem A, Denberg TD, Fitterman N, Schuur JD; Clinical Guidelines Committee of the American College of Physicians. Evaluation of patients with suspected acute pulmonary embolism: best practice advice from the Clinical Guidelines Committee of the American College of Physicians. Ann Intern Med. 2015;163:701-11. [PMID: 26414967]

van Dongen CJ, van den Belt AG, Prins MH, Lensing AW. Fixed dose subcutaneous low molecular weight heparins versus adjusted dose unfractionated heparin for venous thromboembolism. Cochrane Database Syst Rev. 2004:CD001100. [PMID: 15495007]

Hematologic Issues in Pregnancy

Kamel H, Navi BB, Sriram N, Hovsepian DA, Devereux RB, Elkind MS. Risk of a thrombotic event after the 6-week postpartum period. N Engl J Med. 2014;370:1307-15. [PMID: 24524551] doi:10.1056/NEJMoa1311485

Klings ES, Machado RF, Barst RJ, Morris CR, Mubarak KK, Gordeuk VR, et al; American Thoracic Society Ad Hoc Committee on Pulmonary Hypertension of Sickle Cell Disease. An official American Thoracic Society clinical practice guideline: diagnosis, risk stratification, and management of pulmonary hypertension of sickle cell disease. Am J Respir Crit Care Med. 2014;189:727-40. [PMID: 24628312] doi:10.1164/rccm.201401-0065ST

Malinowski AK, Shehata N, D'Souza R, Kuo KH, Ward R, Shah PS, et al. Prophylactic transfusion for pregnant women with sickle cell disease: a systematic review and meta-analysis. Blood. 2015;126:2424-35; quiz 2437. [PMID: 26302758] doi:10.1182/blood-2015-06-649319

Scully M, Thomas M, Underwood M, Watson H, Langley K, Camilleri RS, et al; collaborators of the UK TTP Registry. Thrombotic thrombocytopenic purpura and pregnancy: presentation, management, and subsequent pregnancy outcomes. Blood. 2014;124:211-9. [PMID: 24859360] doi:10.1182/blood-2014-02-553131

Yawn BP, Buchanan GR, Afenyi-Annan AN, Ballas SK, Hassell KL, James AH, et al. Management of sickle cell disease: summary of the 2014 evidence-based report by expert panel members. JAMA. 2014;312:1033-48. [PMID: 25203083] doi:10.1001/jama.2014.10517

Issues in Oncology

Kesselheim AS, Avorn J, Sarpatwari A. The high cost of prescription drugs in the united states: origins and prospects for reform. JAMA. 2016;316:858-71. [PMID: 27552619] doi:10.1001/jama.2016.11237

Khalil DN, Smith EL, Brentjens RJ, Wolchok JD. The future of cancer treatment: immunomodulation, CARs and combination immunotherapy. Nat Rev Clin Oncol. 2016;13:273-90. [PMID: 26977780] doi:10.1038/nrclinonc.2016.25

Saltz LB. Perspectives on cost and value in cancer care [Editorial]. JAMA Oncol. 2016;2:19-21. [PMID: 26501848] doi:10.1001/jamaoncol.2015.4191

Breast Cancer

Finch AP, Lubinski J, Møller P, Singer CF, Karlan B, Senter L, et al. Impact of oophorectomy on cancer incidence and mortality in women with a BRCA1 or BRCA2 mutation. J Clin Oncol. 2014;32:1547-53. [PMID: 24567435] doi:10.1200/JCO.2013.53.2820

Finn RS, Crown JP, Lang I, Boer K, Bondarenko IM, Kulyk SO, et al. The cyclin-dependent kinase 4/6 inhibitor palbociclib in combination with letrozole versus letrozole alone as first-line treatment of oestrogen receptor-positive, HER2-negative, advanced breast cancer (PALOMA-1/TRIO-18): a randomised phase 2 study. Lancet Oncol. 2015;16:25-35. [PMID: 25524798] doi:10.1016/S1470-2045(14)71159-3

Francis PA, Regan MM, Fleming GF, Láng I, Ciruelos E, Bellet M, et al; SOFT Investigators. Adjuvant ovarian suppression in premenopausal breast cancer. N Engl J Med. 2015;372:436-46. [PMID: 25495490] doi:10.1056/NEJMoa1412379

Goss PE, Ingle JN, Pritchard KI, Robert NJ, Muss H, Gralow J, et al. Extending aromatase-inhibitor adjuvant therapy to 10 years. N Engl J Med. 2016;375:209-19. [PMID: 27264120] doi:10.1056/NEJMoa1604700

Hartmann LC, Degnim AC, Santen RJ, Dupont WD, Ghosh K. Atypical hyperplasia of the breast-risk assessment and management options. N Engl J Med. 2015;372:78-89. [PMID: 25551530] doi:10.1056/NEJMsr1407164

Hartmann LC, Lindor NM. The role of risk-reducing surgery in hereditary breast and ovarian cancer. N Engl J Med. 2016;374:454-68. [PMID: 26840135] doi:10.1056/NEJMra1503523

Hughes KS, Schnaper LA, Bellon JR, Cirrincione CT, Berry DA, McCormick B, et al. Lumpectomy plus tamoxifen with or without irradiation in women age 70 years or older with early breast cancer: long-term follow-up of CALGB 9343. J Clin Oncol. 2013;31:2382-7. [PMID: 23690420] doi:10.1200/JCO.2012.45.2615

McLornan DP, List A, Mufti GJ. Applying synthetic lethality for the selective targeting of cancer. N Engl J Med. 2014;371:1725-35. [PMID: 25354106] doi:10.1056/NEJMra1407390

Narod SA, Iqbal J, Giannakeas V, Sopik V, Sun P. Breast cancer mortality after a diagnosis of ductal carcinoma in situ. JAMA Oncol. 2015;1:888-96. [PMID: 26291673] doi:10.1001/jamaoncol.2015.2510

Rugo HS, Rumble RB, Macrae E, Barton DL, Connolly HK, Dickler MN, et al. Endocrine therapy for hormone receptor-positive metastatic breast cancer: American Society of Clinical Oncology Guideline. J Clin Oncol. 2016;34:3069-103. [PMID: 27217461] doi:10.1200/JCO.2016.67.1487

Solin LJ, Gray R, Hughes LL, et al. Surgical excision without radiation for ductal carcinoma in situ of the breast: 12-year results from the ECOG-ACRIN E5194 study. J Clin Oncol. 2015 Nov 20;33(33):3938-44. [PMID: 26371148]

Sparano JA, Gray RJ, Makower DF, Pritchard KI, Albain KS, Hayes DF, et al. Prospective validation of a 21-gene expression assay in breast cancer. N Engl J Med. 2015;373:2005-14. [PMID: 26412349] doi:10.1056/NEJMoa1510764

Swain SM, Baselga J, Kim SB, Ro J, Semiglazov V, Campone M, et al; CLEOPATRA Study Group. Pertuzumab, trastuzumab, and docetaxel in HER2-positive metastatic breast cancer. N Engl J Med. 2015;372:724-34. [PMID: 25693012] doi:10.1056/NEJMoa1413513

Ovarian Cancer

Beral V, Gaitskell K, Hermon C, Moser K, Reeves G, Peto R; Collaborative Group On Epidemiological Studies Of Ovarian Cancer. Menopausal hormone use and ovarian cancer risk: individual participant meta-analysis of 52 epidemiological studies. Lancet. 2015;385:1835-42. [PMID: 25684585] doi:10.1016/S0140-6736(14)61687-1

Cress RD, Chen YS, Morris CR, Petersen M, Leiserowitz GS. Characteristics of long-term survivors of epithelial ovarian cancer. Obstet Gynecol. 2015;126:491-7. [PMID: 26244529] doi:10.1097/AOG.0000000000000981

Finch AP, Lubinski J, Møller P, Singer CF, Karlan B, Senter L, et al. Impact of oophorectomy on cancer incidence and mortality in women with a BRCA1 or BRCA2 mutation. J Clin Oncol. 2014;32:1547-53. [PMID: 24567435] doi:10.1200/JCO.2013.53.2820

Hartmann LC, Lindor NM. The role of risk-reducing surgery in hereditary breast and ovarian cancer. N Engl J Med. 2016;374:454-68. [PMID: 26840135] doi:10.1056/NEJMra1503523

Jacobs IJ, Menon U, Ryan A, Gentry-Maharaj A, Burnell M, Kalsi JK, et al. Ovarian cancer screening and mortality in the UK Collaborative Trial of Ovarian Cancer Screening (UKCTOCS): a randomised controlled trial. Lancet. 2016;387:945-956. [PMID: 26707054] doi:10.1016/S0140-6736(15)01224-6

Jelovac D, Armstrong DK. Recent progress in the diagnosis and treatment of ovarian cancer. CA Cancer J Clin. 2011;61:183-203. [PMID: 21521830] doi:10.3322/caac.20113

Kaufman B, Shapira-Frommer R, Schmutzler RK, Audeh MW, Friedlander M, Balmaña J, et al. Olaparib monotherapy in patients with advanced cancer and a germline BRCA1/2 mutation. J Clin Oncol. 2015;33:244-50. [PMID: 25366685] doi:10.1200/JCO.2014.56.2728

Menon U, Ryan A, Kalsi J, Gentry-Maharaj A, Dawnay A, Habib M, et al. Risk algorithm using serial biomarker measurements doubles the number of screen-detected cancers compared with a single-threshold rule in the United Kingdom Collaborative Trial of Ovarian Cancer Screening. J Clin Oncol. 2015;33:2062-71. [PMID: 25964255] doi:10.1200/JCO.2014.59.4945

Pujade-Lauraine E, Hilpert F, Weber B, Reuss A, Poveda A, Kristensen G, et al. Bevacizumab combined with chemotherapy for platinum-resistant recurrent ovarian cancer: The AURELIA open-label randomized phase III trial. J Clin Oncol. 2014;32:1302-8. [PMID: 24637997] doi:10.1200/JCO.2013.51.4489

Tewari D, Java JJ, Salani R, Armstrong DK, Markman M, Herzog T, et al. Long-term survival advantage and prognostic factors associated with intraperitoneal chemotherapy treatment in advanced ovarian cancer: a gynecologic oncology group study. J Clin Oncol. 2015;33:1460-6. [PMID: 25800756] doi:10.1200/JCO.2014.55.9898

Wright AA, Bohlke K, Armstrong DK, Bookman MA, Cliby WA, Coleman RL, et al. Neoadjuvant Chemotherapy for Newly Diagnosed, Advanced Ovarian Cancer: Society of Gynecologic Oncology and American Society of Clinical Oncology Clinical Practice Guideline. J Clin Oncol. 2016;34:3460-73. [PMID: 27502591] doi:10.1200/JCO.2016.68.6907

Cervical Cancer

Monk BJ, Tewari KS, Koh WJ. Multimodality therapy for locally advanced cervical carcinoma: state of the art and future directions. J Clin Oncol. 2007;25:2952-65. [PMID: 17617527]

Tewari KS, Sill MW, Long HJ 3rd, Penson RT, Huang H, Ramondetta LM, et al. Improved survival with bevacizumab in advanced cervical cancer. N Engl J Med. 2014;370:734-43. [PMID: 24552320] doi:10.1056/NEJMoa1309748

Tsu V, Jerónimo J. Saving the world's women from cervical cancer. N Engl J Med. 2016;374:2509-11. [PMID: 27355529] doi:10.1056/NEJMp1604113

Gastroenterological Malignancies

Ahn DH, Williams TM, Goldstein DA, El-Rayes B, Bekaii-Saab T. Adjuvant therapy for pancreas cancer in an era of value based cancer care. Cancer Treat Rev. 2016;42:10-7. [PMID: 26620819] doi:10.1016/j.ctrv.2015.11.004

Allegra CJ, Rumble RB, Hamilton SR, Mangu PB, Roach N, Hantel A, et al. Extended ras gene mutation testing in metastatic colorectal carcinoma to predict response to anti-epidermal growth factor receptor monoclonal antibody therapy: American Society of Clinical Oncology Provisional Clinical Opinion Update 2015. J Clin Oncol. 2016;34:179-85. [PMID: 26438111] doi:10.1200/JCO.2015.63.9674

André T, de Gramont A, Vernerey D, Chibaudel B, Bonnetain F, Tijeras-Raballand A, et al. Adjuvant fluorouracil, leucovorin, and oxaliplatin in stage II to III colon cancer: updated 10-year survival and outcomes according to BRAF mutation and mismatch repair status of the MOSAIC study. J Clin Oncol. 2015;33:4176-87. [PMID: 26527776] doi:10.1200/JCO.2015.63.4238

Benjamin RS, Casali PG. Adjuvant imatinib for GI stromal tumors: when and for how long? J Clin Oncol. 2016;34:215-8. [PMID: 26644523] doi:10.1200/JCO.2015.64.0102

Brenner H, Kloor M, Pox CP. Colorectal cancer. Lancet. 2014;383:1490-1502. [PMID: 24225001] doi:10.1016/S0140-6736(13)61649-9

Julie DR, Goodman KA. Advances in the management of anal cancer. Curr Oncol Rep. 2016;18:20. [PMID: 26905274] doi:10.1007/s11912-016-0503-3

Kahi CJ, Boland CR, Dominitz JA, Giardiello FM, Johnson DA, Kaltenbach T, et al; United States Multi-Society Task Force on Colorectal Cancer. Colonoscopy Surveillance After Colorectal Cancer Resection: Recommendations of the US Multi-Society Task Force on Colorectal Cancer. Gastroenterology. 2016;150:758-768.e11. [PMID: 26892199] doi:10.1053/j.gastro.2016.01.001

Patel SA, Ryan DP, Hong TS. Combined modality therapy for rectal cancer. Cancer J. 2016;22:211-7. [PMID: 27341601] doi:10.1097/PPO.0000000000000193

Primrose JN, Perera R, Gray A, Rose P, Fuller A, Corkhill A, et al; FACS Trial Investigators. Effect of 3 to 5 years of scheduled CEA and CT follow-up to detect recurrence of colorectal cancer: the FACS randomized clinical trial. JAMA. 2014;311:263-70. [PMID: 24430319] doi:10.1001/jama.2013.285718

Raj N, Reidy-Lagunes D. Systemic therapies for advanced pancreatic neuroendocrine tumors. Hematol Oncol Clin North Am. 2016;30:119-33. [PMID: 26614372] doi:10.1016/j.hoc.2015.09.005

Rustgi AK, El-Serag HB. Esophageal carcinoma. N Engl J Med. 2014;371:2499-509. [PMID: 25539106] doi:10.1056/NEJMra1314530

Smith JJ, D'Angelica MI. Surgical management of hepatic metastases of colorectal cancer. Hematol Oncol Clin North Am. 2015;29:61-84. [PMID: 25475573] doi:10.1016/j.hoc.2014.09.003

Lung Cancer

Brunelli A, Kim AW, Berger KI, Addrizzo-Harris DJ. Physiologic evaluation of the patient with lung cancer being considered for resectional surgery: diagnosis and management of lung cancer, 3rd ed: American College of Chest Physicians evidence-based clinical practice guidelines. Chest. 2013;143:e166S-e190S. [PMID: 23649437] doi:10.1378/chest.12-2395Burdett S, Pignon JP, Tierney J, et al; Non-Small Cell Lung Cancer Collaborative Group. Adjuvant chemotherapy for resected early-stage non-small cell lung cancer. Cochrane Database Syst Rev. 2015 Mar 2;(3):CD011430. [PMID: 25730344]

Curran WJ Jr, Paulus R, Langer CJ, Komaki R, Lee JS, Hauser S, et al. Sequential vs. concurrent chemoradiation for stage III non-small cell lung cancer: randomized phase III trial RTOG 9410. J Natl Cancer Inst. 2011;103:1452-60. [PMID: 21903745] doi:10.1093/jnci/djr325

Ettinger DS, Wood DE, Akerley W, Bazhenova LA, Borghaei H, Camidge DR, et al. NCCN guidelines insights: non-small cell lung cancer, version 4.2016. J Natl Compr Canc Netw. 2016;14:255-64. [PMID: 26957612]

Khullar OV, Liu Y, Gillespie T, et al. Survival after sublobar resection versus lobectomy for clinical stage IA lung cancer: an analysis from the National Cancer Data Base. J Thorac Oncol. 2015 Nov;10(11):1625-33. [PMID: 26352534]

Pignon JP, Tribodet H, Scagliotti GV, Douillard JY, Shepherd FA, Stephens RJ, et al; LACE Collaborative Group. Lung adjuvant cisplatin evaluation: a pooled analysis by the LACE Collaborative Group. J Clin Oncol. 2008;26:3552-9. [PMID: 18506026] doi:10.1200/JCO.2007.13.9030

Scagliotti GV, Parikh P, von Pawel J, Biesma B, Vansteenkiste J, Manegold C, et al. Phase III study comparing cisplatin plus gemcitabine with cisplatin plus pemetrexed in chemotherapy-naive patients with advanced-stage non-small-cell lung cancer. J Clin Oncol. 2008;26:3543-51. [PMID: 18506025] doi:10.1200/JCO.2007.15.0375

Soria JC, Mauguen A, Reck M, Sandler AB, Saijo N, Johnson DH, et al; meta-analysis of bevacizumab in advanced NSCLC collaborative group. Systematic review and meta-analysis of randomised, phase II/III trials adding bevacizumab to platinum-based chemotherapy as first-line treatment in patients with advanced non-small-cell lung cancer. Ann Oncol. 2013;24:20-30. [PMID: 23180113] doi:10.1093/annonc/mds590

Wang EH, Corso CD, Rutter CE, Park HS, Chen AB, Kim AW, et al. Postoperative radiation therapy is associated with improved overall survival in incompletely resected stage II and III non-small-cell lung cancer. J Clin Oncol. 2015;33:2727-34. [PMID: 26101240] doi:10.1200/JCO.2015.61.1517

Head and Neck Cancer

Adelstein D, Gillison ML, Pfister DG, Spencer S, Adkins D, Brizel DM, et al. NCCN guidelines insights: head and neck cancers, version 2.2017. J Natl Compr Canc Netw. 2017;15:761-770. [PMID: 28596256] doi:10.6004/jnccn.2017.0101

Bonner JA, Harari PM, Giralt J, Cohen RB, Jones CU, Sur RK, et al. Radiotherapy plus cetuximab for locoregionally advanced head and neck cancer: 5-year survival data from a phase 3 randomised trial, and relation between cetuximab-induced rash and survival. Lancet Oncol. 2010;11:21-8. [PMID: 19897418] doi:10.1016/S1470-2045(09)70311-0

Chen QY, Wen YF, Guo L, Liu H, Huang PY, Mo HY, et al. Concurrent chemoradiotherapy vs radiotherapy alone in stage II nasopharyngeal carcinoma:

phase III randomized trial. J Natl Cancer Inst. 2011;103:1761-70. [PMID: 22056739] doi:10.1093/jnci/djr432

Cohen EE, Karrison TG, Kocherginsky M, Mueller J, Egan R, Huang CH, et al. Phase III randomized trial of induction chemotherapy in patients with N2 or N3 locally advanced head and neck cancer. J Clin Oncol. 2014;32:2735-43. [PMID: 25049329] doi:10.1200/JCO.2013.54.6309

Goodwin WJ Jr. Salvage surgery for patients with recurrent squamous cell carcinoma of the upper aerodigestive tract: when do the ends justify the means? Laryngoscope. 2000;110:1-18. [PMID: 10714711]

Hitt R, Grau JJ, López-Pousa A, Berrocal A, García-Girón C, Irigoyen A, et al; Spanish Head and Neck Cancer Cooperative Group (TTCC). A randomized phase III trial comparing induction chemotherapy followed by chemoradiotherapy versus chemoradiotherapy alone as treatment of unresectable head and neck cancer. Ann Oncol. 2014;25:216-25. [PMID: 24256848] doi:10.1093/annonc/mdt461

Ho AS, Kraus DH, Ganly I, Lee NY, Shah JP, Morris LG. Decision making in the management of recurrent head and neck cancer. Head Neck. 2014;36:144-51. [PMID: 23471843] doi:10.1002/hed.23227

Schwartz DL, Ford E, Rajendran J, Yueh B, Coltrera MD, Virgin J, et al. FDG-PET/CT imaging for preradiotherapy staging of head-and-neck squamous cell carcinoma. Int J Radiat Oncol Biol Phys. 2005;61:129-36. [PMID: 15629603]

Tandon S, Shahab R, Benton JI, Ghosh SK, Sheard J, Jones TM. Fine-needle aspiration cytology in a regional head and neck cancer center: comparison with a systematic review and meta-analysis. Head Neck. 2008;30:1246-52. [PMID: 18528906] doi:10.1002/hed.20849

Vermorken JB, Mesia R, Rivera F, Remenar E, Kawecki A, Rottey S, et al. Platinum-based chemotherapy plus cetuximab in head and neck cancer. N Engl J Med. 2008;359:1116-27. [PMID: 18784101] doi:10.1056/NEJMoa0802656

Genitourinary Cancer

Bolla M, Van Tienhoven G, Warde P, Dubois JB, Mirimanoff RO, Storme G, et al. External irradiation with or without long-term androgen suppression for prostate cancer with high metastatic risk: 10-year results of an EORTC randomised study. Lancet Oncol. 2010;11:1066-73. [PMID: 20933466] doi:10.1016/S1470-2045(10)70223-0

Chen RC, Rumble RB, Loblaw DA, Finelli A, Ehdaie B, Cooperberg MR, et al. Active surveillance for the management of localized prostate cancer (Cancer Care Ontario Guideline): American Society of Clinical Oncology clinical practice guideline endorsement. J Clin Oncol. 2016;34:2182-90. [PMID: 26884580] doi:10.1200/JCO.2015.65.7759

Hall MC, Chang SS, Dalbagni G, Pruthi RS, Seigne JD, Skinner EC, et al. Guideline for the management of nonmuscle invasive bladder cancer (stages Ta, T1, and Tis): 2007 update. J Urol. 2007;178:2314-30. [PMID: 17993339]

James ND, Sydes MR, Clarke NW, Mason MD, Dearnaley DP, Spears MR, et al; STAMPEDE investigators. Addition of docetaxel, zoledronic acid, or both to first-line long-term hormone therapy in prostate cancer (STAMPEDE): survival results from an adaptive, multiarm, multistage, platform randomised controlled trial. Lancet. 2016;387:1163-77. [PMID: 26719232] doi:10.1016/S0140-6736(15)01037-5

Motzer RJ, Escudier B, McDermott DF, George S, Hammers HJ, Srinivas S, et al; CheckMate 025 Investigators. Nivolumab versus everolimus in advanced renal-cell carcinoma. N Engl J Med. 2015;373:1803-13. [PMID: 26406148] doi:10.1056/NEJMoa1510665

NCCN Clinical Guidelines in Oncology. Prostate Cancer. Version 2.2017. NCCN. org. https://www.nccn.org/professionals/physician_gls/pdf/prostate.pdf. Accessed February 17, 2018.

Nielsen M, Qaseem A; High Value Care Task Force of the American College of Physicians. Hematuria as a marker of occult urinary tract cancer: advice for high-value care from the American College of Physicians. Ann Intern Med. 2016;164:488-97. [PMID: 26810935]

Ravaud A, Motzer RJ, Pandha HS, George DJ, Pantuck AJ, Patel A, et al; S-TRAC Investigators. Adjuvant Sunitinib in High-Risk Renal-Cell Carcinoma after Nephrectomy. N Engl J Med. 2016;375:2246-2254. [PMID: 27718781]

Sweeney CJ, Chen YH, Carducci M, Liu G, Jarrard DF, Eisenberger M, et al. Chemohormonal therapy in metastatic hormone-sensitive prostate cancer. N Engl J Med. 2015;373:737-46. [PMID: 26244877] doi:10.1056/NEJMoa1503747

Travis LB, Fosså SD, Schonfeld SJ, McMaster ML, Lynch CF, Storm H, et al. Second cancers among 40,576 testicular cancer patients: focus on long-term survivors. J Natl Cancer Inst. 2005;97:1354-65. [PMID: 16174857]

Lymphoid Malignancies

Ansell SM. Hodgkin lymphoma: diagnosis and treatment. Mayo Clin Proc. 2015;90:1574-83. [PMID: 26541251] doi:10.1016/j.mayocp.2015.07.005

Burger JA, Tedeschi A, Barr PM, Robak T, Owen C, Ghia P, et al; RESONATE-2 Investigators. Ibrutinib as initial therapy for patients with chronic lymphocytic leukemia. N Engl J Med. 2015;373:2425-37. [PMID: 26639149] doi:10.1056/NEJMoa1509388

Casulo C, Friedberg J. Treating Burkitt lymphoma in adults. Curr Hematol Malig Rep. 2015;10:266-71. [PMID: 26013028] doi:10.1007/s11899-015-0263-4

Cheah CY, Seymour JF, Wang ML. Mantle cell lymphoma. J Clin Oncol. 2016;34:1256-69. [PMID: 26755518] doi:10.1200/JCO.2015.63.5904

Getta BM, Park JH, Tallman MS. Hairy cell leukemia: past, present and future. Best Pract Res Clin Haematol. 2015;28:269-72. [PMID: 26614906] doi:10.1016/j.beha.2015.10.015

Kahl BS, Yang DT. Follicular lymphoma: evolving therapeutic strategies. Blood. 2016;127:2055-63. [PMID: 26989204] doi:10.1182/blood-2015-11-624288

Lunning MA, Horwitz S. Treatment of peripheral T-cell lymphoma: are we data driven or driving the data? Curr Treat Options Oncol. 2013;14:212-23. [PMID: 23568456] doi:10.1007/s11864-013-0232-x

Matsuki E, Younes A. Checkpoint inhibitors and other immune therapies for Hodgkin and non-Hodgkin lymphoma. Curr Treat Options Oncol. 2016;17:31. [PMID: 27193488] doi:10.1007/s11864-016-0401-9

Roberts AW, Davids MS, Pagel JM, Kahl BS, Puvvada SD, Gerecitano JF, et al. Targeting BCL2 with venetoclax in relapsed chronic lymphocytic leukemia. N Engl J Med. 2016;374:311-22. [PMID: 26639348] doi:10.1056/NEJMoa1513257

Routledge DJ, Bloor AJ. Recent advances in therapy of chronic lymphocytic leukaemia. Br J Haematol. 2016;174:351-67. [PMID: 27291144] doi:10.1111/bjh.14184

Thanarajasingam G, Bennani-Baiti N, Thompson CA. PET-CT in staging, response evaluation, and surveillance of lymphoma. Curr Treat Options Oncol. 2016;17:24. [PMID: 27032646] doi:10.1007/s11864-016-0399-z

Zucca E, Bertoni F. The spectrum of MALT lymphoma at different sites: biological and therapeutic relevance. Blood. 2016;127:2082-92. [PMID: 26989205] doi:10.1182/blood-2015-12-624304

Cancer of Unknown Primary Site

Fizazi K, Greco FA, Pavlidis N, Daugaard G, Oien K, Pentheroudakis G; ESMO Guidelines Committee. Cancers of unknown primary site: ESMO Clinical Practice Guidelines for diagnosis, treatment and follow-up. Ann Oncol. 2015;26 Suppl 5:v133-8. [PMID: 26314775] doi:10.1093/annonc/mdv305

Samadder NJ, Smith KR, Hanson H, Pimentel R, Wong J, Boucher K, et al. Familial risk in patients with carcinoma of unknown primary. JAMA Oncol. 2016;2:340-6. [PMID: 26863281] doi:10.1001/jamaoncol.2015.4265

Varadhachary GR, Raber MN. Cancer of unknown primary site. N Engl J Med. 2014;371:757-65. [PMID: 25140961] doi:10.1056/NEJMra1303917

Melanoma

Larkin J, Chiarion-Sileni V, Gonzalez R, Grob JJ, Cowey CL, Lao CD, et al. Combined nivolumab and ipilimumab or monotherapy in untreated melanoma. N Engl J Med. 2015;373:23-34. [PMID: 26027431] doi:10.1056/NEJMoa1504030

Lee DY, Lau BJ, Huynh KT, Flaherty DC, Lee JH, Stern SL, et al. Impact of completion lymph node dissection on patients with positive sentinel lymph node biopsy in melanoma. J Am Coll Surg. 2016;223:9-18. [PMID: 27236435] doi:10.1016/j.jamcollsurg.2016.01.045

Long GV, Weber JS, Infante JR, Kim KB, Daud A, Gonzalez R, et al. Overall survival and durable responses in patients with BRAF V600-mutant metastatic melanoma receiving dabrafenib combined with trametinib. J Clin Oncol. 2016;34:871-8. [PMID: 26811525] doi:10.1200/JCO.2015.62.9345

Morton DL, Thompson JF, Cochran AJ, Mozzillo N, Nieweg OE, Roses DF, et al; MSLT Group. Final trial report of sentinel-node biopsy versus nodal observation in melanoma. N Engl J Med. 2014;370:599-609. [PMID: 24521106] doi:10.1056/NEJMoa1310460

Weber J, Mandala M, Del Vecchio M, Gogas HJ, Arance AM, Cowey CL, et al; CheckMate 238 Collaborators. Adjuvant nivolumab versus ipilimumab in resected stage III or IV melanoma. N Engl J Med. 2017. [PMID: 28891423] doi:10.1056/NEJMoa1709030

Oncologic Urgencies and Emergencies

Howard SC, Jones DP, Pui CH. The tumor lysis syndrome. N Engl J Med. 2011;364:1844-54. [PMID: 21561350] doi:10.1056/NEJMra0904569

Lin X, DeAngelis LM. Treatment of brain metastases. J Clin Oncol. 2015;33:3475-84. [PMID: 26282648] doi:10.1200/JCO.2015.60.9503

Patchell RA, Tibbs PA, Regine WF, Payne R, Saris S, Kryscio RJ, et al. Direct decompressive surgical resection in the treatment of spinal cord compression caused by metastatic cancer: a randomised trial. Lancet. 2005;366:643-8. [PMID: 16112300]

Wilson LD, Detterbeck FC, Yahalom J. Clinical practice. Superior vena cava syndrome with malignant causes. N Engl J Med. 2007;356:1862-9. [PMID: 17476012]

Effects of Cancer Therapy and Survivorship

Ganz PA, Earle CC, Goodwin PJ. Journal of Clinical Oncology update on progress in cancer survivorship care and research. J Clin Oncol. 2012;30:3655-6. [PMID: 23008327] doi:10.1200/JCO.2012.45.3886

Glaspy J. Current status of use of erythropoietic agents in cancer patients. Semin Thromb Hemost. 2014;40:306-12. [PMID: 24676903] doi:10.1055/s-0034-1370768

Hesketh PJ, Bohlke K, Lyman GH, Basch E, Chesney M, Clark-Snow RA, et al; American Society of Clinical Oncology. Antiemetics: American Society of Clinical Oncology focused guideline update. J Clin Oncol. 2016;34:381-6. [PMID: 26527784] doi:10.1200/JCO.2015.64.3635

Mulder RL, Kremer LC, Hudson MM, Bhatia S, Landier W, Levitt G, et al; International Late Effects of Childhood Cancer Guideline Harmonization Group. Recommendations for breast cancer surveillance for female survivors of childhood, adolescent, and young adult cancer given chest radiation: a report from the International Late Effects of Childhood Cancer Guideline Harmonization Group. Lancet Oncol. 2013;14:e621-9. [PMID: 24275135] doi:10.1016/S1470-2045(13)70303-6

Navari RM, Qin R, Ruddy KJ, Liu H, Powell SF, Bajaj M, et al. Olanzapine for the prevention of chemotherapy-induced nausea and vomiting. N Engl J Med. 2016;375:134-42. [PMID: 27410922] doi:10.1056/NEJMoa1515725

Nolan CP, DeAngelis LM. Neurologic complications of chemotherapy and radiation therapy. Continuum (Minneap Minn). 2015;21:429-51. [PMID: 25837905] doi:10.1212/01.CON.0000464179.81957.51

Rowland JH, Bellizzi KM. Cancer survivorship issues: life after treatment and implications for an aging population. J Clin Oncol. 2014;32:2662-8. [PMID: 25071099] doi:10.1200/JCO.2014.55.8361

Runowicz CD, Leach CR, Henry NL, Henry KS, Mackey HT, Cowens-Alvarado RL, et al. American Cancer Society/American Society of Clinical Oncology Breast Cancer Survivorship Care Guideline. J Clin Oncol. 2016;34:611-35. [PMID: 26644543] doi:10.1200/JCO.2015.64.3809

Smith TJ, Bohlke K, Lyman GH, Carson KR, Crawford J, Cross SJ, et al; American Society of Clinical Oncology. Recommendations for the use of WBC growth factors: American Society of Clinical Oncology clinical practice guideline update. J Clin Oncol. 2015;33:3199-212. [PMID: 26169616] doi:10.1200/JCO.2015.62.3488

White L, Ybarra M. Neutropenic fever. Emerg Med Clin North Am. 2014;32:549-61. [PMID: 25060249] doi:10.1016/j.emc.2014.04.002

Hematology and Oncology Self-Assessment Test

This self-assessment test contains one-best-answer multiple-choice questions. Please read these directions carefully before answering the questions. Answers, critiques, and bibliographies immediately follow these multiple-choice questions. The American College of Physicians (ACP) is accredited by the Accreditation Council for Continuing Medical Education (ACCME) to provide continuing medical education for physicians.

The American College of Physicians designates MKSAP 18 Hematology and Oncology for a maximum of 33 *AMA PRA Category 1 Credits*™. Physicians should claim only the credit commensurate with the extent of their participation in the activity.

Successful completion of the CME activity, which includes participation in the evaluation component, enables the participant to earn up to 33 medical knowledge MOC points in the American Board of Internal Medicine's Maintenance of Certification (MOC) program. It is the CME activity provider's responsibility to submit participant completion information to ACCME for the purpose of granting MOC credit.

Earn Instantaneous CME Credits or MOC Points Online

Print subscribers can enter their answers online to earn instantaneous CME credits or MOC points. You can submit your answers using online answer sheets that are provided at mksap.acponline.org, where a record of your MKSAP 18 credits will be available. To earn CME credits or to apply for MOC points, you need to answer all of the questions in a test and earn a score of at least 50% correct (number of correct answers divided by the total number of questions). Please note that if you are applying for MOC points, you must also enter your birth date and ABIM candidate number.

Take either of the following approaches:

- Use the printed answer sheet at the back of this book to record your answers. Go to mksap.acponline.org, access the appropriate online answer sheet, transcribe your answers, and submit your test for instantaneous CME credits or MOC points. There is no additional fee for this service.

- Go to mksap.acponline.org, access the appropriate online answer sheet, directly enter your answers, and submit your test for instantaneous CME credits or MOC points. There is no additional fee for this service.

Earn CME Credits or MOC Points by Mail or Fax

Pay a $20 processing fee per answer sheet and submit the printed answer sheet at the back of this book by mail or fax, as instructed on the answer sheet. Make sure you calculate your score and enter your birth date and ABIM candidate number, and fax the answer sheet to 215-351-2799 or mail the answer sheet to Member and Customer Service, American College of Physicians, 190 N. Independence Mall West, Philadelphia, PA 19106-1572, using the courtesy envelope provided in your MKSAP 18 slipcase. You will need your 10-digit order number and 8-digit ACP ID number, which are printed on your packing slip. Please allow 4 to 6 weeks for your score report to be emailed back to you. Be sure to include your email address for a response.

If you do not have a 10-digit order number and 8-digit ACP ID number, or if you need help creating a username and password to access the MKSAP 18 online answer sheets, go to mksap.acponline.org or email custserv@acponline.org.

CME credits and MOC points are available from the publication date of July 31, 2018, until July 31, 2021. You may submit your answer sheet or enter your answers online at any time during this period.

Hematology Questions

Item 1

A 34-year-old woman is evaluated for a rash on her lower extremities that appeared 3 days ago. She also reports easy bruising for the past week and bleeding when she brushes her teeth. Her medical history is otherwise unremarkable, and she takes no medications.

On physical examination, vital signs are normal. Petechiae are noted on the lower extremities, and ecchymoses are present on her right thigh and on her abdomen. No hepatomegaly, splenomegaly, or lymphadenopathy is noted.

Laboratory studies:

Hemoglobin	12.8 g/dL (128 g/L)
Leukocyte count	6600/µL (6.6 × 10⁹/L) with a normal differential
Mean corpuscular volume	82 fL
Platelet count	28,000/µL (28 × 10⁹/L)
Hepatitis C antibody	Negative

Large and giant platelets are seen on the peripheral blood smear, but no schistocytes or platelet clumping is noted.

Which of the following laboratory tests should be performed?

(A) Antiplatelet antibodies
(B) HIV testing
(C) Lupus anticoagulant
(D) Vitamin B$_{12}$ level

Item 2

A 68-year-old man is evaluated for epistaxis, gum bleeding, and easy bruising of 3 months' duration. Medical history is notable for anxiety, depression, and hyperlipidemia. Medications are atorvastatin, citalopram, a multivitamin, and ginkgo biloba.

On physical examination, vital signs are normal; BMI is 21. Scattered petechiae and several small ecchymoses are visible on the anterior thigh. The examination is otherwise normal.

Laboratory studies:

Activated partial thrombo-plastin time (aPTT)	Normal
Hemoglobin	14.8 g/dL (148 g/L)
Leukocyte count	4200/µL (4.2 × 10⁹/L)
Platelet count	245,000/µL (245 × 10⁹/L)
Prothrombin time (PT)	Normal
Thrombin time	Normal

Which of the following is the most appropriate diagnostic test to perform next?

(A) Fibrinogen level
(B) Mixing studies for PT and aPTT
(C) Peripheral blood smear review
(D) Platelet Function Analyzer-100
(E) Serum protein electrophoresis

Item 3

A 59-year-old woman arrives at the emergency department with left lower leg swelling of 2 weeks' duration and shortness of breath of 1 week's duration that has worsened during the past 6 hours. She reports no chest pain or hemoptysis. She has no history of recent travel, surgery, malignancy, or immobilization. She takes no medications.

On physical examination, temperature is 37.7 °C (99.9 °F), blood pressure is 140/85 mm Hg, pulse rate is 102/min, and respiration rate is 19/min. Oxygen saturation is 95% breathing ambient air. Edema of the left lower extremity is noted.

Laboratory studies show an elevated D-dimer level.

CT angiography shows a right subsegmental pulmonary embolism.

The patient's Pulmonary Embolism Severity Index score is 59.

It is determined the patient can be safely treated as an outpatient.

Which of the following is the most appropriate treatment?

(A) Apixaban
(B) Dabigatran
(C) Edoxaban
(D) Low-molecular-weight heparin

Item 4

A 52-year-old woman with a recent diagnosis of adenocarcinoma is seen for follow-up to discuss management plans. Medical history is notable for an 80-pack-year history of smoking. She takes no medications.

On physical examination, temperature is 37.2 °C (99.0 °F), blood pressure is 110/75 mm Hg, pulse rate is 99/min, and respiration rate is 20/min. Oxygen saturation is 95% breathing ambient air. Temporal wasting is noted. Pulmonary examination reveals decreased breath sounds in the right upper lobe. The remainder of the examination is unremarkable.

Laboratory studies:

Hemoglobin	10.6 g/dL (106 g/L)
Leukocyte count	9700/µL (9.7 × 10⁹/L)
Mean corpuscular volume	87 fL
Iron studies	
Ferritin	430 ng/mL (430 µg/L)
Iron	30 µg/dL (5 µmol/L)
Total iron-binding capacity	200 µg/dL (36 µmol/L)
Transferrin saturation	15%

A peripheral blood smear is normal. A chest radiograph shows a right upper lung mass and bilateral hilar and mediastinal lymphadenopathy. She will begin chemotherapy for the non–small cell lung cancer.

Which of the following is the most appropriate treatment for this patient's anemia?

(A) Erythropoietin
(B) Oral ferrous sulfate
(C) Parenteral iron sucrose
(D) No treatment

Item 5

A 74-year-old man is evaluated in follow-up for myelodysplastic syndrome diagnosed 3 months ago. Cytogenetic studies and fluorescence in-situ hybridization showed deletion of 5q. It was determined he has low-risk MDS by the Revised International Prognostic Scoring System. He requires erythrocyte transfusions every 2 weeks to prevent symptomatic anemia. He takes no medications.

On physical examination, pulse rate is 120/min, and respiration rate is 24/min; other vital signs are normal. Skin pallor is noted. Cardiac examination reveals tachycardia.

Laboratory studies show a hemoglobin level of 6.5 g/dL (65 g/L), leukocyte count of 2500/µL (2.5×10^9/L), and platelet count of 220,000/µL (220×10^9/L).

Which of the following is the most appropriate treatment?

(A) Allogeneic hematopoietic stem cell transplantation
(B) Antithymocyte globulin and cyclosporine
(C) Imatinib
(D) Lenalidomide

Item 6

A 45-year-old man is evaluated for shortness of breath with exertion and lower extremity edema of 6 months' duration. He reports no chest pain, fever, or cough. He takes no medications.

On physical examination, vital signs are normal. Jugular venous distention is noted. Cardiopulmonary examination reveals crackles at the base of the lungs. He also has 1+ lower extremity edema.

Laboratory studies are remarkable for eosinophilia, with an absolute eosinophil count of 2500/µL (2.5×10^9/L). A review of the medical record shows an eosinophil count of 2900/µL (2.9×10^9/L) 1 year ago.

An electrocardiogram shows sinus rhythm with low-voltage QRS and nonspecific ST changes. An echocardiogram shows findings compatible with a restrictive cardiomyopathy.

Which of the following is the most appropriate initial management?

(A) Evaluation for helminth infection
(B) Fat pad biopsy
(C) Prednisone
(D) Repeat laboratory evaluation in 3 months

Item 7

A 30-year-old man is evaluated for worsening exertional dyspnea. One week ago, he developed fever, sore throat, and cough. Those symptoms have resolved, but he has become more easily fatigued and short of breath. He had cholecystectomy 2 years ago because of symptomatic cholelithiasis; at that time, he was noted to be anemic and was diagnosed with hereditary spherocytosis. His only medication is a folate supplement.

On physical examination, he is pale but in no distress. Temperature is 37.0 °C (98.7 °F), blood pressure is 100/60 mm Hg, pulse rate is 116/min, and respiratory rate is 16/min. Oxygen saturation is 98% breathing ambient air. The spleen is palpable 3 cm below the left costal margin. Other examination findings are normal.

Laboratory studies:

Hemoglobin	7 g/dL (70 g/L)
Leukocyte count	5600/µL (5.6×10^9/L), with a normal differential
Mean corpuscular hemoglobin concentration	40 g/dL (400 g/L)
Platelet count	213,000/µL (213×10^9/L)
Reticulocyte count	1% of erythrocytes
Bilirubin	
Total	6.2 mg/dL (106 µmol/L)
Indirect	5.6 mg/dL (95.8 µmol/L)

Spherocytes are seen on the peripheral blood smear. A direct antiglobulin test is negative.

Which of the following is the most appropriate management?

(A) Erythropoiesis-stimulating agent
(B) Prednisone
(C) Splenectomy
(D) Observation

Item 8

A 64-year-old man is evaluated in the hospital for progressive shortness of breath and hypoxia 18 hours after undergoing surgery for an obstructing colonic adenocarcinoma with known liver metastases. Medical history is also notable for hypertension treated with hydrochlorothiazide.

On physical examination, vital signs are normal. Oxygen saturation is 92% breathing ambient air. The abdominal dressing is clean and dry. The examination is otherwise unremarkable.

CT angiography shows a left lower lobe pulmonary embolism.

Which of the following is the most appropriate treatment?

(A) Dabigatran
(B) Enoxaparin
(C) Fondaparinux
(D) Rivaroxaban
(E) Warfarin

Item 9

A 39-year-old woman is evaluated for new-onset nonproductive cough and dyspnea on exertion. She is pregnant at 32 weeks' gestation. Medical history is unremarkable. Her only medication is a prenatal vitamin.

On physical examination, temperature is 37.0 °C (98.6 °F), blood pressure is 105/62 mm Hg, pulse rate is 100/min, and respiration rate is 22/min. Oxygen saturation is 86% breathing ambient air. Cardiopulmonary examination is normal. She has a gravid uterus and 1+ edema of the lower extremities without calf tenderness.

Laboratory studies:

Hemoglobin	12.1 g/dL (121 g/L)
Leukocyte count	4800/µL (4.8×10^9/L)
Platelet count	189,000/µL (189×10^9/L)
Urinalysis	Normal

Doppler ultrasonography of both legs is negative for deep venous thrombosis.

Which of the following is the most appropriate diagnostic test to perform next?

(A) CT angiography

(B) D-dimer assay

(C) Magnetic resonance pulmonary angiography

(D) Pulmonary function testing

(E) Ventilation-perfusion lung scan

Item 10

A 52-year-old woman undergoes perioperative evaluation. She has osteoarthritis of the right hip since sustaining injuries in a motor vehicle accident 15 years ago and is scheduled for elective hip arthroplasty in the next few months. Medical history is otherwise notable for type 2 diabetes mellitus. She is up to date on routine health care. Her last menstrual period was 5 weeks ago. Medications are ibuprofen and metformin.

On physical examination, vital signs are normal. She has painful and limited range of motion in the right hip.

Laboratory studies:

Hemoglobin	10 g/dL (100 g/L)
Mean corpuscular volume	81 fL
Platelet count	223,000/μL (223 × 10⁹/L)
Creatinine	1 mg/dL (88.4 μmol/L)
Hemoglobin A$_{1c}$	7.5%

Which of the following is the most appropriate test to perform next?

(A) Hemoglobin electrophoresis

(B) Iron studies

(C) Vitamin B$_{12}$ level

(D) No further evaluation

Item 11

A 55-year-old man is evaluated in the emergency department for abrupt loss of consciousness after a fall. Medical history is notable for atrial fibrillation. He has otherwise been well without additional medical problems. Medications are warfarin and metoprolol.

On physical examination, temperature is 37 °C (98.6 °F), blood pressure is 135/85 mm Hg, pulse rate is 83/min and irregular, and respiration rate is 16/min. The patient is obtunded without localizing neurologic findings. Cardiac examination reveals an irregularly irregular rhythm. The remainder of the examination is unremarkable.

Head CT scan shows a large subdural hematoma.

Laboratory studies show a hemoglobin level of 13 g/dL (130 g/L), platelet count of 183,000/μL (183 × 10⁹/L), and INR of 3.0.

Intravenous vitamin K is administered, and plans are made for emergent neurosurgery.

Which of the following is the most appropriate treatment?

(A) Cryoprecipitate

(B) Four-factor prothrombin complex concentrate

(C) Fresh frozen plasma

(D) Idarucizumab

Item 12

A 50-year-old woman undergoes follow-up evaluation for a right iliofemoral deep venous thrombosis diagnosed 6 weeks ago by Doppler ultrasonography. She reports no new symptoms and notes her right leg edema is improving. She has no history of travel, surgery, or immobility. She indicates feeling well before her diagnosis, with no shortness of breath. She had a normal screening colonoscopy 3 months ago and a normal mammogram and Pap smear 6 months ago. Medical history is otherwise unremarkable. Her only medication is rivaroxaban.

On physical examination, vital signs are normal. She has mild edema of the right lower extremity. The examination is otherwise unremarkable.

Which of the following is the most appropriate diagnostic test to perform next?

(A) Abdominal and pelvic CT

(B) Chest CT

(C) Repeat lower extremity Doppler ultrasonography

(D) No additional testing

Item 13

A 35-year-old man is evaluated in the emergency department for fever and epistaxis. He has been experiencing malaise for several weeks and fever, chills, and anorexia for the past 3 days. Today he developed epistaxis. He takes no medications.

On physical examination, temperature is 38.8 °C (100.4 °F), blood pressure is 105/70 mm Hg, pulse rate is 110/min, and respiration rate is 24/min. He is diaphoretic. Dried blood is noted in the nares, and gingival bleeding is present. No lymphadenopathy or hepatosplenomegaly is noted. He has petechiae bilaterally on the lower extremities.

Laboratory studies:

Activated partial thromboplastin time	60 s
Hemoglobin	9.8 g/dL (98 g/L)
Leukocyte count	3600/μL (3.6 × 10⁹/L) with 20% neutrophils, 3% bands, 35% lymphocytes, 23% monocytes, and 18% "atypical" cells
Platelet count	17,000/μL (17 × 10⁹/L)
Prothrombin time	24 s
Fibrinogen	93 mg/dL (0.93 g/L)

The peripheral blood smear shows immature leukocytes with prominent granules in the cytoplasm.

Which of the following is the most likely diagnosis?

(A) Acute promyelocytic leukemia

(B) Aplastic anemia

(C) Chronic granulocytic leukemia

(D) Immune thrombocytopenic purpura

Item 14

A 67-year-old woman undergoes follow-up evaluation for an elevated globulin fraction of total serum protein level. She has no symptoms. Medical history is notable for hypertension treated with hydrochlorothiazide and atorvastatin.

On physical examination, vital signs are normal. No lymphadenopathy or hepatosplenomegaly is noted.

Laboratory studies:

Hemoglobin	14.5 g/dL (145 g/L)
Leukocyte count	7000/µL (7×10^9/L)
Platelet count	300,000/µL (300×10^9/L)
Calcium	9.1 mg/dL (2.3 mmol/L)
Creatinine	0.8 mg/dL (70.7 µmol/L)

Serum protein electrophoresis and immunofixation show an IgG monoclonal spike of 0.7 g/dL. Serum free light chain assay and 24-hour urine protein electrophoresis are normal.

Skeletal survey shows no lytic lesions.

Which of the following is the most appropriate management?

(A) Kidney biopsy
(B) MRI of the cervical, thoracic, and lumbar spine
(C) Repeat laboratory studies in 6 months
(D) Serum β_2-microglobulin I measurement

Item 15

A 65-year-old woman is evaluated for recurrent sinusitis. She has felt unwell for the past year, experiencing six episodes of sinusitis requiring antibiotic treatment and two courses of oral glucocorticoids. The most recent culture of the sinus drainage grew *Haemophilus influenzae*. Laboratory studies obtained 6 months ago showed mild anemia but were otherwise unremarkable. CT imaging revealed changes consistent with chronic sinusitis.

On physical examination, temperature is 38.0 °C (100.4 °F), and all other vital signs are normal. Nasal examination reveals left sinus ostia purulent drainage. She has no nasal polyps. Palpation of the maxillary sinuses elicits tenderness.

Laboratory studies:

Hemoglobin	9 g/dL (90 g/L)
Leukocyte count	4500/µL (4.5×10^9/L) with lymphocyte count of 400/µL (normal 1000-3000/µL)
Absolute neutrophil count	1500/µL (1.5×10^9/L)
Platelet count	100,000/µL (100×10^9/L)
Calcium	9.1 mg/dL (2.3 mmol/L)
Creatinine	0.8 mg/dL (70.7 µmol/L)
Immunoglobulins	
IgG	300 mg/dL (3 g/L)
IgA	Undetectable
IgM	Undetectable

Serum protein electrophoresis shows a monoclonal spike. Skeletal survey shows multiple lytic bone lesions.

A bone marrow biopsy specimen shows 25% plasma cells. Plans are made to begin therapy for her plasma cell malignancy.

Which of the following is the most appropriate immediate management to prevent recurrent infection?

(A) Acyclovir
(B) Granulocyte colony-stimulating factor
(C) Fluconazole
(D) Intravenous immune globulin

Item 16

A 53-year-old man is evaluated for tea-colored urine. He reports no other symptoms. He was hospitalized 2 weeks ago with melena. Upper gastrointestinal endoscopy and colonoscopy at the time did not show a bleeding source, but he stabilized after the transfusion of one unit of blood. He was discharged 10 days ago and has returned to work. Medical history is otherwise significant for trauma sustained in a motor vehicle accident 5 years ago, requiring multiple surgeries. He takes no medications.

On physical examination, temperature is 37.8 °C (100.1 °F), and other vital signs are normal, with no postural blood pressure or pulse changes. Scleral icterus is noted. The stool guaiac test result is negative. The remainder of the examination is unremarkable.

Laboratory studies:

	Current	10 Days Ago
Hemoglobin	6.9 g/dL (69 g/L)	8 g/dL (80 g/L)
Bilirubin		
Total	5 mg/dL (34.2 µmol/L)	1.1 mg/dL (18.8 µmol/L)
Direct	0.7 mg/dL (12 µmol/L)	–
Urinalysis	4+ blood, 2-3 erythrocytes/hpf, 1 leukocyte/hpf	–

Which of the following is the most appropriate next step in the management of this patient?

(A) Direct antiglobulin (Coombs) test
(B) Flow cytometry
(C) Repeat upper and lower endoscopy
(D) Transfusion of one unit of blood

Item 17

A 31-year-old woman arrives at the hospital in labor at 39 weeks' gestation of an otherwise uncomplicated first pregnancy. Her labor fails to progress after 20 hours; a cesarean section delivers a healthy female infant. A few minutes after the procedure, the patient begins to have heavy vaginal bleeding. Placental abruption is diagnosed and appropriately managed with fluid resuscitation and transfusion of 3 units of blood.

On physical examination, temperature is 36.7 °C (98.0 °F), blood pressure is 98/63 mm Hg, pulse rate is 102/min, and respiration rate is 22/min. Moderate bleeding persists.

Laboratory studies:

Activated partial thromboplastin time	38 s
D-dimer	Elevated
Hemoglobin	7.1 g/dL (71 g/L)
Platelet count	83,000/µL (83 × 10⁹/L)
Prothrombin time	17.9 s
Fibrinogen	75 mg/dL (0.75 g/L)

Infusion of which of the following is the most appropriate management?

(A) Albumin

(B) Cryo-poor plasma

(C) Cryoprecipitate

(D) Platelets

Item 18

A 22-year-old woman is evaluated in the emergency department for a 2-day history of progressive fatigue and shortness of breath. Medical history is significant for sickle cell disease diagnosed at age 6 years. Her sickle cell disease is under good control with rare crisis. Medications are hydroxyurea and folic acid.

On physical examination, temperature and blood pressure are normal, pulse rate is 125/min, and respiration rate is 25/min. Oxygen saturation is 93% breathing ambient air. Lungs are clear without wheezing. Other examination findings are unremarkable.

Laboratory studies:

Hemoglobin	4 g/dL (40 g/L)
Leukocyte count	13,000/µL (13 × 10⁹/L)
Platelet count	500,000/µL (500 × 10⁹/L)
Reticulocyte count	0.1% of erythrocytes

Chest radiograph is normal.

Which of the following is the most likely diagnosis?

(A) Aplastic anemia

(B) Hyperhemolysis syndrome

(C) Myelodysplastic syndrome

(D) Parvovirus B19 infection

Item 19

A 76-year-old woman arrives for follow-up consultation regarding a recent diagnosis of essential thrombocythemia. She was hospitalized 5 days ago for a cerebrovascular accident. Evaluation at the time showed a platelet count of 660,000/µL (660 × 10⁹/L). Results of iron studies, *JAK2 V617F* mutation testing, and polymerase chain reaction for *BCR-ABL* were normal. No secondary cause of thrombocythemia was found. Medical history is also notable for type 2 diabetes mellitus and dyslipidemia. Medications are low-dose aspirin, metformin, and atorvastatin.

On physical examination, vital signs are normal. She displays slight left hemiparesis. The spleen tip is palpable.

A bone marrow biopsy specimen showed hypercellularity with increased numbers of enlarged megakaryocytes.

Which of the following is the most appropriate management?

(A) Add clopidogrel

(B) Add hydroxyurea

(C) Change aspirin to clopidogrel

(D) Perform plateletpheresis

Item 20

A 28-year-old woman undergoes follow-up consultation regarding a pre-employment physical examination. She reports feeling well, with no recent illness. Medical history is notable for gastroesophageal reflux disease. Her only medication is omeprazole. She is black.

On physical examination, vital signs and other examination findings are normal.

Laboratory studies:

Hemoglobin	13.2 g/dL (132 g/L)
Leukocyte count	1867/µL (1.87 × 10⁹/L) with 75% neutrophils, 20% lymphocytes, and 5% monocytes
Absolute neutrophil count	1400/µL (1.4 × 10⁹/L)
Platelet count	258,000/µL (258 × 10⁹/L)

A peripheral blood smear shows decreased neutrophils, normal lymphocytes, normochromic erythrocytes, and normal platelets.

Which of the following is the most likely diagnosis?

(A) Autoimmune neutropenia

(B) Benign ethnic neutropenia

(C) Cyclical neutropenia

(D) Drug-induced neutropenia

Item 21

A 52-year-old man is evaluated in the emergency department for decreased exercise tolerance and yellowing of the eyes for the past 3 days. He was diagnosed with leprosy 6 days ago and began antibacterial therapy 4 days ago. His complete blood count at that time was normal. He is a Haitian immigrant. Medications are dapsone, rifampicin, and clofazimine.

On physical examination, temperature is 36.7 °C (98.0 °F), blood pressure is 125/75 mm Hg, pulse rate is 100/min, and respiration rate is 18/min. He has icteric sclerae. Cardiac examination reveals a grade 2/6 systolic flow murmur. Multiple raised erythematous papules with decreased sensation are noted on the back and hands. No organomegaly is observed.

Laboratory studies:

Haptoglobin	Undetectable
Hemoglobin	5.6 g/dL (56 g/L)
Leukocyte count	5600/µL (5.6 × 10⁹/L)
Platelet count	223,000/µL (223 × 10⁹/L)
Reticulocyte count	12% of erythrocytes

CONT.

Examination of the peripheral blood smear shows bite cells. The direct antiglobulin (Coombs) test is negative.

Which of the following is the most appropriate immediate management?

(A) Administer prednisone

(B) Administer rituximab

(C) Discontinue dapsone

(D) Measure ADAMTS13 activity

(E) Measure glucose-6-phosphate dehydrogenase level

Item 22

An 80-year-old woman is evaluated for fatigue and exertional dyspnea developing over several months. Medical history is significant for longstanding hypertension, but she has not been adherent with her medications.

On physical examination, vital signs are normal except for blood pressure of 180/110 mm Hg. She is frail, with pallor of mucous membranes and nail beds. The remainder of the examination is normal.

Laboratory studies:

Hemoglobin	9 g/dL (90 g/L)
Leukocyte count	8700/µL (8.7 × 10⁹/L), with a normal differential
Mean corpuscular volume	85 fL
Platelet count	380,000 (380 × 10⁹/L)
Reticulocyte count	1% of erythrocytes
Creatinine	1.8 mg/dL (159 µmol/L)
Folate	8 ng/mL (18.1 nmol/L)
Iron studies	
Ferritin	120 ng/mL (120 µg/L)
Iron	70 µg/dL (13 µmol/L)
Total iron-binding capacity	250 µg/dL (44.8 µmol/L)
Vitamin B₁₂	540 pg/mL (399 pmol/L)

Peripheral blood smear shows normal erythrocyte morphology.

On kidney ultrasonography, kidneys are small bilaterally, with echographic features suggesting chronic kidney disease.

Which of the following is the most likely cause of this patient's anemia?

(A) Erythropoietin deficiency

(B) Inflammation

(C) Iron deficiency

(D) Myelodysplastic syndrome

Item 23

A 61-year-old man is evaluated for worsening symptoms of edema and dizziness with standing over the past 6 months. His only medication is as-needed acetaminophen.

On physical examination, temperature is 37.0 °C (98.6 °F), blood pressure is 105/60 mm Hg sitting and 80/50 mm Hg standing, pulse rate is 105/min, and respiration rate is 18/min. Indentations are noted on the sides of the

tongue, which appears enlarged. Jugular venous distention is noted. Cardiopulmonary examination reveals decreased breath sounds at the lung bases and an S₃ gallop. Dependent edema is present.

On laboratory evaluation, the serum creatinine level is 1.5 mg/dL (132.6 µmol/L); 24-hour urine collection shows 3.5 g of albumin. Serum protein electrophoresis shows an IgG λ spike of 1.2 g/dL (0.012 g/L).

Echocardiography shows increased thickening of the left ventricular wall and significant diastolic dysfunction. Left ventricular ejection fraction is 51%.

Which of the following is the most appropriate diagnostic test to perform next?

(A) Abdominal fat pad biopsy

(B) Cardiac catheterization

(C) Kidney biopsy

(D) Tilt table test

Item 24

A 28-year-old woman is evaluated for decreased exercise tolerance and ice cravings for the past several weeks. Medical history is notable for Crohn colitis diagnosed 6 years ago. Her symptoms flared 3 months ago with increased abdominal pain and diarrhea, and she began therapy with azathioprine and infliximab. Her only other medication is ferrous sulfate tablets, 325 mg once daily, which she has been taking for 6 weeks after being diagnosed with iron deficiency anemia; her hemoglobin level at that time was 8.2 g/dL (82 g/L).

On physical examination, vital signs are normal. She is thin, with pale conjunctivae and nail beds. Cardiac examination reveals a grade 2/6 systolic flow murmur. The remainder of the examination is unremarkable.

Laboratory studies show a hemoglobin level of 7.5 g/dL (75 g/L) and a serum ferritin level of 1 ng/mL (1 µg/L).

Which of the following is the most appropriate treatment?

(A) Intravenous iron preparation

(B) Oral iron in a liquid preparation

(C) Oral iron tablets three times daily

(D) Sustained-release iron preparation

Item 25

A 74-year-old man undergoes follow-up evaluation for anemia found on preoperative assessment. He reports a 3-month history of night sweats but no headaches, vision changes, or shortness of breath. He is scheduled to have hip replacement surgery. Medical history is significant for hypertension. His only medication is hydrochlorothiazide.

On physical examination, vital signs are normal. Funduscopic examination is normal. No lymphadenopathy is present in the cervical, axillary, or inguinal regions. Hepatosplenomegaly is noted on abdominal examination.

Laboratory studies:

Hemoglobin	8.4 g/dL (84 g/L)
Leukocyte count	7000/µL (7 × 10⁹/L) with normal differential
Mean corpuscular volume	102 fL
Platelet count	300,000/µL (300 × 10⁹/L)
Reticulocyte count	1.9% of erythrocytes
Calcium	9.4 mg/dL (2.4 mmol/L)
Creatinine	1.1 mg/dL (97.2 µmol/L)

Serum protein electrophoresis with immunofixation shows an IgM spike of 330 mg/dL (3.3 g/L).

CT scan of the chest and abdomen shows hepatomegaly and splenomegaly. Prominent lymph nodes are seen in the para-aortic and celiac regions, the largest of which is 2.1 cm.

Which of the following is the most appropriate diagnostic test to perform next?

(A) Bone marrow biopsy

(B) CT imaging–guided needle biopsy of a para-aortic lymph node

(C) Excisional biopsy of a para-aortic lymph node

(D) Serum viscosity testing

Item 26

A 53-year-old man is evaluated for fatigue and arthralgia for the past 2 years. He indicates multiple joints in the hands and lower extremities are involved, but the pain is not exacerbated by joint use and is partially relieved with ibuprofen. He typically consumes two beers per day. His only medication is ibuprofen.

On physical examination, vital signs are normal. The right second and third metacarpophalangeal (MCP) joints are swollen. The examination is otherwise unremarkable.

Hand radiographs show hook-like osteophytes in the MCP joints.

Which of the following is the most appropriate test to perform next?

(A) *HFE* genotyping

(B) Liver biopsy

(C) Rheumatoid factor and anti–cyclic citrullinated peptide antibodies

(D) Transferrin saturation and serum ferritin level

Item 27

A 45-year-old man is evaluated in the hospital for worsening pain and progressive swelling of the left lower extremity that began abruptly approximately 12 hours ago. Medical history is otherwise noncontributory, and he takes no other medications.

On physical examination, pulse rate is 112/min; other vital signs are normal. He has erythema and marked edema of the entire left lower extremity. The left foot appears cyanotic, with decreased sensation, absent arterial pulses, and delayed capillary refill. The physical examination is otherwise unremarkable.

Doppler ultrasonography of the left lower extremity shows extensive ileofemoral deep venous thrombosis.

Which of the following is the most appropriate management?

(A) Alteplase

(B) Argatroban

(C) Rivaroxaban

(D) Unfractionated heparin

(E) Unfractionated heparin plus inferior vena cava filter insertion

Item 28

A 68-year-old man is evaluated in the emergency department for fatigue and exertional dyspnea. He has a 5-year history of chronic lymphocytic leukemia, which has not required therapy. He takes no medications.

On physical examination, temperature is 37 °C (98.6 °F), blood pressure is 123/82 mm Hg, pulse rate is 108/min, and respiration rate is 18/min. Oxygen saturation is 95% breathing ambient air. Cervical, axillary, and inguinal lymphadenopathy and splenomegaly are present.

Laboratory studies:

Hemoglobin	5 g/dL (50 g/L)
Leukocyte count	35,000/µL (35 × 10⁹/L) with 85% lymphocytes, 15% neutrophils
Platelet count	180,000/µL (180 × 10⁹/L)
Reticulocyte count	10% of erythrocytes

A direct antiglobulin test result is positive for IgG and C3. The patient is group A-positive and crossmatch incompatible with 5 units of group A-positive blood.

Glucocorticoid therapy is started.

Which of the following is the most appropriate management?

(A) Avoid transfusion until a compatible unit can be found

(B) Begin plasma exchange therapy

(C) Transfuse crossmatch-incompatible blood

(D) Transfuse O-negative uncrossmatched blood

Item 29

A 73-year-old man undergoes follow-up evaluation after autologous hematopoietic stem cell transplantation (HSCT) 3 weeks ago for multiple myeloma. He had induction chemotherapy 1 year ago. He is doing well, without fever, chills, cough, or localizing symptoms of infection. Medications are acyclovir and omeprazole.

On physical examination, vital signs are normal; BMI is 20. He weighs 2.5 kg (6 lb) less than he did 2 months ago before HSCT. Alopecia is noted.

In the next 30 days, this patient is at increased risk for which of the following treatment-related complications?

(A) Acute graft-versus-host disease

(B) Infection

(C) Lymphoma

(D) Myelodysplastic syndrome

Item 30

A 60-year-old man is evaluated for an asymptomatic elevation of serum protein. Medical history is unremarkable, and he takes no medications.

On physical examination, vital signs are normal. Neurologic examination reveals no deficits.

Laboratory studies:

Hemoglobin	14 g/dL (140 g/L)
Leukocyte count	7000/µL (7 × 10⁹/L)
Platelet count	300,000/µL (300 × 10⁹/L)
Calcium	9.4 mg/dL (2.4 mmol/L)
Creatinine	1.1 mg/dL (97.2 µmol/L)

Serum protein electrophoresis and immunofixation show an IgA spike of 3.5 g/dL. Skeletal survey findings are negative.

Which of the following is the most appropriate next test?

(A) Bone scan
(B) CT of the chest, abdomen, and pelvis
(C) Whole body MRI
(D) No further testing

Item 31

A 70-year-old man is evaluated in the emergency department for headache, confusion, and weakness. Medical history is significant for ischemic cardiomyopathy with heart failure and mural thrombus. Medications are lisinopril, carvedilol, spironolactone, furosemide, and warfarin.

On physical examination, the patient is disoriented. Temperature and respiration rate are normal, blood pressure is 160/90 mm Hg, and pulse rate is 88/min. The examination is otherwise unremarkable.

Laboratory studies show an INR of 7.5.

CT scan of the head shows left intraparenchymal hemorrhage.

In addition to vitamin K administration, which of the following is the most appropriate treatment?

(A) Fresh frozen plasma
(B) Idarucizumab
(C) Prothrombin complex concentrate
(D) Recombinant activated factor VII

Item 32

A 76-year-old woman is evaluated for worsening fatigue. She reports no additional symptoms. Medical history is significant for myelodysplastic syndrome diagnosed 3 years ago, which has required the transfusion of 1 to 2 units of blood every 5 to 6 weeks to maintain a hemoglobin level of approximately 8 g/dL (80 g/L); she has exertional dyspnea when the hemoglobin level drops below 7 g/dL (70 g/L).

On physical examination, vital signs are normal. The abdomen is soft. Conjunctival pallor is noted. The examination is otherwise noncontributory.

Laboratory studies show a hemoglobin level of 7.5 g/dL (75 g/L) and a serum ferritin level of 1638 ng/mL (1638 µg/L).

Which of the following is the most appropriate management?

(A) Begin deferasirox
(B) Begin succimer
(C) Perform therapeutic phlebotomy
(D) Withhold transfusion until hemoglobin level is 6 g/dL (60 g/L)

Item 33

A 63-year-old man is evaluated for increasing fatigue and exertional dyspnea over the past 5 months. Medical history is notable for diabetes mellitus, hypertension, and chronic kidney disease. Medications are insulin glargine, metformin, enalapril, aspirin, and atorvastatin.

On physical examination, vital signs are normal. Pallor is noted. Examination findings are otherwise normal.

Laboratory studies show a hemoglobin level of 9.5 g/dL (90 g/L) (11 g/dL [110 g/L] 1 year ago), reticulocyte count of 1% of erythrocytes, and serum creatinine level of 2.0 mg/dL (176.8 µmol/L) (1.6 mg/dL [141.4 µmol/L] 1 year ago). Serum haptoglobin, iron, ferritin, and folate levels; total iron-binding capacity; vitamin B₁₂ level; and liver chemistry studies are normal.

The stool guaiac test result is negative for occult blood.

Which of the following is the most appropriate next step in management?

(A) Darbepoetin administration for a target hemoglobin level of 11 g/dL (110 g/L)
(B) Darbepoetin administration for a target hemoglobin level of 14 g/dL (140 g/L)
(C) Oral iron supplementation and repeat hemoglobin level in 1 month
(D) Parenteral iron supplementation and repeat hemoglobin level in 1 month

Item 34

A 67-year-old woman arrives at the emergency department with hematuria of 3 days' duration. She has no other sites of bleeding. Medical history is significant for recently diagnosed nonvalvular paroxysmal atrial fibrillation and hypertension. Medications are hydrochlorothiazide and dabigatran.

On physical examination, vital signs are normal and other examination findings are unremarkable.

A urine sample is grossly bloody.

Laboratory studies:

Activated partial thromboplastin time	58 s
Hemoglobin	12.8 g/dL (128 g/L)
Prothrombin time	12 s
Creatinine	1.1 mg/dL (97.2 µmol/L)
Urinalysis	pH 5.0; 4+ blood; no protein. On microscopic examination, erythrocytes were too numerous to count. No casts or dysmorphic erythrocytes observed.

In addition to discontinuing dabigatran, which of the following is the most appropriate immediate management?

CONT.

(A) Four-factor prothrombin complex concentrate

(B) Fresh frozen plasma

(C) Idarucizumab

(D) Vitamin K

(E) Observation

Item 35

A 32-year-old man undergoes preoperative consultation for a hip replacement. He has an 18-month history of hip pain secondary to avascular necrosis of the left hip. He also has sickle cell disease, requiring three to four hospitalizations per year for vaso-occlusive crisis. Medications are ibuprofen, hydroxyurea, and folic acid.

On physical examination, vital signs are normal. Cardiac examination reveals a grade 2/6 systolic flow murmur. He has left hip pain with abduction.

Laboratory studies show a hemoglobin level of 5.8 g/dL (58 g/L; baseline, 5-6.5 g/dL [50-65 g/L]).

Which of the following is the most appropriate preoperative transfusion management for this patient?

(A) Exchange transfusion to 30% hemoglobin S

(B) Exchange transfusion to 50% hemoglobin S

(C) Simple transfusion to a target hemoglobin level of 10 g/dL (100 g/L)

(D) Simple transfusion to a target hemoglobin level of 12 g/dL (120 g/L)

(E) No transfusion

Item 36

A 32-year-old woman is evaluated for a painful rash occurring bilaterally on her lower extremities, which began 2 days ago. She was admitted to the hospital 5 days ago for diagnosis and treatment of pulmonary embolism with heparin and warfarin. Her father had a pulmonary embolism after a long airplane ride. Her medical history is otherwise unremarkable, and she takes no other medications.

On physical examination, vital signs are normal. She has nonblanchable macules and papules and areas of cutaneous necrosis in an angulated reticular pattern on the lower legs; findings on the feet are shown (see top of next column). The examination is otherwise unremarkable.

Laboratory studies show a normal complete blood count, a normal peripheral blood smear, and an INR of 4.

Which of the following is the most likely diagnosis?

(A) Factor V Leiden mutation

(B) Plasminogen activator inhibitor 1 deficiency

(C) Protein C deficiency

(D) Prothrombin gene mutation

Item 37

A 25-year-old woman is evaluated in the emergency department for mild shortness of breath and right lateral chest

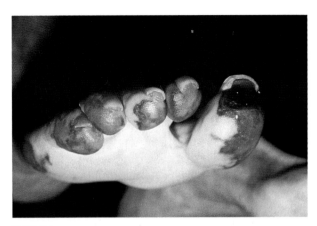

ITEM 36

pain of 2 days' duration. She reports no orthopnea or lower extremity edema. Medical history is unremarkable other than anxiety related to meeting the demands of her new job as an engineer. She takes no medications.

On physical examination, she is in no apparent distress. Vital signs are normal. Oxygen saturation is 99% breathing ambient air. The lungs are clear to auscultation. No peripheral edema is noted.

Her Wells Criteria for Pulmonary Embolism score is 0.

A complete blood count, electrocardiogram, and chest radiograph are normal.

Which of the following tests should be performed next to rule out pulmonary embolism?

(A) CT angiography of the chest

(B) D-dimer

(C) Echocardiography

(D) No further testing

Item 38

A 35-year-old man is evaluated for a 6-month history of night sweats, malaise, and weight loss of 11.3 kg (25 lb). He reports no fevers or other localizing symptoms. His only medication is acetaminophen.

On physical examination, vital signs are normal. Abdominal examination reveals splenomegaly. The remainder of the examination is noncontributory.

Laboratory studies show a hemoglobin level of 12.5 g/dL (125 g/L); a leukocyte count of 55,000/μL (55 × 10⁹/L), with 87% neutrophils, 2% myelocytes, 1% metamyelocytes, 0.5% basophils, 7% lymphocytes, and 2.5% monocytes; and a platelet count of 450,000/μL (450 × 10⁹/L).

Polymerase chain reaction for *BCR-ABL* fusion gene is positive. A bone marrow biopsy specimen shows hypercellular marrow with myeloid hyperplasia and 1% myeloid blasts.

Which of the following is the most appropriate treatment?

(A) Bone marrow transplantation

(B) Idarubicin and cytarabine

(C) Imatinib

(D) Vancomycin and levofloxacin

Item 39

A 24-year-old man with progressive fatigue and intermittent dark urine over several months is evaluated in the emergency department for exertional dyspnea, abdominal pain, and red urine.

On physical examination, he is pale. Temperature is 37.0 °C (98.6 °F), blood pressure is 110/70 mm Hg, pulse rate is 112/min, and respiration rate is 16/min. Oxygen saturation is 98% breathing ambient air. Scattered petechiae are visible on the skin. The abdomen is not distended and is diffusely tender to palpation without guarding. Bowel sounds are normal. The remainder of the examination is normal.

Laboratory studies:

Haptoglobin	Undetectable
Hemoglobin	7.2 g/dL (72 g/L)
Leukocyte count	1200/µL (1.2 × 10⁹/L) with 70% neutrophils and 30% lymphocytes
Mean corpuscular volume	84 fL
Platelet count	23,000/µL (23 × 10⁹/L)
Reticulocyte count	8% of erythrocytes
Lactate dehydrogenase	500 U/L
Urinalysis	4+ blood; 0-1 erythrocytes/hpf; 0 leukocytes/hpf

The peripheral blood smear shows normal-appearing erythrocytes without spherocytes, schistocytes, agglutinated erythrocytes, or immature-appearing leukocytes.

Which of the following is the most appropriate next test?

(A) Direct antiglobulin test
(B) Flow cytometry
(C) Methylmalonic acid measurement
(D) Quantitative and functional levels of C1 esterase inhibitor

Item 40

A 43-year-old man with chronic alcoholic liver disease is hospitalized after massive vomiting of blood. Medical history is notable for alcohol dependence. He takes no medications.

On physical examination, temperature is normal, blood pressure is 102/68 mm Hg, pulse rate is 118/min, and respiration rate is 22/min. He is jaundiced and has spider angiomata on the anterior chest. The liver is palpable but not tender.

Laboratory studies:

Activated partial thromboplastin time	45 s
Prothrombin time	17.8 s
Hemoglobin	9.8 g/dL (98 g/L)
Platelet count	42,000/µL (42 × 10⁹/L)
D-dimer	5800 µg/mL (5800 mg/L)
Fibrinogen	66 mg/dL (0.6 g/L)

He receives volume resuscitation with fluids, erythrocyte and platelet transfusions, and vitamin K.

Which of the following should also be provided to manage this patient's coagulopathy?

(A) Activated factor VII concentrate
(B) ε-Aminocaproic acid
(C) Cryoprecipitate
(D) Four-factor prothrombin concentrate

Item 41

A 73-year-old man is admitted to the hospital with right lower lobe pneumonia. He has stage III colonic adenocarcinoma and underwent colonic resection 2 months ago. He has begun combination chemotherapy.

On physical examination, temperature is 38.5 °C (101.3 °F), blood pressure is 110/50 mm Hg, pulse rate is 103/min, and respiration rate is 24/min. Oxygen saturation is 98% breathing ambient air. Crackles are heard in the right lower lobe. The examination is otherwise noncontributory.

Which of the following is the most appropriate venous thromboembolism prophylaxis intervention?

(A) Aspirin
(B) Enoxaparin
(C) Graduated compression stockings
(D) Intermittent pneumatic compression
(E) Warfarin

Item 42

A 22-year-old woman is seen for a routine prenatal evaluation; she is 10 weeks pregnant. This is her second pregnancy; the first pregnancy was uncomplicated. Medical history is notable for sickle cell disease requiring one to two hospitalizations per year for painful events. She has no history of stroke or acute chest syndrome. Her only medication is a folic acid supplement.

On physical examination, vital signs are normal. Cardiac examination reveals a grade 2/6 systolic flow murmur. She has a gravid uterus.

Laboratory studies show a hemoglobin level of 6.4 g/dL (64 g/L; baseline, 5-7 g/dL [50-70 g/L]), leukocyte count of 11,500/µL (11.5 × 10⁹/L), and platelet count of 279,000/µL (279 × 10⁹/L).

Which of the following is the most appropriate treatment?

(A) Clopidogrel
(B) Exchange transfusion throughout pregnancy
(C) Hydroxyurea
(D) Simple transfusion throughout pregnancy
(E) Expectant care

Item 43

A 22-year-old woman undergoes routine evaluation for chronic anemia, which was diagnosed 6 years ago. Medical history is otherwise unremarkable, but a maternal aunt also has anemia. Her only medication is a combination oral contraceptive pill. On physical examination, vital signs are normal. No hepatosplenomegaly is noted.

Laboratory studies:

Hemoglobin	10 g/dL (100 g/L)
Mean corpuscular volume	67 fL
Iron studies	
Ferritin	200 ng/mL (200 µg/L)
Iron	150 µg/dL (27 µmol/L)
Total iron-binding capacity	340 µg/dL (61 µmol/L)

Hemoglobin electrophoresis reveals a normal pattern of migration of hemoglobin A and normal levels of hemoglobin A_2 and hemoglobin F.

Which of the following is the most likely diagnosis?

(A) Inflammatory anemia
(B) Iron deficiency
(C) α-Thalassemia silent carrier
(D) α-Thalassemia trait
(E) β-Thalassemia minor

Item 44

A 61-year-old woman undergoes routine evaluation. She reports no recent changes in her medications. She has a history of idiopathic deep venous thrombosis. Her only medication is warfarin, initiated 2 months ago.

On physical examination, vital signs are normal, and the examination is unremarkable.

She has an INR of 7.2.

In addition to withholding warfarin, which of the following is the most appropriate management?

(A) Administer fresh frozen plasma
(B) Administer prothrombin complex concentrate
(C) Administer vitamin K
(D) Remeasure INR in 2 days

Item 45

A 36-year-old woman is evaluated for a severe headache. She is at 36 weeks' gestation with her first pregnancy. Her only medication is a prenatal vitamin.

On physical examination, temperature is 37.0 °C (98.7 °F), blood pressure is 160/100 mm Hg, pulse rate is 100/min, and respiration rate is 16/min. Oxygen saturation is 98% breathing ambient air. Neurologic examination is nonfocal. Cardiopulmonary examination is normal. She has a gravid uterus and 2+ edema of the lower extremities. No petechiae or ecchymoses are seen.

Laboratory studies:

Hemoglobin	11.9 g/dL (119 g/L)
Leukocyte count	12,700/µL (12.7 × 10⁹/L)
Platelet count	52,000/µL (52 × 10⁹/L)
Alanine aminotransferase	50 U/L
Aspartate aminotransferase	52 U/L
Creatinine	1.2 mg/dL (106 µmol/L)
Urinalysis	3+ proteinuria

The peripheral smear shows occasional fragmented erythrocytes without platelet clumping.

Which of the following is the most appropriate management?

(A) Eculizumab
(B) Emergent delivery
(C) High-dose dexamethasone
(D) Plasma exchange

Item 46

A 28-year-old woman is evaluated preoperatively; she is scheduled for elective repair of an umbilical hernia. Medical history is notable for heavy menstrual periods and 5 days of bleeding after extraction of wisdom teeth. Her only medication is an oral contraceptive.

On physical examination, vital signs and other findings are normal.

Laboratory studies show a normal complete blood count. The activated partial thromboplastin time and prothrombin time are normal. The Platelet Function Analyzer-100 result is prolonged.

Which of the following is the most likely diagnosis?

(A) Congenital hemophilia A
(B) Factor XI deficiency
(C) Lupus anticoagulant
(D) von Willebrand disease

Item 47

A 24-year-old woman is evaluated for severe pain in her arms and legs of 5 hours' duration. Medical history is notable for lifelong mild anemia and four episodes of similar pain without precipitating factors, each episode resolving in 3 to 4 days. She has a cousin with sickle cell disease. She takes no medications.

On physical examination, vital signs are normal. She has normal range of motion in all joints with no skeletal deformities.

Laboratory studies:

Hemoglobin	11.2 g/dL (112 g/L)
Mean corpuscular volume	76 fL
Hemoglobin electrophoresis	
Hemoglobin A	33%
Hemoglobin A_2	4%
Hemoglobin S	63%
Hemoglobin F	0%

Which of the following is the most likely diagnosis?

(A) Hemoglobin E disease
(B) Hemoglobin S β-thalassemia
(C) Hemoglobin SS disease
(D) Sickle cell trait

Item 48

A 55-year-old man is evaluated in the emergency department for hematemesis. He has had intermittent epigastric

CONT.

discomfort for the past few weeks that does not vary with meals. He does not smoke cigarettes, drink alcohol, or take any medications.

On physical examination, temperature is 37 °C (98.6 °F), blood pressure is 118/68 mm Hg without postural changes, pulse rate is 110/min, and respiration rate is 18/min. Physical examination findings are unrevealing.

Laboratory studies show a hemoglobin level of 8.0 g/dL (80 g/L), platelet count of 130,000/µL (130 × 10⁹/L), and prothrombin time of 10 s.

Crystalloid resuscitation is initiated, and the patient undergoes upper endoscopy, which reveals an 8-mm duodenal ulcer with a clean ulcer base without active arterial bleeding.

Which of the following is the most appropriate management?

(A) Continue crystalloid resuscitation
(B) Packed red blood cell transfusion
(C) Plasma transfusion
(D) Platelet transfusion

Item 49

A 22-year-old man with sickle cell anemia (SCA) is seen 1 week after hospitalization for acute chest syndrome that required critical care and treatment with exchange transfusion and noninvasive assisted ventilation. He has not had any previous pulmonary or any other major complications from his SCA and typically has two to three episodes of acute pain events yearly. He reports he has returned to his usual level of activity and has no pulmonary symptoms and no pain. His only medication is folate, 1 mg/d.

On physical examination, vital signs are normal. He appears pale. Cardiac examination reveals a grade 3/4 systolic flow murmur. The remainder of the examination, including pulmonary examination, is unremarkable.

Laboratory studies:

Hemoglobin	8.4 g/dL (84 g/L)
Leukocyte count	14,000/µL (14 × 10⁹/L)
Mean corpuscular volume	86 fL
Platelet count	325,000 (325 × 10⁹/L)
Reticulocyte count	8% of erythrocytes

Which of the following is the most appropriate management?

(A) Folate supplementation of 4 mg/d
(B) Hydroxyurea
(C) Incentive spirometry
(D) Monthly exchange transfusions
(E) Monthly simple transfusions

Item 50

An 81-year-old woman is evaluated for a 1-year history of headaches, redness of the face, and itching. She indicates being otherwise capable of performing her daily activities on her farm. She reports no shortness of breath,

chest pain, or difficulty sleeping. Medical history is significant for hypertension; she has never smoked and does not drink alcohol. Her only medication is hydrochlorothiazide.

On physical examination, vital signs are normal except for a blood pressure of 160/90 mm Hg; BMI is 19. Abdominal examination shows splenomegaly.

Laboratory studies:

Erythropoietin	Undetectable
Hemoglobin	17.5 g/dL (175 g/L)
Leukocyte count	11,000/µL (11 × 10⁹/L)
Platelet count	400,000/µL (400 × 10⁹/L)

Which of the following is the most appropriate diagnostic test to perform next?

(A) Calreticulin mutation testing
(B) *JAK2 V617F* mutation testing
(C) Polymerase chain reaction for *BCR-ABL*
(D) Sleep study

Item 51

A 42-year-old man is admitted to the hospital with an acute change in mental status and fever of 2 days' duration. Medical history is noncontributory, and he takes no medications.

On physical examination, temperature is 38.2 °C (100.8 °F), blood pressure is 108/70 mm Hg, pulse rate is 104/min, and respiration rate is 18/min. Oxygen saturation is 96% breathing ambient air. He is agitated and disoriented to place and time. Petechiae are noted on his shins. The remainder of the examination is normal.

Laboratory studies:

Haptoglobin	20 mg/dL (200 mg/L)
Hemoglobin	10.2 g/dL (102 g/L)
Leukocyte count	9800/µL (9.8 × 10⁹/L)
Platelet count	44,000/µL (44 × 10⁹/L)
Reticulocytes	6.8% of erythrocytes
Creatinine	1.4 mg/dL (123.8 µmol/L)
Lactate dehydrogenase	1600 U/L

The direct antiglobulin (Coombs) test is negative.

Therapy should be immediately initiated pending results of which of the following studies?

(A) ADAMTS13 activity
(B) Coagulation studies
(C) Peripheral blood smear
(D) Stool culture and testing for Shiga toxin

Item 52

A 27-year-old woman arrives to establish primary care. She feels well. Her last menstrual period was 2 weeks ago, and menses are regular. Medical history is significant for acute lymphoblastic leukemia diagnosed at 5 years of age. She received treatment for 2 years and has been leukemia free since the completion of therapy. She takes no medications.

On physical examination, vital signs are normal; BMI is 27. Other examination findings are unremarkable.

Complete blood counts performed within the past year were normal.

The patient will arrange a treatment summary to be transferred to the office.

Which of the following is the most appropriate test to obtain next in this patient?

(A) Bone marrow biopsy

(B) Estrogen and progesterone levels

(C) Exercise stress test

(D) Lipid profile and fasting blood glucose

(E) Whole genome sequencing

Item 53

A 78-year-old woman is hospitalized from an outpatient infusion clinic for progressive shortness of breath. She was receiving a transfusion of one unit of blood. She reports no chest pain, cough, dizziness, or palpitations. Medical history is notable for heart failure, hypertension, and myelodysplastic syndrome with symptomatic anemia requiring transfusion approximately every 3 weeks. Medications are low-dose aspirin, metoprolol, lisinopril, hydrochlorothiazide, and azacytidine.

On physical examination, temperature is 36.7 °C (98.0 °F), blood pressure is 153/76 mm Hg (pretransfusion, 123/71 mm Hg), pulse rate is 94/min (pretransfusion, 65/min), and respiration rate is 32/min (pretransfusion, 20/min). Oxygen saturation is 85% breathing ambient air. Jugular venous pressure is 10 cm H_2O. An S_3 is present on cardiac examination. Bilateral crackles are heard on pulmonary examination.

A chest radiograph shows moderate pulmonary vascular congestion with a small left pleural effusion.

Which of the following is the most likely diagnosis?

(A) Acute hemolytic transfusion reaction

(B) Anaphylactic reaction

(C) Transfusion-associated circulatory overload

(D) Transfusion-related acute lung injury

Item 54

A 24-year-old man is admitted to the hospital for fever, chest pain, shortness of breath, and cough of 3 days' duration. He is homozygous for hemoglobin S (Hb SS). Medications are folate and hydroxyurea.

On physical examination, temperature is 38.9 °C (102 °F), blood pressure is 100/70 mm Hg, pulse rate is 110/min, and respiration rate is 22/min. Oxygen saturation is 90% breathing 40% oxygen. He appears ill. Cardiopulmonary examination reveals a grade 2/6 systolic flow murmur and crackles in the lower lung fields bilaterally. The remainder of the examination is unremarkable.

Laboratory studies show a hemoglobin level of 7.8 g/dL (78 g/L) and a leukocyte count of 22,000/µL $(22 \times 10^9/L)$.

Bilateral lower lobe infiltrates are seen on a chest radiograph. The patient receives intravenous saline, prophylactic doses of low-molecular-weight heparin, and ceftriaxone and levofloxacin. Incentive spirometry is begun. Six hours later, he has worsening hypoxia and respiratory distress requiring intubation and mechanical ventilation. A repeat chest radiograph shows worsening infiltrates.

Which of the following is the most appropriate management?

(A) CT pulmonary angiography

(B) Exchange transfusion

(C) Intravenous amphotericin

(D) Intravenous full-dose unfractionated heparin

(E) Lower extremity Doppler ultrasonography

Item 55

A 77-year-old woman is evaluated in the emergency department with a 3-day history of progressive abdominal pain and fever. Medical history is notable for atrial fibrillation. Her only medication is dabigatran; she took her last dose 16 hours ago.

On physical examination, temperature is 39.1 °C (102.3 °F), blood pressure is 90/55 mm Hg, pulse rate is 115/min, and respiration rate is normal. She has abdominal guarding with rebound tenderness. The examination is otherwise unremarkable.

Laboratory studies show an activated partial thromboplastin time of greater than 100 seconds and a serum creatinine level of 1.7 mg/dL (150 µmol/L).

CT scan of the abdomen shows a complete large bowel obstruction.

Emergency surgery is planned.

Which of the following is the most appropriate management of the patient's anticoagulation?

(A) Dialysis

(B) Fresh frozen plasma

(C) Idarucizumab

(D) Prothrombin complex concentrate

Item 56

A 56-year-old man is brought to the emergency department after being found lying unresponsive in the local train station. Medical history is significant for chronic alcohol dependence. He is homeless. The patient is a frequent visitor to the emergency department for minor trauma and ailments; his last visit was 6 months ago. Until that time, the patient lived in various shelters and received at least one nutritious meal per day. His whereabouts and living circumstances since that time are unknown. His medical history is otherwise not significant, and at his last visit to the emergency department, he was taking no medications.

On physical examination, vital signs are normal. The patient is disheveled, cachectic, and malodorous. He moans in response to painful stimuli and moves all extremities. He has poor dentition. Hepatomegaly is noted.

Laboratory studies:

Hemoglobin	7.4 g/dL (74 g/L)
Leukocyte count	4200/μL (4.2×10⁹/L)
Mean corpuscular volume	110 fL
Platelet count	97,000/μL (97×10⁹/L)
Reticulocyte count	1% of erythrocytes
Blood alcohol level	500 mg/dL (108 mmol/L)

Hypersegmented neutrophils are seen on the peripheral blood smear.

Which of the following is the most likely cause of this patient's anemia?

(A) Cobalamin deficiency

(B) Folate deficiency

(C) Inflammatory anemia

(D) Iron deficiency

Item 57

A 59-year-old man is evaluated for progressive fatigue of 3 months' duration and recent worsening of his chronic back pain. He also reports swelling of his lower extremities. He does not indicate problems with urination. Medical history is notable for chronic low back pain. His only medication is acetaminophen as needed.

On physical examination, vital signs are normal. Deep palpation of the lower back elicits pain. He has 1+ edema of the lower extremities.

Laboratory studies:

Hemoglobin	8 g/dL (80 g/L)
Leukocyte count	4000/μL (4×10⁹/L)
Platelet count	300,000/μL (300×10⁹/L)
Albumin	2.7 g/dL (27 g/L)
Calcium	13.4 mg/dL (3.4 mmol/L)
Creatinine	2.1 mg/dL (186 μmol/L)
Protein, total	9.2 g/dL (92 g/L)

A radiograph of the lumbar spine shows compression fracture of the L1 vertebral body.

Which of the following is the most appropriate diagnostic test to perform next?

(A) Bone scan

(B) Prostate-specific antigen measurement

(C) Serum parathyroid hormone measurement

(D) Serum protein electrophoresis and free light chain analysis

Item 58

A 67-year-old woman is evaluated for slowly worsening fatigue and exertional dyspnea of several months' duration, with more recent yellowing of the skin. Medical history is notable for Hashimoto thyroiditis diagnosed 30 years ago. Her only medication is levothyroxine.

On physical examination, temperature is 36.7 °C (98.0 °F), blood pressure is 125/75 mm Hg, pulse rate is 100/min, and respiration rate is 18/min. Jaundice is noted. The remainder of the examination is noncontributory.

Laboratory studies:

Hemoglobin	6.2 g/dL (62 g/L)
Leukocyte count	3100/μL (3.1 × 10⁹/L), with a normal differential
Mean corpuscular volume	110 fL
Platelet count	94,000 (94×10⁹/L)
Bilirubin	
Total	6.2 mg/dL (106 μmol/L)
Direct	1.0 mg/dL (17.1 μmol/L)
Lactate dehydrogenase	400 U/L

A peripheral blood smear shows macrocytic erythrocytes with rare nucleated erythrocytes and scattered, six-lobed neutrophils. A direct antiglobulin (Coombs) test is negative.

Which of the following should be obtained next?

(A) Bone marrow biopsy

(B) Cobalamin and folate levels

(C) Flow cytometry

(D) Glucose-6-phosphate dehydrogenase level

Item 59

A 68-year-old man notes 3 days of melena and the recent onset of epistaxis and easy bruising. He had no bleeding problems until the past week. He has advanced ischemic cardiomyopathy and had a left ventricular assist device (LVAD) placed 3 months ago. He had no bleeding history before LVAD implantation surgery, and his preoperative coagulation studies were normal. Medications are atorvastatin, carvedilol, lisinopril, spironolactone, and warfarin initiated after LVAD placement.

On physical examination, other than a pulse rate of 112/min, vital signs are normal. Oxygen saturation is 94% breathing ambient air. He has crusted blood in the left nares, scattered ecchymoses, and multiple petechiae. The surgical scar on the anterior chest appears well healed. Stool for fecal occult blood is strongly positive. The remainder of the examination is normal.

Laboratory studies:

Activated partial thromboplastin time	40 s
Hemoglobin	8.0 mg/dL (80 g/L)
Platelet count	130,000/μL (130×10⁹/L)
Prothrombin time	19 s
INR	2.0
Platelet Function Analyzer-100	Prolonged
Aminotransferases	Normal
Fibrinogen	350 mg/dL (3.5 g/L)

Which of the following is the most likely cause of this patient's new bleeding symptoms?

(A) Acquired von Willebrand disease

(B) Coagulopathy of liver disease

(C) Dysfibrinogenemia

(D) Immune thrombocytopenic purpura

Item 60

An 81-year-old man is evaluated for increasing fatigue. He has no other symptoms to report. Medical history is significant for diabetes mellitus and hypertension. He does not drink alcohol or smoke. Medications are metformin and lisinopril.

On physical examination, vital signs are normal. The examination is unremarkable.

Laboratory studies:

Hemoglobin	8.5 g/dL (85 g/L)
Leukocyte count	3100/µL (3.1 × 10⁹/L) with 35% neutrophils, 45% lymphocytes, 20% monocytes
Mean corpuscular volume	105 fL
Platelet count	120,000/µL (120 × 10⁹/L)

Serum levels of vitamin B$_{12}$ and folate are normal. Peripheral blood smear is shown.

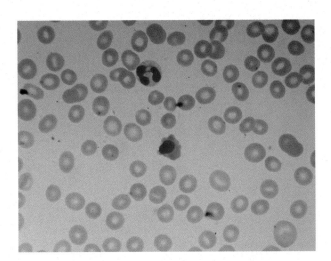

Which of the following is the most appropriate diagnostic test to perform next to evaluate this patient's anemia?

(A) *BCR-ABL* testing
(B) Bone marrow biopsy
(C) Immunoelectrophoresis
(D) *JAK2* mutation testing

Item 61

A 24-year-old woman is evaluated for an episode of syncope. She is in her sixth month of pregnancy. She reports exertional dyspnea and occasional chest pain. She has sickle cell disease characterized by acute pain events occurring four to five times per year, typically not requiring hospitalization. She had an episode of acute chest syndrome 1 year ago, at which time she received exchange transfusion. Medications are a prenatal multivitamin and folic acid supplement.

On physical examination, temperature is 37 °C (98.7 °F), blood pressure is 90/60 mm Hg, pulse rate is 110/min, and respiration rate is 20/min. Oxygen saturation is 98% breathing ambient air. Cardiac examination reveals a parasternal heave. The pulmonic component of the S$_2$ is accentuated, and a holosystolic murmur that increases with inspiration is heard at the apex. Other examination findings are normal.

Electrocardiography reveals right axis deviation, a tall R wave in lead V1, and inverted T waves in V1 to V3.

Laboratory studies:

Hemoglobin	8.2 g/dL (82 g/L)
Leukocyte count	13,600/µL (13.6 × 10⁹/L)
Platelet count	385,000/µL (385 × 10⁹/L)
Reticulocytes	7% of erythrocytes

Which of the following is the most appropriate diagnostic test to perform next?

(A) Cardiac MRI
(B) Echocardiography
(C) Exercise stress test
(D) Thoracic aortography

Item 62

A 71-year-old man is evaluated for headaches of 2 months' duration. He reports no shortness of breath and has a good energy level. Medical history is significant for hypertension, hypothyroidism, and hypogonadism; he has never smoked. Medications are lisinopril, levothyroxine, and testosterone injections.

On physical examination, vital signs are normal except for a blood pressure of 160/92 mm Hg; BMI is 19. He has facial plethora. Cardiopulmonary examination is normal. No hepatosplenomegaly is noted.

Laboratory studies:

Erythropoietin	40 mU/mL (40 U/L)
Hematocrit	56%
Hemoglobin	18.9 g/dL (189 g/L)
Leukocyte count	7000/µL (7 × 10⁹/L) with normal differential
Platelet count	300,000/µL (300 × 10⁹/L)

Which of the following is the most likely cause of this patient's findings?

(A) Levothyroxine
(B) Lisinopril
(C) Polycythemia vera
(D) Testosterone

Item 63

A 59-year-old man is evaluated in the hospital for swelling of his left leg. He was admitted 5 days ago with deep venous thrombosis of the right lower extremity and bilateral pulmonary emboli. Therapy with low-molecular-weight heparin (LMWH) was initiated on hospital day 1. Medical history is significant for chronic heart failure, with a hospitalization 1 month ago for pulmonary edema. Other medications are lisinopril, furosemide, and metoprolol.

On physical examination, temperature is 38.1 °C (100.6 °F), blood pressure is 132/84 mm Hg, pulse rate is 104/min, and respiration rate is 24/min. Oxygen saturation is 91% breathing ambient air. The right and left legs are swollen to midthigh.

Laboratory studies show a hemoglobin level of 12.8 g/dL (128 g/L), leukocyte count of 11,200/µL (11.2 × 10⁹/L), and platelet count of 78,000/µL (78 × 10⁹/L) (at admission, 168,000/µL [168 × 10⁹/L]).

Doppler ultrasonography discloses a new left femoral vein thrombosis.

Which of the following is the most appropriate management?

(A) Discontinue LMWH and begin argatroban

(B) Discontinue LMWH and begin unfractionated heparin

(C) Insert an inferior vena cava retrievable filter

(D) Overlap LMWH and warfarin for 5 days

Item 64

An 18-year-old man is evaluated in the emergency department for abdominal cramping and bloody diarrhea of 6 days' duration. Medical history is unremarkable, and he takes no medications.

On physical examination, temperature is 37.0 °C (98.6 °F), blood pressure is 98/60 mm Hg, pulse rate is 100/min, and respiration rate is 16/min. Oxygen saturation is normal breathing ambient air. His abdomen is tender, without guarding or organomegaly. The examination is otherwise unremarkable.

Laboratory studies:

Haptoglobin	Undetectable
Hemoglobin	6.1 g/dL (61 g/L)
Leukocyte count	6800/µL (6.8 × 10⁹/L)
Platelet count	37,000/µL (37 × 10⁹/L)
Reticulocytes	9.8% of erythrocytes
Creatinine	3.6 mg/dL (318 µmol/L)
Urinalysis	3+ blood; 3+ protein; 0-2 erythrocytes/hpf; 0-2 leukocytes/hpf; several granular casts

The peripheral blood smear shows schistocytes and scant platelets without clumps. The direct antiglobulin (Coombs) test is negative.

What is the most likely diagnosis?

(A) Atypical hemolytic uremic syndrome

(B) Hemolytic uremic syndrome

(C) Immune hemolytic anemia and thrombocytopenia

(D) Rapidly progressive glomerulonephritis

Item 65

A 62-year-old woman is evaluated for mild anemia noted on routine complete blood counts over the past 6 months. Medical history is notable for a mechanical bileaflet mitral valve placed 14 years ago and essential hypertension diagnosed 15 years ago. Medications are warfarin, atenolol, and lisinopril.

On physical examination, vital signs are normal. Cardiac examination reveals crisp mechanical valve sounds without murmur. The remainder of the examination is noncontributory.

Laboratory studies:

Haptoglobin	Undetectable
Hemoglobin	10.6 g/dL (106 g/L)
Mean corpuscular volume	86 fL
Reticulocyte count	9% of erythrocytes
Lactate dehydrogenase	400 U/L

The peripheral blood smear shows normochromic normocytic erythrocytes with rare schistocytes. Leukocyte and platelet counts are normal.

Echocardiography reveals normal valve function.

Which of the following is the most likely diagnosis?

(A) Drug-induced hemolysis

(B) Gastrointestinal blood loss

(C) Glucose-6-phosphate dehydrogenase deficiency

(D) Valve hemolysis

Item 66

A 54-year-old man undergoes follow-up evaluation for deep venous thrombosis after a left hip replacement 2 months ago. He is feeling well, his swelling has improved, and he reports no pain. His only medication is rivaroxaban.

On physical examination, vital signs are normal. The examination is otherwise unremarkable.

Which of the following is the most appropriate management?

(A) Completion of 3-month course of anticoagulation

(B) D-dimer measurement

(C) Extended anticoagulation

(D) Thrombophilia evaluation

Item 67

A 32-year-old woman is evaluated in the emergency department for extremely heavy menstrual bleeding. She reports she is on the third day of her menstrual cycle and is changing her pad or tampon every 2 hours with "clots." Medications are a daily multivitamin and ibuprofen as needed for cramps.

On physical examination, vital signs are normal. She has no ecchymoses, petechiae, or splenomegaly.

Laboratory studies:

Hemoglobin	10.5 g/dL (105 g/L)
Leukocyte count	Normal
Mean corpuscular volume	72 fL
Platelet count	68,000/µL (68 × 10⁹/L)

Review of the peripheral blood smear shows platelet clumps. A repeat platelet count performed on blood obtained in a heparinized container is normal.

In addition to iron deficiency anemia, which of the following is the most likely diagnosis?

(A) Essential thrombocythemia

(B) Immune thrombocytopenic purpura

(C) Myelodysplastic syndrome

(D) Pseudothrombocytopenia

Item 68

A 62-year-old man arrives for follow-up consultation for multiple myeloma diagnosed 3 weeks ago. A skeletal survey showed multiple lytic lesions in the spine and pelvis, but the patient's vertebral height was maintained. MRI showed abnormalities in the vertebral bodies but no evidence of spinal cord compression. Myeloma therapy was begun with borte-zomib, lenalidomide, and dexamethasone. Medical history is otherwise unremarkable. He takes no other medications.

On physical examination, vital signs are normal. The lower spine is nontender to palpation. The remainder of the physical examination is unremarkable.

Laboratory studies show a serum calcium level of 9.1 mg/dL (2.3 mmol/L) and a serum creatinine level of 0.8 mg/dL (70.7 µmol/L); a complete blood count and serum electrolyte levels are normal.

Which of the following is the most appropriate management of this patient's lytic bone lesions?

(A) Dual-energy x-ray absorptiometry
(B) Radiation therapy
(C) Zoledronic acid
(D) Current myeloma treatment

Item 69

A 32-year-old woman is hospitalized with progressive exertional dyspnea. She has noted dark urine for the last week and yellowing of her skin for several days. Medical history is unremarkable, and she takes no medications.

On physical examination, temperature is 36.7 °C (98.0 °F), blood pressure is 100/70 mm Hg, pulse rate is 100/min, and respiration rate is 18/min. Icteric sclera and skin are noted. Cardiac examination reveals a grade 2/6 systolic flow murmur. No lymphadenopathy or hepatosplenomegaly is present. The remainder of the examination is noncontributory.

Laboratory studies:

Haptoglobin	Undetectable
Hemoglobin	4.8 g/dL (48 g/L)
Leukocyte count	8200/µL (8.2 × 10⁹/L)
Mean corpuscular volume	134 fL
Platelet count	230,000 (230 × 10⁹/L)
Reticulocyte count	12% of erythrocytes
Bilirubin	
Total	6.7 mg/dL (114.6 µmol/L)
Direct	1.2 mg/dL (20.5 µmol/L)
Lactate dehydrogenase	660 U/L
Urinalysis	Dipstick positive for 4+ blood; 0-1 leukocytes/hpf, and 0 erythrocytes/hpf

A peripheral blood smear shows erythrocyte agglutination. A direct antiglobulin (Coombs) test is positive for C3. Diagnostic testing for *Mycoplasma* and Epstein-Barr virus is negative.

Which of the following is the most appropriate treatment?

(A) Intravenous immune globulin
(B) Prednisone
(C) Rituximab
(D) Splenectomy

Item 70

A 24-year-old woman is admitted to the hospital with a right lower lobe pulmonary embolism. Her mother experienced a deep venous thrombosis 25 years ago. Weight-based intravenous heparin is initiated.

On physical examination, temperature and blood pressure are normal, pulse rate is 120/min, and respiration rate is 19/min. Oxygen saturation is 91% breathing ambient air. The examination is otherwise unremarkable.

Despite appropriately increasing doses of heparin, her activated partial thromboplastin time remains in the normal range.

Which of the following is the most likely diagnosis?

(A) Antiphospholipid antibody syndrome
(B) Antithrombin deficiency
(C) Factor V Leiden
(D) Protein C deficiency

Item 71

A 64-year-old woman is evaluated in the emergency department for large ecchymoses, bleeding gums, and a hematoma extending from her upper thigh to her knee. Medical history is significant for chronic lymphocytic leukemia, which has been asymptomatic and managed expectantly. She has experienced no previous bleeding symptoms and has no family history of bleeding disorders. She takes no medications.

On physical examination, other than a pulse rate of 104/min, vital signs are normal. Ecchymoses are present on her arms and legs. Small cervical and axillary lymph nodes are palpable. Other examination findings are normal.

Laboratory studies:

Activated partial thromboplastin time (aPTT)	88 s
aPTT with mixing study	64 s
Hemoglobin	10.8 g/dL (108 g/L)
Leukocyte count	65,000/µL (65 × 10⁹/L)
Platelet count	215,000/µL (215 × 10⁹/L)
Prothrombin time	11.5 s
Factor VIII	1%

Administration of which of the following is the most appropriate management?

(A) Activated factor VII
(B) Cryoprecipitate
(C) Desmopressin
(D) Fresh frozen plasma

Item 72

A 74-year-old man is noted to have prolonged bleeding from venipuncture sites and new ecchymoses. He was admitted to the hospital 2 weeks ago for antibiotic treatment of a lung abscess. He developed *Clostridium difficile*-related diarrhea 1 week ago. His oral intake has been poor. Medical history is notable for hyperlipidemia. Medications are ampicillin-sulbactam, oral vancomycin, atorvastatin, and low-dose subcutaneous low-molecular-weight heparin.

On physical examination, temperature is 38.2 °C (100.8 °F), blood pressure is 115/68 mm Hg, pulse rate is 96/min, and respiration rate is 24/min. He is thin and chronically ill appearing. On pulmonary examination, crackles are heard at the right lung base. The remainder of the examination is normal.

Laboratory studies:

Activated partial thromboplastin time	30 s
Hemoglobin	11.8 g/dL (118 g/L)
Prothrombin time	22 s
Alanine aminotransferase	54 U/L
Aspartate aminotransferase	56 U/L
Factor V	100%
Factor VIII	100%
Factor X	24%

Which of the following is the most appropriate management?

(A) Administer vitamin K

(B) Discontinue atorvastatin

(C) Discontinue heparin and repeat tests in 24 hours

(D) Transfuse fresh frozen plasma

Item 73

A 26-year-old man undergoes follow-up evaluation after hospitalization for deep venous thrombosis last week. He reports no recent travel, surgery, or immobilization. He has a sister who was diagnosed with an unprovoked deep venous thrombosis 1 year ago at 35 years of age. Medical history is otherwise unremarkable. His only medication is rivaroxaban.

On physical examination, vital signs are normal. The examination is otherwise unremarkable.

The possibility of an inherited thrombophilia is discussed with the patient. After reviewing the risks and benefits of additional testing, he would like to be further evaluated for a possible thrombophilia.

Which of the following is the ideal testing strategy?

(A) Test now

(B) Test in 2 months

(C) Test a saved blood sample obtained during hospitalization but before anticoagulation

(D) Temporarily stop rivaroxaban in 1 year and test 2 weeks later

Item 74

A 35-year-old woman arrives at the emergency department with epigastric abdominal pain of 3 months' duration, which has worsened during the past week. She also reports fatigue. Medical history is significant for a deep venous thrombosis that occurred 4 years ago, which was treated with 6 months of anticoagulation. She takes no medications.

On physical examination, vital signs are normal, except for a pulse rate of 105/min. She has mildly diffuse abdominal tenderness. The physical examination is otherwise noncontributory.

Laboratory studies:

Haptoglobin	110 mg/dL (1100 mg/L)
Hemoglobin	11 g/dL (110 g/L)
Leukocyte count	3800/µL (3.8 × 10⁹/L)
Mean corpuscular volume	80 fL
Platelet count	252,000/µL (252 × 10⁹/L)
Alkaline phosphatase	158 U/L
Bilirubin	
Total	3.5 mg/dL (59.9 µmol/L)
Direct	3.0 mg/dL (51.3 µmol/L)
γ-Glutamyltransferase	120 U/L

Prothrombin and activated partial thromboplastin times are normal. Testing for hepatitis B and C are negative.

A triphasic CT scan of the abdomen shows occlusion of the hepatic veins, ascites, splenomegaly, and abdominal varices; no cirrhosis is seen.

Which of the following is the most appropriate diagnostic test to perform next?

(A) α-Fetoprotein

(B) Factor VIII level

(C) Flow cytometry for CD 55/59

(D) *JAK2 V617F* mutation

Item 75

A 28-year-old woman is evaluated for severe anemia. She was admitted to the hospital 5 days ago for Lyme-related meningoencephalitis. Her only medication is intravenous ceftriaxone.

On physical examination, temperature is 36.7 °C (98.0 °F), blood pressure is 110/70 mm Hg, pulse rate is 100/min, and respiration rate is 15/min. She is alert and oriented. She has icteric sclera. Cardiac examination is normal, and no lymphadenopathy or organomegaly is noted.

Laboratory studies:

Hemoglobin	6.5 g/dL (65 g/L)
Leukocyte count	11,000/µL (11 × 10⁹/L)
Platelet count	145,000 (145 × 10⁹/L)
Reticulocyte count	10% of erythrocytes
Lactate dehydrogenase	400 U/L

The peripheral blood smear shows occasional spherocytes. A direct antiglobulin (Coombs) test is positive for IgG.

Which of the following is the most likely diagnosis?

(A) Cold agglutinin disease

(B) Drug-induced hemolysis

(C) Glucose-6-phosphate dehydrogenase deficiency

(D) Lyme-induced hemolysis

Item 76

A 68-year-old woman is hospitalized with fatigue, anorexia, and myalgia worsening over the last week. She underwent laparotomy 4 weeks ago for trauma sustained in a motor vehicle accident, which necessitated a splenectomy.

She received 3 units of blood as well as pneumococcal, haemophilus, and meningococcal vaccination; she was discharged on postoperative day 8. Hemoglobin level at discharge was 11 mg/dL (110 g/L). Her only medication is acetaminophen as needed for pain.

On physical examination, temperature is 38.6 °C (101.5 °F), blood pressure is 138/63 mm Hg, pulse rate is 92/min, and respiration rate is 18/min. The examination is otherwise noncontributory.

Laboratory studies:

Hemoglobin	9.9 g/dL (99 g/L)
Leukocyte count	10,100/μL (10.1 × 10⁹/L) with 82% neutrophils, 2% bands, 11% lymphocytes, 3% monocytes, and 2% atypical lymphocytes
Platelet count	92,000/μL (92 × 10⁹/L)
Reticulocyte count	8% of erythrocytes
Alkaline phosphatase	833 U/L
Alanine aminotransferase	140 U/L
Aspartate aminotransferase	134 U/L

Blood cultures are obtained. Peripheral blood smear is shown.

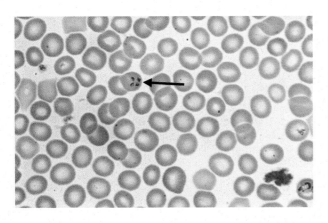

Which of the following transfusion-transmitted diseases is the most likely diagnosis?

(A) Babesiosis
(B) Bacterial infection
(C) Cytomegalovirus
(D) West Nile virus
(E) Zika virus

Item 77

A 32-year-old woman is evaluated for urinary frequency and dysuria. She is at 10 weeks' gestation with her first pregnancy. Medical history is notable for chronic immune thrombocytopenic purpura diagnosed 6 years ago. Her only medication is a prenatal vitamin.

On physical examination, blood pressure is 110/60 mm Hg; vital signs are otherwise normal. She has a gravid uterus. No petechiae or ecchymoses are noted.

Laboratory studies:

Hemoglobin	12.2 g/dL (122 g/L)
Leukocyte count	9800/μL (9.8 × 10⁹/L)
Platelet count	40,000/μL (40 × 10⁹/L); normally 60,000-80,000/μL (60-80 × 10⁹/L)
Aminotransferase levels	Normal
Urinalysis	Nitrite +, leukocyte esterase +, small blood; no protein

A peripheral blood smear shows large and giant platelets but no clumps or schistocytes.

In addition to treating this patient's urinary tract infection, which of the following is the most appropriate management?

(A) Begin intravenous immune globulin
(B) Begin prednisone
(C) Transfuse platelets
(D) Monitor platelet count

Oncology Questions

Item 78

A 65-year-old woman is evaluated for new-onset hemoptysis. Her medical history is significant for a 40-pack-year smoking history. She takes no medications.

On physical examination, vital signs are normal. BMI is 29. Oxygen saturation is normal breathing ambient air. Digital clubbing is present.

CT scan of the chest, abdomen, and pelvis shows a large left hilar mass; there are no other pulmonary lesions, and there is no evidence of metastatic disease. Bronchoscopy with biopsy reveals small cell lung cancer. Brain MRI shows no metastatic disease.

Which of the following is the most appropriate treatment?

(A) Chemotherapy alone
(B) Chemotherapy followed by radiation
(C) Combined chemotherapy and radiation
(D) Radiation alone

Item 79

A 77-year-old man is evaluated for a 6-month history of worsening urinary frequency and nocturia. He takes no medications.

On physical examination, vital signs are normal. BMI is 22. Digital rectal examination reveals a firm, enlarged prostate.

Laboratory studies reveal a serum prostate-specific antigen level of 18.5 ng/mL (18.5 μg/L). Biopsy of the prostate reveals adenocarcinoma with bilateral gland involvement; the Gleason score is 8.

MRI of the pelvis shows evidence of focal extension beyond the prostate capsule. Bone and CT scans are negative for metastatic disease.

Which of the following is the most appropriate management?

(A) Brachytherapy
(B) Gonadotropin-releasing hormone agonist
(C) Gonadotropin-releasing hormone agonist plus radiation
(D) Radiation

Item 80

A 59-year-old woman is hospitalized with a biopsy-confirmed poorly differentiated squamous cell carcinoma of the base of tongue. Her medical history is significant for a 30-pack-year smoking history and moderate to heavy alcohol use. She takes no medications.

On physical examination, vital signs are normal. BMI is 24. Right-sided lymphadenopathy is present on palpation. There is a large mass on the right base of the tongue extending across the midline, nearly obstructing the airway.

Laboratory studies are notable for a serum creatinine level of 1.8 mg/dL (159.12 µmol/L).

CT scan of the neck shows a very large mass on the right base of the tongue that crosses the midline, extending into the extrinsic muscles of the tongue and adjacent to the carotid artery. Multiple enlarged right-sided cervical lymph nodes are noted, with the largest being 3.5 cm. Enlarged nodes are also noted on the left side. CT scan of the chest is negative.

Which of the following is the most appropriate treatment?

(A) Bevacizumab
(B) Cetuximab plus radiation
(C) Cisplatin plus radiation
(D) Radiation alone

Item 81

A 29-year-old woman diagnosed with stage IA cervical cancer is evaluated during a follow-up visit. The patient would like to preserve fertility. She has no other medical problems and takes no medications.

On physical examination, vital signs are normal. The general physical examination is normal.

Which of the following is the most appropriate management?

(A) Conization
(B) Neoadjuvant chemotherapy
(C) Radiation therapy
(D) Radical hysterectomy

Item 82

A 48-year-old woman is evaluated during a follow-up visit for breast cancer. At age 43 years, she was diagnosed with low-risk, stage IIA invasive ductal cancer. The cancer was estrogen receptor positive, progesterone receptor positive, and *HER2* negative. She has completed 5 years of tamoxifen and has tolerated it well. She continues to have menstrual periods. She takes no other medications.

On physical examination, vital signs are normal. There are well-healed incisions of the right breast and axilla. There are no breast masses.

Which of the following is the most appropriate management?

(A) Continue tamoxifen for 5 more years
(B) Stop tamoxifen

(C) Stop tamoxifen; begin anastrozole
(D) Stop tamoxifen; begin leuprolide and anastrozole

Item 83

A 22-year-old man is evaluated for a mass on the left side of his neck. He has not experienced fevers, night sweats, or weight loss. He takes no medications.

On physical examination, all vital signs are normal. A left supraclavicular lymph node is enlarged to 4 cm, and axillary lymphadenopathy is noted bilaterally. There is no hepatosplenomegaly.

A biopsy specimen of the supraclavicular lymph node reveals Hodgkin lymphoma, nodular sclerosis subtype.

Laboratory results, including complete blood count, biochemical profile, and serum lactate dehydrogenase, are normal.

CT scan and PET scan show mediastinal lymphadenopathy, with nodes up to 4 cm in size, and left supraclavicular and bilateral axillary lymphadenopathy. No infradiaphragmatic disease is observed.

Which of the following is the most appropriate initial management?

(A) Bone marrow biopsy
(B) Chemotherapy
(C) Radiation therapy
(D) Staging laparotomy and splenectomy

Item 84

A 42-year-old woman is evaluated during a follow-up visit. She was diagnosed 4 years ago with stage IIIA high-grade serous ovarian cancer, with a deleterious *BRCA1* germline mutation found on genetic testing. She was treated with total abdominal hysterectomy, bilateral salpingo-oophorectomy, and chemotherapy with intravenous and intraperitoneal cisplatin and paclitaxel. Her cancer recurred 18 months after she completed chemotherapy, and she underwent two additional sequential chemotherapies, including carboplatin and paclitaxel, cisplatin and gemcitabine, and bevacizumab. The cancer is progressing on her current treatment. Her performance status is good (Eastern Cooperative Oncology Group = 1). The patient is still taking chemotherapy medications.

On physical examination, vital signs are normal. Abdominal distention with lateral dullness is present. The remainder of the examination is normal.

Laboratory studies reveal a serum CA-125 value of 145 U/mL (145 kU/L) (1 month ago, 82 U/mL [82 kU/L]).

CT scans of the chest, abdomen, and pelvis show increased size and number of peritoneal masses and increasing ascites. There are no pleural effusions.

In addition to stopping the current chemotherapy regimen, which of the following is the most appropriate treatment?

(A) High-dose chemotherapy with hematopoietic stem cell transplantation
(B) Oral (poly adenosine diphosphate-ribose) polymerase inhibitor
(C) Repeat intraperitoneal cisplatin chemotherapy
(D) Supportive care

Item 85

A 38-year-old woman is evaluated. She has just been diagnosed with hormone receptor–negative, *HER2*-positive stage II infiltrating ductal breast cancer. She takes no medications. Neoadjuvant chemotherapy with docetaxel, trastuzumab, and pertuzumab is planned; a port has been placed, and treatment is to start next week. The patient has a 2-year-old daughter and has very recently decided that she wishes to conceive again.

On physical examination, vital signs are normal. A 2.5-cm left breast mass is noted, with no regional lymphadenopathy.

Which of the following is the most appropriate management?

(A) Advise against any further pregnancies

(B) Cancel chemotherapy and proceed with mastectomy and radiation therapy

(C) Delay chemotherapy until counseled by a fertility specialist

(D) Proceed with chemotherapy

Item 86

A 62-year-old woman is evaluated during a follow-up visit for recently diagnosed stage IIIA high-grade serous ovarian cancer. She underwent total abdominal hysterectomy and bilateral salpingo-oophorectomy and completed six cycles of chemotherapy with cisplatin and paclitaxel. The patient's paternal aunt was diagnosed with breast cancer at age 52 years. There is no personal or family history of any other cancers. She takes no medications.

On physical examination, vital signs and the remainder of the examination are normal.

Laboratory studies reveal a serum CA-125 value of 14 U/mL (14 kU/L) after chemotherapy (383 U/mL [383 kU/L] at diagnosis).

Which of the following is the most appropriate test to perform next?

(A) Chest radiography annually

(B) CT of the abdomen and pelvis in 3 months

(C) Genetic testing for *BRCA1* and *BRCA2* mutations

(D) Genetic testing for Lynch mutations

Item 87

A 65-year-old man is evaluated for persistent dyspepsia despite treatment with antacid therapy. He also has recent weight loss of 3 kg (6.6 lb) and development of epigastric abdominal pain. He does not smoke or drink alcohol. He takes no medications other than antacids.

On physical examination, vital signs are normal. There is epigastric tenderness but no abdominal masses, no hepatosplenomegaly, and no lymphadenopathy.

The endoscopic biopsy specimen shows evidence of mucosa-associated lymphoid tissue (MALT) lymphoma involving the stomach. Immunohistochemical stains for *Helicobacter pylori* are positive.

A CT scan shows thickening of the gastric wall but no abdominal or other lymphadenopathy.

Which of the following is the most appropriate management?

(A) Combination therapy with rituximab and chemotherapy

(B) Gastrectomy

(C) PET

(D) Proton pump inhibitor and antibiotic therapy

(E) Radiation therapy

Item 88

A 55-year-old woman is evaluated in the office for a recent diagnosis of lobular carcinoma in situ and atypical lobular hyperplasia. She wishes to discuss options to decrease her risk of breast cancer. The patient is postmenopausal. Her medical history is significant for a left calf deep venous thrombosis at 25 years of age concurrent with oral contraceptive use. She takes no medications.

On physical examination, vital signs are normal. There is a healed left upper breast incision. The remainder of the examination is normal.

Which of the following is the most appropriate preventive measure for this patient?

(A) Exemestane

(B) High-dose vitamin D

(C) Low-fat diet

(D) Raloxifene

(E) Tamoxifen

Item 89

A 74-year-old man is evaluated for a 4-month history of increasing fatigue. He also reports increased dyspnea climbing stairs. He takes no medications.

On physical examination, vital signs are normal. The remainder of the physical examination is unremarkable.

Laboratory studies reveal a hemoglobin level of 8.8 g/dL (88 g/L) and a mean corpuscular volume of 70 fL.

A colonoscopy, performed to the ileocecal valve, identifies a fungating mass at the hepatic flexure. A biopsy specimen shows moderately differentiated invasive adenocarcinoma.

Which of the following is the most appropriate test to perform next?

(A) Contrast-enhanced CT scan of the chest, abdomen, and pelvis

(B) CT colonography

(C) Liver MRI scan

(D) Whole body PET/CT scan

Item 90

A 57-year-old postmenopausal woman is evaluated following the diagnosis of right breast ductal carcinoma in situ after lumpectomy. Pathologic findings showed a grade 3 ductal carcinoma in situ spanning 2.5 cm with negative margins that is estrogen receptor–positive; lymph nodes were not sampled. She has received primary breast radiation therapy. She takes no medications.

On physical examination, vital signs are normal. There is a healed right breast incision. There are no breast masses or lymphadenopathy.

Which of the following is the most appropriate management to decrease the risk of ipsilateral and contralateral breast cancer?

(A) Initiate anastrozole

(B) Initiate raloxifene

(C) Initiate tamoxifen plus docetaxel

(D) Obtain 21-gene recurrence score testing

Item 91

A 62-year-old woman is evaluated for a 3-month history of worsening cough and a 2-week history of shortness of breath. She has lost 9.1 kg (20.0 lb). She quit smoking 25 years ago. She takes no medications.

On physical examination, vital signs are normal. Oxygen saturation is 94% breathing ambient air. Pulmonary examination reveals decreased breath sounds in the left lower lung field.

CT scan of the chest shows a large left pleural effusion, multiple right-sided lung nodules, and hypodense lesions in the upper portion of the liver. Bone scan reveals metastatic lesions involving the ribs and thoracic spine. Brain MRI shows no metastatic disease.

Thoracentesis is performed and cytologic findings confirm adenocarcinoma.

Which of the following is the most appropriate management?

(A) Erlotinib

(B) Prophylactic cranial irradiation

(C) Radiation to the metastatic lesion on the thoracic spine

(D) Systemic chemotherapy

(E) Test for activating mutations

Item 92

A 60-year-old man is seen for a routine evaluation. His family history is notable for prostate cancer in his father. He takes no medications.

On physical examination, vital signs are normal. The remainder of the examination is normal.

After discussion of the benefits and harms of prostate cancer screening, the patient wishes to proceed with screening.

Laboratory studies reveal a serum prostate-specific antigen level of 5.1 ng/mL (5.1 µg/L).

Biopsy of the prostate reveals cancer in two cores of the right lobe (Gleason score, 6), with less than 10% cancer in each core.

Which of the following is the most appropriate management?

(A) Active surveillance

(B) Bone scan

(C) Leuprolide

(D) Observation

Item 93

A 61-year-old woman is evaluated for follow-up of stage IVA hypopharyngeal squamous cell carcinoma, which was treated with combined cisplatin and radiation therapy 1 year ago. She has xerostomia and some dysphagia since completing therapy. She has a 30-pack-year smoking history and quit smoking 1 year ago. She takes no medications.

On physical examination, vital signs are normal. BMI is 21. There is chronic induration of the right neck and limitation in neck range of motion, findings that have been noted on previous examinations. There is no palpable lymphadenopathy.

Laboratory studies reveal a normal thyroid-stimulating hormone level.

Recent laryngoscopy identified no evidence of recurrent cancer or new primary cancer.

Which of the following is the most appropriate screening or surveillance test to perform next?

(A) Head and neck CT scan

(B) Low-dose chest CT scan

(C) PET/CT scan

(D) Thyroid ultrasonography

Item 94

A 23-year-old woman is evaluated for swollen glands on the left side of her neck, which have persisted for 6 weeks. She has not had fevers, night sweats, or weight loss. Fine-needle aspiration of a cervical lymph node performed 1 week ago yielded no evidence of malignancy on either cytologic evaluation or flow cytometry. She takes no medications.

On physical examination, all vital signs are normal. There are multiple left cervical and supraclavicular nodes measuring up to 3 cm in size, which are firm and rubbery. The chest is clear to auscultation. There is no hepatosplenomegaly.

Laboratory results, including complete blood count with differential, are normal.

Which of the following is the most appropriate management?

(A) Core lymph node biopsy

(B) PET/CT scan

(C) Surgical lymph node biopsy

(D) Observation

Item 95

A 61-year-old man is hospitalized after several days of productive cough, fatigue, and fever. He quit smoking 10 years ago. He takes no medications.

CONT.

On physical examination, temperature is 39.2 °C (102.6 °F), blood pressure is 110/75 mm Hg, pulse rate is 110/min, and respiration rate is 24/min. Oxygen saturation is 90% breathing 2 L/min of oxygen through nasal cannula. Pulmonary examination reveals crackles in the right lower lung field. He has good performance status.

Chest radiograph shows right lower lobe pneumonia and a right hilar mass. CT scan of the chest and abdomen confirms an endobronchial lesion and right hilar mass, multiple lytic bone lesions, and a right adrenal mass. Bronchoscopy with biopsy confirms squamous cell carcinoma. Bone scan confirms multiple osseous metastatic lesions. Brain MRI shows no metastatic disease.

In addition to platinum-based chemotherapy, which of the following is most likely to improve outcome in this patient?

(A) Palliative care consultation

(B) PET/CT scan

(C) Prophylactic cranial irradiation

(D) Test for epidermal growth factor receptor mutation

Item 96

A 42-year-old woman has follow-up evaluation for stage II colon cancer that was diagnosed 3 years ago. Her tumor was found to be deficient in the mismatch repair protein MLH1. Genetic evaluation showed that she had Lynch syndrome, a germline mutation of one of the DNA mismatch repair genes. Nine months later, she developed recurrent disease with liver and lung metastases. Analysis of her tumor at that time revealed a *KRAS* mutation. She was treated initially with 5-fluorouracil, leucovorin, and oxaliplatin (FOLFOX) and then with irinotecan, each with only a short duration of tumor control and subsequent progression of disease. She reports that she has been able to maintain her full-time job and has been walking more than a mile daily. She takes no medications.

On physical examination, vital signs and the remainder of the examination are normal.

Which of the following is the most appropriate treatment?

(A) An epidermal growth factor receptor inhibitor

(B) An immune checkpoint inhibitor

(C) Dual antibody therapy targeting vascular endothelial growth factor and endothelial growth factor receptor

(D) No further chemotherapy; palliation care only

Item 97

A 69-year-old man with previously untreated chronic lymphocytic leukemia returns to the office after his third hospitalization this year for pneumonia. He received the pneumococcal conjugate vaccine at age 65 years and the polysaccharide vaccine at age 66 years. He is taking no medications.

On physical examination, vital signs are normal. He has diffuse lymphadenopathy with nodes up to 2.5 cm in size and a palpable spleen below his left costal margin. The chest is clear to auscultation.

Laboratory studies:

Leukocyte count	34,000/µL (34 × 10^9/L) with 91% lymphocytes, 5% neutrophils, 3% monocytes, and 1% bands
Platelet count	118,000/µL (118 × 10^9/L)
Hemoglobin	12.2 g/dL (122 g/L)

Which of the following is the most appropriate management?

(A) Assess immunoglobulin levels

(B) Start bendamustine and rituximab

(C) Start granulocyte colony-stimulating factor (G-CSF) injections

(D) Start ibrutinib

Item 98

A 69-year-old man is evaluated on routine follow-up. He has a history of stage IIIC sigmoid colon cancer that was resected 18 months ago. He received postoperative chemotherapy and has been followed expectantly since that time. He takes no medications.

On physical examination, vital signs are normal. Examination is notable for a liver edge palpable 2 cm below the right costal margin.

He is now found to have a new elevation in serum carcinoembryonic antigen level.

A contrast-enhanced CT scan of the chest, abdomen and pelvis shows numerous hypodense lesions up to 4 cm in diameter in the liver and lungs. Previous postoperative CT scan results were normal.

Which of the following is the most appropriate diagnostic test to perform next?

(A) Multi-gene sequencing of tumor

(B) Needle biopsy of most accessible lesion

(C) PET/CT scan

(D) *RAS* mutation status of primary tumor

Item 99

A 70-year-old woman is evaluated for a 1-month history of worsening productive cough with 1 week of blood-tinged sputum. Her appetite is decreased, and she has lost 10 lb (4.5.kg); but her performance status is otherwise normal, and she takes no medications.

On physical examination, vital signs are normal. The remainder of the physical examination, including the pulmonary examination, is normal. BMI is 27. Oxygen saturation is normal on ambient air.

CT scan of the chest, abdomen, and pelvis reveals a 4-cm left upper lobe mass, ipsilateral mediastinal lymphadenopathy, and a 4-cm adrenal mass. CT-guided biopsy of the lung mass confirms adenocarcinoma; mutation testing results are negative. Brain MRI shows no metastatic disease.

Repeat CT scan after six cycles of carboplatin and pemetrexed chemotherapy reveals a reduction in size of the lung mass, stable lymphadenopathy, and significant reduction in size of the adrenal mass. Her appetite remains diminished, but her weight is stable. The cough and sputum production have resolved.

Which of the following is the most appropriate treatment?

(A) Carboplatin and gemcitabine for four more cycles
(B) Erlotinib maintenance chemotherapy
(C) Pemetrexed maintenance chemotherapy
(D) Radiation

Item 100

A 70-year-old man is evaluated for a 2-month history of persistent hoarse voice. He has a 50-pack-year smoking history. His medical history is otherwise normal, and he takes no medications.

On physical examination, vital signs and other findings are normal.

Laryngoscopy shows a small mass on the right vocal cord without fixation or limitation in mobility. CT scan of the neck shows a small lesion on the right vocal cord with no evidence of left-sided involvement, cartilage involvement, or lymphadenopathy.

Which of the following is the most appropriate treatment?

(A) Chemotherapy plus radiation
(B) Partial laryngectomy
(C) Radiation therapy
(D) Total laryngectomy, chemotherapy, and radiation

Item 101

A 55-year-old woman is evaluated for rectal bleeding and pain with defecation that had increased during the past 3 months. She takes no medications.

On physical examination, vital signs are normal. BMI is 19. The rectal examination reveals a brown stool sample that is guaiac positive. The remainder of the physical examination is unremarkable.

Hemoglobin level is 12.5 g/dL (125 g/L). Leukocyte count, platelet count, and liver chemistry test results are normal.

A colonoscopy to the ileocecal valve identifies a fungating mass 8 cm from the anal verge, and a biopsy specimen shows adenocarcinoma. An MRI of the pelvis shows a nonobstructing tumor invading into the muscularis but not through the full thickness of the rectal wall (T2). No abnormal lymph nodes are seen. Contrast-enhanced CT scans of the chest and abdomen are normal.

Which of the following is the most appropriate treatment?

(A) Chemotherapy
(B) Radiation therapy
(C) Radiation therapy plus chemotherapy
(D) Radiation therapy plus chemotherapy followed by surgery
(E) Surgery

Item 102

A 26-year-old woman is hospitalized with a temperature of 38 °C (101.5 °F) 10 days after her first cycle of chemotherapy with rituximab, cyclophosphamide, doxorubicin, vincristine and prednisone (R-CHOP) for diffuse large B-cell lymphoma. Other than fever, she has no symptoms of infection.

On physical examination, temperature is 38.6 °C (101.5 °F). The remainder of the vital signs and physical examination are normal.

Pertinent laboratory results are a leukocyte count of 1100/µL (1.1×10^9/L) with 10% neutrophils, platelet count of 144,000/µL (144×10^9/L), and hemoglobin level of 11.2 g/dL (112 g/L). Blood and urine culture results are pending. Chest radiographic findings are negative.

Empiric broad-spectrum antibiotics are initiated.

Which of the following is the most appropriate additional management?

(A) Reduce the doses of cyclophosphamide and doxorubicin
(B) Start granulocyte colony-stimulating factor (G-CSF) now
(C) Start G-CSF on day 2 of her subsequent cycles of therapy
(D) Start levofloxacin prophylaxis before next cycles of therapy

Item 103

A 50-year-old woman is evaluated for nausea and abdominal discomfort that have been present and increasing for the past 3 to 4 months. She takes no medications.

On physical examination, vital signs are normal. BMI is 24. The abdominal examination reveals no masses, tenderness, or organomegaly.

An esophagogastroscopy identifies a discrete 8-cm mass in the pylorus. The biopsy specimen shows a gastrointestinal stromal tumor (GIST). Immunohistochemical stain for the *KIT* gene is strongly positive.

Contrast-enhanced CT scans of the chest, abdomen, and pelvis confirm the mass and do not identify any other abnormal findings.

The patient undergoes a distal gastrectomy. Pathologic findings confirm a GIST and further note a high mitotic rate (10 mitoses per 50 high-power fields). Margins of resection and all lymph nodes examined are free of tumor.

Which of the following is the most appropriate management?

(A) Intravenous rituximab
(B) Oral imatinib
(C) Radiation therapy
(D) Observation without further therapy

Item 104

A 36-year-old woman is hospitalized with a 2-week history of gradually worsening dyspnea on exertion, facial swelling, and a sensation of head fullness. She has had fatigue, night sweats, and a 4.5-kg (10-lb) weight loss over the past

2 months. Her medical history is otherwise unremarkable, and she takes no medications.

On physical examination, vital signs are normal. She is not in respiratory distress and has no stridor. She has facial and neck edema, and her face appears flushed. There is no lymphadenopathy. Lungs are clear on auscultation. Cardiac and abdominal examinations are normal.

A CT scan of the chest done in the emergency department shows an 8.5-cm right mediastinal mass with compression of the superior vena cava. There is no evidence of thrombosis. There are no other areas of lymphadenopathy and no lung masses.

Which of the following is the most appropriate next step in management?

(A) Dexamethasone
(B) Mediastinoscopy
(C) Percutaneous intravascular stent placement
(D) Urgent radiation therapy

Item 105

A 49-year-old man is evaluated for a 1-month history of a painless enlarging left neck mass. His medical history is unremarkable, and he takes no medications.

On physical examination, vital signs are normal. BMI is 26. On palpation, there is a 2-cm left anterior cervical lymph node near the angle of the mandible.

Laryngoscopy shows a left-sided tonsil cancer. Biopsy of the tonsil reveals moderately differentiated squamous cell carcinoma that is positive for p16 (human papillomavirus). CT scan of the neck reveals a cystic left-sided cervical lymph node; a left tonsil mass is noted. CT scan of the chest is negative.

Postoperative pathology reveals a 2.5-cm tonsil cancer with negative margins and 3/26 positive cervical nodes, one with extracapsular extension.

Which of the following is the most appropriate treatment?

(A) Cisplatin alone
(B) Cisplatin plus human papillomavirus vaccine
(C) Cisplatin plus radiation
(D) Radiation alone

Item 106

A 65-year-old man is evaluated for an episode of hemoptysis. His medical history is significant for a 30-pack-year smoking history; he quit smoking 1 year ago. He takes no medications.

On physical examination, vital signs are normal. BMI is 28. Oxygen saturation is 96% breathing ambient air.

CT scan of the chest identifies a 3.5-cm spiculated mass in the right lower lobe and an enlarged hilar lymph node. PET/CT scans and brain MRI scans show no evidence of metastatic disease.

Surgery is performed and reveals a 3.2-cm, poorly differentiated adenocarcinoma with negative margins, two hilar lymph nodes positive for metastatic adenocarcinoma, and negative mediastinal lymph nodes.

Which of the following is the most appropriate management?

(A) Adjuvant chemoradiation
(B) Adjuvant chemotherapy
(C) Adjuvant radiation
(D) Observation

Item 107

A 77-year-old man is evaluated in the office for weight loss and failure to thrive. He reports that he spends most of the day in a bed or chair and rarely leaves the house, and then only for short times and with considerable assistance. His appetite has been poor, and his abdominal girth has expanded. He estimates that his weight has dropped about 9 kg (20 lb) from his baseline. He takes no medications.

On physical examination, vital signs are normal. BMI is 17. He is frail, fatigued, and cachectic. Marked bitemporal wasting is noted. The sclerae are icteric. Breath sounds are diminished at bases bilaterally. The liver edge is palpable below the rib cage in the midcostal line. The abdomen is distended. There is 2+ dependent edema. The remainder of the examination is normal.

Laboratory studies:

Albumin	1.9 g/dL (19 g/L)
Alkaline phosphatase	353 U/L
Bilirubin	3.1 mg/dL (17.1 µmol/L)
Complete blood count	Hemoglobin 10 g/dL (100 g/L), with normochromic normocytic indices, normal leukocyte and platelet counts
Creatinine	0.5 mg/dL (44.2 µmol/L)

A contrast-enhanced CT scan of the chest, abdomen, and pelvis shows extensive hypodense lesions replacing more than 50% of the liver, and ascites and abdominal carcinomatosis. A diagnostic paracentesis is performed and cytologic findings show moderately differentiated adenocarcinoma.

Which of the following is the most appropriate management?

(A) Combination chemotherapy targeted at a gastrointestinal primary tumor
(B) Combination chemotherapy targeted at a germ cell tumor
(C) Hepatic arterial embolization
(D) Supportive management and hospice care

Item 108

A 58-year-old woman is evaluated for a 6-month history of headache and facial redness. Her medical history is unremarkable, and she takes no medications.

On physical examination, she is afebrile. Blood pressure is 160/95 mm Hg, pulse rate is 96/min, and respiration rate is 20/min. BMI is 28. Oxygen saturation is normal. Facial plethora and palmar erythema are present. There is no hepatomegaly or splenomegaly on palpation.

Laboratory studies:

Erythropoietin	Markedly elevated
Hemoglobin	18.1 g/dL (181 g/L)
Leukocyte count	5400/μL (5.4×10⁹/L) with a normal differential
Liver chemistry tests	Normal
Platelet count	250,000/μL (250×10⁹/L)
Urinalysis	Normal

Which of the following is the most appropriate diagnostic test to perform next?

(A) Bone marrow biopsy

(B) Chest radiography

(C) CT scan of the abdomen

(D) *JAK2* mutation testing

Item 109

A 71-year-old man is evaluated during a follow-up appointment for stage II rectal cancer that was resected 3 years ago. He takes no medications.

On physical examination, vital signs are normal. BMI is 23. The liver edge is palpable 3 cm below the xiphisternum.

A surveillance CT scan shows three new hypodense lesions in the left lobe of the liver consistent with metastatic disease. The largest lesion is 4 cm. No other abnormal findings are found on a contrast-enhanced CT scan of the chest, abdomen, and pelvis.

Which of the following is the most appropriate management?

(A) Hepatic arterial embolization

(B) Needle biopsy of the most accessible liver lesion

(C) Palliative chemotherapy

(D) Resection of all lesions

Item 110

A 66-year-old woman is evaluated for a lump in her left axilla. She is otherwise feeling well and takes no medications. On physical examination, vital signs are normal. A firm, 2-cm mass is palpable in the left axilla. The right axilla is normal. Bilateral breast examination results are normal. The remainder of the physical examination is unremarkable.

Mammography and an MRI scan of the breasts show the enlarged left axillary node but no other abnormal findings.

An excisional biopsy of the axillary node reveals a moderately differentiated adenocarcinoma that is estrogen receptor negative, progesterone receptor negative, and *HER2* negative (1+).

A CT scan of the chest, abdomen, and pelvis shows no abnormal findings. A bone scan is normal.

Which of the following is the most appropriate management?

(A) Left axillary dissection and management as primary breast cancer

(B) Letrozole

(C) Radiation therapy to the left axilla

(D) Observation with no further therapy at this time

Item 111

A 37-year-old man is evaluated in the hospital for rapidly enlarging axillary and supraclavicular lymphadenopathy. He is HIV positive. His only medication is efavirenz-emtricitabine-tenofovir.

On physical examination, vital signs are normal. A left supraclavicular lymph node is enlarged to 5 cm, and a left axillary node is enlarged to 6 cm. The remainder of the physical examination is normal.

Laboratory studies:

Creatinine	1.7 mg/dL (150.3 mmol/L)
Hemoglobin	8.6 g/dL (86 g/L)
Lactate dehydrogenase	2459 U/L
Leukocyte count	2600/μL (2.6×10⁹/L)
Platelet count	110,000/μL (110×10⁹/L)
Urate	13.3 mg/dL (0.78 mmol/L)

Biopsy of the node shows CD20-positive Burkitt lymphoma.

A CT scan of the chest, abdomen, and pelvis without contrast identifies mesenteric and retroperitoneal lymphadenopathy and splenomegaly. There is no hydronephrosis.

Before starting chemotherapy, which of the following is the most appropriate treatment?

(A) Allopurinol and intravenous hydration

(B) High-dose glucocorticoid therapy

(C) Radiation therapy

(D) Rasburicase and intravenous hydration

Item 112

A 32-year-old woman is evaluated during a follow-up visit for management of stage IIIA left breast cancer (3.5-cm, grade 3 invasive ductal carcinoma; estrogen receptor positive, progesterone receptor positive, and *HER2* negative; four positive axillary lymph nodes). She has completed neoadjuvant chemotherapy, lumpectomy, and axillary dissection as well as primary breast radiation. She resumed menstruation after completing chemotherapy, and her estradiol levels are in the premenopausal range. She takes no medications.

On physical examination, vital signs are normal. There are healed incisions on the left breast and axilla. There are no breast masses.

Which of the following is the most appropriate treatment?

(A) An aromatase inhibitor

(B) Leuprolide

(C) Leuprolide and an aromatase inhibitor

(D) Tamoxifen

Item 113

A 55-year-old woman is evaluated during a follow-up examination. She completed six cycles of chemotherapy with rituximab plus cyclophosphamide, doxorubicin, vincristine, and prednisone (R-CHOP) for stage III diffuse large B-cell lymphoma with bulky retroperitoneal lymphadenopathy. She takes no medications.

The results of the physical examination are unremarkable, with no findings of lymphadenopathy or abdominal masses.

CT scan shows a decrease in the confluent retroperitoneal nodal mass, from 15 cm × 17 cm before chemotherapy to 5 cm × 4 cm. PET scan shows no metabolic activity of the mass. No other areas of disease are noted.

Which of the following is the most appropriate management?

(A) Autologous stem cell transplant

(B) CT-guided biopsy of the residual mass

(C) Radiation therapy to the site of residual disease

(D) Surgical biopsy of the residual mass

(E) Observation by serial CT scanning

Item 114

A 55-year-old woman is evaluated to discuss additional cancer therapy. She was recently diagnosed with stage IIIB ovarian high-grade serous carcinoma. She underwent surgical staging, total abdominal hysterectomy, salpingo-oophorectomy, and debulking, with residual tumor size less than 1 cm. Genetic testing was negative for *BRCA1* and *BRCA2* mutations. She takes no medications.

On physical examination, vital signs are normal. There is a healing midline abdominal incision. The remainder of the examination is normal.

Her performance status is excellent (Eastern Cooperative Oncology Group performance status = 0).

Which of the following is the most appropriate treatment?

(A) High-dose chemotherapy with hematopoietic stem cell transplantation

(B) Intravenous and intraperitoneal cisplatin and paclitaxel chemotherapy

(C) Intravenous cisplatin and paclitaxel chemotherapy

(D) Olaparib

Item 115

A 61-year-old woman has a follow-up evaluation for the incidental discovery of several hypodense lesions in both lobes of her liver and a 2.5-cm mesenteric mass during CT imaging for nephrolithiasis. She has fully recovered from the nephrolithiasis and now feels entirely well. She does not have abdominal pain, a change in either appetite or bowel habits, hot flushes, or facial flushing. She takes no medications.

On physical examination, vital signs and the remainder of the examination are normal.

Complete blood count and liver chemistry test results are normal.

A needle biopsy of an accessible liver lesion shows a well-differentiated low-grade neuroendocrine tumor, with a low rate of mitotic figures.

Which of the following is the most appropriate management?

(A) Begin hormonal therapy with a somatostatin analogue

(B) Hepatic artery embolization

(C) No immediate intervention; repeat CT scan in 3 months

(D) Surgery to remove primary tumor

(E) Systemic chemotherapy

Item 116

A 40-year-old woman is evaluated in the office following a recent diagnosis of stage IIA breast cancer. Pathologic findings showed a 2.5-cm, grade 2 invasive ductal carcinoma with no lymphatic or vascular invasion and negative margins. The cancer was estrogen receptor positive, progesterone receptor positive, and *HER2* negative. Two sentinel nodes were negative. The 21-gene recurrence score is 8 (low risk of recurrence). She takes no medications.

She is seeking advice about adjuvant systemic therapy. The patient is premenopausal and has no family history of breast or ovarian cancer.

On physical examination, vital signs are normal. There is a healed right-upper outer breast incision and healed right axillary incision. The remainder of the examination is normal.

Laboratory studies show normal findings on complete blood count, basic metabolic panel, and liver chemistry tests.

In addition to primary breast radiation, which of the following is the most appropriate treatment?

(A) Adjuvant chemotherapy

(B) Adjuvant chemotherapy followed by tamoxifen

(C) Ovarian suppression and anastrozole

(D) Tamoxifen

Item 117

A 75-year-old man is evaluated for a 3-month history of worsening urinary hesitancy, decreased stream, and a sense of incompletely emptying his bladder. His medical history is significant for COPD, hypertension, and stroke. He has dyspnea with minimal exertion. His medications are ipratropium bromide, salmeterol, fluticasone, amlodipine, atorvastatin, and aspirin.

On physical examination, there is evidence of mild muscle wasting. His respiration rate is 18/min; other vital signs are normal. Oxygen saturation is 92% breathing ambient air. Pulmonary examination reveals decreased breath sounds throughout both lung fields. Digital rectal examination reveals an enlarged prostate without any palpable nodules.

Laboratory studies reveal a serum prostate-specific antigen level of 6 ng/mL (6 µg/L).

Biopsy of the prostate confirms prostate cancer with a Gleason score of 6. The patient begins therapy with tamsulosin, and his voiding symptoms improve.

Which of the following is the most appropriate management of his prostate cancer?

(A) Active surveillance

(B) Androgen deprivation therapy

(C) Bone scan

(D) Radiation

(E) Observation

Item 118

A 40-year-old woman is evaluated during a follow-up visit after a recent diagnosis of stage IIB left breast cancer. She has postoperative left breast pain but no other symptoms. She takes no medications.

On physical examination, vital signs are normal. There is a healed left breast incision and a healed left axillary incision. The remainder of the examination is normal.

Results from a complete blood count and chemistry panel, including liver chemistry tests and serum alkaline phosphatase levels, are normal.

Which of the following is the most appropriate imaging study to perform next?

(A) Bone scan
(B) CT of the chest, abdomen, and pelvis
(C) PET scan
(D) No imaging studies

Item 119

A 67-year-old man is evaluated for fatigue and anemia of approximately 2 month's duration. He has no other symptoms and takes no medications.

On physical examination, vital signs are normal. Petechiae are noted on the lower extremities, and there is conjunctival pallor. The spleen is palpable 4 cm below the costal margin. There is no lymphadenopathy and no hepatomegaly.

Laboratory studies:

Hemoglobin	10.4 g/dL (104 g/L)
Leukocyte count	2200/µL (2.2 × 10⁹/L) with 63% lymphocytes, 34% segmented neutrophils, 3% monocytes
Platelet count	73,000/µL (73 × 10⁹/L)

Flow cytometry of peripheral blood confirms kappa-restricted CD20+ B cells expressing CD11c, CD25, and CD103.

Peripheral blood smear is shown below:

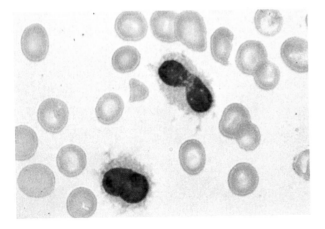

Which of the following is the most appropriate treatment?

(A) Cladribine
(B) Interferon alfa
(C) Rituximab
(D) Splenectomy
(E) Observation

Item 120

A 43-year-old woman with a 7-year history of relapsing follicular lymphoma is evaluated for fevers, night sweats, and a rapidly enlarging right inguinal nodal mass. Her lymphoma has been treated on multiple occasions. Her current relapse began 1 year ago with diffuse lymphadenopathy; however, the onset of her symptoms and the right inguinal node enlargement is recent. She takes no medications.

On physical examination, all vital signs are normal. There is diffuse cervical and axillary lymphadenopathy bilaterally. The left inguinal node is enlarged to 2 cm; the right inguinal node is enlarged to 5 cm. There is no splenomegaly.

Laboratory results are significant only for a serum lactate dehydrogenase level of 6420 U/L.

Which of the following is the most appropriate management?

(A) Biopsy of the right inguinal lymph node
(B) Oral idelalisib
(C) Radiation therapy to the right inguinal node
(D) Repeat a course of chemotherapy

Item 121

A 58-year-old woman is evaluated for a palpable mass in her right groin. She takes no medications.

On physical examination, vital signs are normal. A hard, fixed, 3-cm lymph node is palpated in the right inguinal region. Careful inspection of the perianal skin, vulva, vagina, and cervix shows no findings. The remainder of the physical examination is normal.

A biopsy of the enlarged node demonstrates poorly differentiated carcinoma.

A contrast-enhanced CT scan of the chest, abdomen, and pelvis shows the enlarged inguinal node and no other abnormal findings.

Which of the following is the most appropriate diagnostic test to perform next?

(A) Anoscopy
(B) Bone scan
(C) Colonoscopy and upper endoscopy
(D) PET scan
(E) Serum CEA, CA-15-3, and CA-125

Item 122

A 53-year-old man is evaluated after a hemicolectomy for a well-differentiated adenocarcinoma of the descending colon. Final pathologic findings showed a well-differentiated adenocarcinoma penetrating into the serosa (T3). Margins of resection were free of tumor. No lymphovascular or perineural invasion was seen. Twenty-seven lymph nodes were identified, and all were free of cancer. He takes no medications.

CT scans of the chest, abdomen, and pelvis showed no evidence of metastatic disease.

On physical examination, vital signs are normal. All other examination findings are normal.

The postoperative carcinoembryonic antigen (CEA) level is normal.

Which of the following is the most appropriate management?

(A) FOLFOX (parenteral 5-fluorouracil, leucovorin, and oxaliplatin)

(B) Oral capecitabine

(C) Radiation therapy

(D) No further treatment

Item 123

A 42-year-old woman is evaluated in the office after care in the emergency department for a new-onset seizure. She has a history of malignant melanoma resected 7 years ago. It had a 3.2-mm depth of invasion by Breslow microstaging. Her only medications are dexamethasone and levetiracetam.

On physical examination, vital signs are normal. There is no lymphadenopathy. Results of the neurologic examination are normal.

Brain MRI shows a 3.5-cm left frontal lesion consistent with metastatic disease. CT scan of the chest, abdomen, and pelvis is negative.

Which of the following is the most appropriate treatment?

(A) Ipilimumab and nivolumab

(B) Stereotactic radiosurgery to the brain lesion

(C) Surgical resection of the brain lesion

(D) Vemurafenib plus cobimetinib

(E) Whole brain radiation therapy

Item 124

A 56-year-old man is evaluated for a 3-month history of anorectal pain with bleeding. Medical history is significant for a long-standing HIV infection for which he is taking appropriate antiretroviral therapy. Viral load is undetectable, with a CD4 T-cell count of 650/µL.

On physical examination, vital signs are normal. The examination is notable for a hard, tender mass palpable in the anal canal. There is no inguinal lymphadenopathy.

Pelvic MRI shows a 3-cm mass in the anal canal and one enlarged 11-mm local-regional lymph node. Contrast-enhanced CT of chest and abdomen are normal.

Which of the following is the most appropriate treatment?

(A) Human papillomavirus (HPV) vaccination

(B) Pelvic radiation therapy

(C) Pelvic radiation therapy and concurrent chemotherapy

(D) Surgery

Item 125

A 65-year-old woman is evaluated during a follow-up visit for breast cancer management. She was diagnosed 6 years ago with stage IIB left breast cancer. Pathologic findings showed a 2.5-cm, grade 3 infiltrating ductal cancer that was estrogen receptor positive, progesterone receptor positive, and *HER2* negative. Three axillary lymph nodes were positive. She received adjuvant chemotherapy followed by 5 years of anastrozole. She takes no other medications. She has had no side effects from the anastrozole, and her bone density has remained normal.

On physical examination, vital signs are normal. There are well-healed incisions of the left breast and axilla. There are no breast masses.

Which of the following is the most appropriate management?

(A) Continue anastrozole; add tamoxifen for an additional 5 years

(B) Continue anastrozole alone for an additional 5 years

(C) Stop anastrozole

(D) Stop anastrozole; begin tamoxifen for an additional 5 years

Item 126

A 55-year-old man is hospitalized for a 6-month history of progressive shortness of breath and cough. He has lost 18.1 kg (40.0 lb). He has been experiencing generalized weakness and has become more inactive. Although he is independent with self-care, he no longer leaves home and spends most of his time in bed because he is too weak to do any household chores and becomes dyspneic with minimal exertion. His medical history is significant for diabetes mellitus, chronic kidney disease, and a 40-pack-year smoking history. He takes basal and prandial insulin and acetaminophen as needed for pain.

On physical examination, he is cachectic and frail. He is afebrile. Blood pressure is 105/60 mm Hg, pulse rate is 92/min, and respiration rate is 24/min. BMI is 20. Oxygen saturation is 93% breathing 2 L/min of oxygen through nasal cannula. Breath sounds are normal. Hepatomegaly is present on palpation.

Laboratory studies reveal a hemoglobin level of 9.2 g/dL (92 g/L), an albumin level of 2.9 g/dL (29 g/L), and a creatinine level of 2.1 mg/dL (185.6 µmol/L).

CT scan of the chest, abdomen, and pelvis shows a large right upper lung mass with associated hilar and mediastinal lymphadenopathy, multiple osseous metastatic lesions, and multiple hepatic lesions. Brain MRI shows no metastatic disease. Liver biopsy findings confirm metastatic adenocarcinoma.

Which of the following is the most appropriate management?

(A) Ablation of liver metastases

(B) Palliative care consultation

(C) Platinum-based chemotherapy

(D) Radiation to the right upper lobe

Item 127

A 60-year-old woman is evaluated in the emergency department for a 4-week history of worsening midthoracic back pain and a 1-week history of leg weakness and numbness in her lower abdomen and legs. She does not have any bowel or bladder incontinence. She has hormone receptor-positive, *HER2*-negative breast cancer that has metastasized to the spine, ribs, and pelvis. Current medications are letrozole and palbociclib. Until this recent deterioration, she has had excellent functional status.

On physical examination, vital signs are normal. She has tenderness to percussion on the T6 vertebra. There is a sensory level at the T8 vertebral body; bilateral, proximal, and distal lower-extremity weakness; hyperactive knee and ankle reflexes; and bilateral plantar extension responses. The remainder of the physical examination is normal.

MRI scans show a large lytic lesion in the T6 vertebral body, with an epidural mass causing compression of the spinal canal.

In addition to intravenous dexamethasone, which of the following is the most appropriate treatment?

(A) Elective radiation therapy

(B) Immediate decompressive surgery

(C) Palliative care only

(D) Urgent radiation therapy

Item 128

A 38-year-old woman seeks advice about decreasing her risk for ovarian cancer. Her mother and maternal grandmother were diagnosed with breast cancer at 40 years of age and 38 years of age, respectively. The patient tested positive for a deleterious *BRCA2* gene mutation and had bilateral prophylactic mastectomies done at age 35 years. She has a 2-year-old son and would like to have at least one other child. She is premenopausal and takes no medications. There is no family history of ovarian cancer.

On physical examination, vital signs are normal. Chest wall and gynecologic examination are normal. The remainder of the examination is normal.

Which of the following is the most appropriate recommendation?

(A) Annual pelvic examination and serum CA-125 screening studies

(B) Bilateral salpingo-oophorectomy by age 40 to 45 years

(C) Bilateral salpingo-oophorectomy now

(D) Long-term oral contraceptive use

Item 129

An 82-year-old woman is evaluated for persistent swellings in her neck, armpit, and groin. She describes no additional symptoms. She has long-standing systolic hypertension for which she takes chlorthalidone.

On physical examination, blood pressure is 154/82 mm Hg. The other vital signs are normal. There are bilateral enlargements of cervical, supraclavicular, axillary, and inguinal lymph nodes. The remainder of the examination is unremarkable.

Laboratory studies:

Hemoglobin	12.5 g/dL (125 g/L)
Leukocyte count	14,000/µL (14 × 10⁹/L) with 66% lymphocytes, 23% segmented neutrophils, 6% monocytes, 1% eosinophils, and 4% bands
Platelet count	174,000/µL (174 × 10⁹/L)

Smudge cells are noted on a peripheral blood smear.

Which of the following is the most appropriate diagnostic test to perform next?

(A) Bone marrow aspiration and biopsy

(B) CT scan of the chest, abdomen, and pelvis

(C) Cytogenetic studies on peripheral blood

(D) Flow cytometry on peripheral blood

Item 130

A 50-year-old woman is evaluated for a 4-month history of left flank pain, worsening despite NSAIDs and now requiring opioid analgesics, and 4-kg (8.8 lb) weight loss. Her medical history is otherwise unremarkable.

On physical examination, the skin and mucous membranes are pale. Vital signs are normal. There is left flank tenderness on palpation. The remainder of the physical examination is unremarkable.

Laboratory studies reveal a hemoglobin level of 10.1 g/dL (101 g/L).

CT scan of the chest, abdomen, and pelvis reveals a 10-cm left kidney mass with radiographic features suggesting renal cell carcinoma and a 1.2-cm single pulmonary nodule.

Which of the following is the most appropriate management?

(A) Left radical nephrectomy

(B) Nivolumab

(C) PET/CT scan

(D) Radiation to the kidney mass

Item 131

A 75-year-old man is evaluated for generalized lymphadenopathy. He is otherwise asymptomatic and takes no medications.

On physical examination, all vital signs are normal. There is generalized lymphadenopathy with nodes 1 cm to 2.5 cm in size in his cervical, supraclavicular, axillary, and inguinal areas bilaterally. There is no hepatosplenomegaly. The remainder of the physical examination is normal.

CT scan of the chest, abdomen, and pelvis shows mediastinal and retroperitoneal nodes that are 1.5 cm to 2.0 cm in size.

Laboratory results, including complete blood count, biochemistry profile, and lactate dehydrogenase level, are normal. Serum urate level is 9.5 mg/dL (0.56 mmol/L).

Left inguinal node biopsy shows follicular lymphoma.

Which of the following is the most appropriate management?

(A) Allopurinol

(B) Radiation therapy

(C) Rituximab plus cyclophosphamide, doxorubicin, vincristine, and prednisone (R-CHOP)

(D) Observation

Item 132

A 27-year-old woman seeks advice on breast cancer screening recommendations. Medical history is significant for stage IIB Hodgkin lymphoma diagnosed at age 19 years, treated with mantle and para-aortic radiation; there has been no evidence of recurrence. The patient is premenopausal and has no family history of breast or ovarian cancer. She takes no medications.

On physical examination, vital signs are normal. BMI is 28. There is a healed right supraclavicular incision from a previous lymph node biopsy. Breast examination findings are normal.

When should this patient begin breast cancer screening?

(A) At age 30 years

(B) At age 40 years

(C) At age 50 years

(D) Now

Item 133

A 32-year-old woman is evaluated after a recent diagnosis of stage IIB right breast cancer. She will be starting neoadjuvant chemotherapy with cyclophosphamide, doxorubicin, and paclitaxel, along with *HER2*-targeted therapy. She has a 1-year-old son and is interested in having more children.

Which of the following is the most appropriate management?

(A) Fertility specialist consultation after chemotherapy

(B) Fertility specialist consultation before chemotherapy

(C) Goserelin during chemotherapy

(D) Recommend against future childbearing

Item 134

A 69-year-old woman is evaluated for 6 months of progressive dysphagia. She has been previously healthy and takes no medications.

On physical examination, vital signs and the remainder of the physical examination are normal.

Results of upper endoscopy and biopsy indicate adenocarcinoma of the gastroesophageal junction. The staging evaluation reveals a T3 tumor on ultrasound and no evidence of distant metastatic disease. The patient's tumor is technically resectable.

Which of the following is the most reasonable treatment strategy?

(A) Adjuvant radiation therapy

(B) Neoadjuvant chemotherapy plus radiation therapy

(C) Palliative chemotherapy

(D) Surgery alone

Item 135

An 81-year-old man is evaluated for a 2-week history of gross hematuria. He is a former cigarette smoker, having quit 15 years ago. He is otherwise healthy and takes no medications.

On physical examination, vital signs and other findings are normal.

An ultrasound of the kidneys, ureters, and bladder is unremarkable.

Cystoscopy reveals a lesion along the bladder wall. Transurethral resection of the bladder tumor reveals high-grade, stage T1 transitional cell carcinoma.

Which of the following is the most appropriate treatment?

(A) Cisplatin-based systemic chemotherapy

(B) Intravesicular bacillus Calmette-Guérin

(C) Intravesicular bacillus Calmette-Guérin followed by partial cystectomy

(D) Partial cystectomy

Item 136

A 70-year-old man is seen for treatment recommendations for newly diagnosed colon cancer metastatic to the liver. He also has a long-standing history of diabetes and heart failure for which he takes metformin and lisinopril. The patient spends most of the day on the couch and is unable to walk across the room, dress himself, or do other basic activities of daily living without becoming dyspneic and fatigued. His appetite is poor.

On physical examination, vital signs are normal. The patient is thin and has obvious muscle wasting. The liver edge is palpable. The examination is otherwise normal.

The patient has read about an ongoing clinical trial of a chemotherapy regimen for metastatic colon cancer that resulted in a response rate of 40% and a progression-free survival of 11 months.

Which of the following would this patient be likely to experience with the treatment given relative to the results reported in this clinical trial?

(A) Comparable efficacy and comparable toxicity

(B) Comparable efficacy but increased toxicity

(C) Decreased efficacy and comparable toxicity

(D) Decreased efficacy and increased toxicity

Item 137

A 62-year-old woman is evaluated for recurrent breast cancer with bone and liver metastases. She was diagnosed with stage IA estrogen receptor–positive, progesterone receptor-positive, *HER2*-negative right breast cancer 8 years ago. She underwent lumpectomy and sentinel lymph-node biopsy and primary breast radiation, and completed 5 years of anastrozole therapy 2 years ago. She presented with right hip pain, with lesions on a bone scan consistent with metastases. Biopsy of a bone lesion shows metastatic adenocarcinoma that is estrogen receptor positive, progesterone receptor positive, and *HER2* negative, consistent with metastatic breast cancer. She takes no medications.

On physical examination, vital signs are normal. Healed incisions of the right breast and axilla are present. Tenderness to palpation of the right lateral hip is noted. The remainder of the examination is normal.

Which of the following is the most appropriate treatment?

(A) Exemestane
(B) Letrozole plus palbociclib
(C) Raloxifene
(D) Tamoxifen

Item 138

A 65-year-old woman is evaluated 3 weeks postoperatively following right hemicolectomy for colon cancer. Pathology of the surgical specimen revealed a 3-cm adenocarcinoma invading into but not through the colonic wall. Four of 17 local-regional lymph nodes examined contained metastatic cancer. All margins of resection were free of tumor. Contrast-enhanced CT scans of the chest, abdomen, and pelvis were unremarkable. She takes no medications.

On physical examination, vital signs are normal. Surgical incisions are fully healed. The remainder of the examination is normal.

Carcinoembryonic antigen (CEA) is 1.7 µg/L (normal is less than 5.0 µg/L).

Which of the following is the most appropriate treatment?

(A) 5-Fluorouracil, leucovorin, and oxaliplatin (FOLFOX)
(B) Radiation therapy
(C) Radiation therapy plus FOLFOX
(D) No further therapy

Item 139

A 78-year-old woman is evaluated for increasing fatigue during the past 2 weeks. She has a 7-year history of chronic lymphocytic leukemia previously treated with bendamustine and rituximab with excellent results. One month ago, after presenting with persistent night sweats, she was diagnosed with relapsed chronic lymphocytic leukemia based on lymphocytosis on a complete blood count and results of peripheral blood flow cytometry. Her hemoglobin level at that time was 12.1 g/dL (121 g/L). She was started on oral ibrutinib.

On physical examination, vital signs are normal. Scleral icterus is noted. The spleen is palpable 3 cm below the costal margin. There is no peripheral lymphadenopathy.

Laboratory studies:

Hemoglobin	7.4 g/dL (74 g/L)
Leukocyte count	22,000/µL (22×10⁹/L) with 79% lymphocytes
Platelet count	122,000/µL (122×10⁹/L)
Reticulocyte count	11% of erythrocytes

Which of the following is the most appropriate management?

(A) Anti-parvovirus IgM antibody assay
(B) Bone marrow aspiration and biopsy

(C) Direct antiglobulin (Coombs) test
(D) Discontinue ibrutinib
(E) Splenectomy

Item 140

A 65-year-old man is evaluated for cough and shortness of breath with exertion for the past 2 months, accompanied by 10 pounds of weight loss. He takes no medications.

On physical examination, vital signs are normal. Examination reveals decreased breath sounds in the lower right lung field.

Chest radiograph reveals right lower lobe opacity, and CT scan of the chest reveals a large right lower lobe mass, liver masses, and a right adrenal mass. These findings are consistent with metastases.

A biopsy of a right lung mass reveals adenocarcinoma. Testing for driver mutations is negative.

Which of the following is the most appropriate diagnostic or screening test to perform next?

(A) Liver biopsy
(B) Programmed cell death ligand 1 expression
(C) PET/CT scan
(D) Pulmonary function testing

Item 141

A 29-year-old man is evaluated for a 2-month history of night sweats, fevers, a sense of abdominal fullness, and fatigue. He takes no medications.

On physical examination, vital signs are normal. The abdomen is distended with diffuse tenderness without rebound or guarding. Bowel sounds are normal. Other examination findings are normal.

Laboratory results, including complete blood count and serum bilirubin, creatinine, alkaline phosphatase, aminotransferase, α-fetoprotein, and β-human chorionic gonadotropin levels, are normal. A contrast-enhanced CT scan of the chest, abdomen, and pelvis shows bulky retroperitoneal lymphadenopathy (the largest mass is 10 cm in diameter) with somewhat smaller but still enlarged mediastinal lymphadenopathy. A biopsy specimen of the most accessible enlarged node shows poorly differentiated carcinoma. A testicular ultrasound is unremarkable.

Which of the following is the most appropriate treatment?

(A) A gastrointestinal cancer chemotherapy regimen
(B) A germ cell chemotherapy regimen
(C) Radiation therapy to the lymphadenopathy
(D) Surgical debulking of the lymphadenopathy

Item 142

A 71-year-old man has a follow-up evaluation. He was recently diagnosed with metastatic melanoma characterized by a *BRAF* V600E mutation for which he was treated with a *BRAF* inhibitor. After treatment, he was found to have major tumor regression at all disease sites. He takes no medications.

On physical examination, vital signs and other findings are normal.

Which of the following best describes the type of tumor marker present in this patient?

(A) Exclusionary predictive marker

(B) Exclusionary prognostic marker

(C) Inclusionary predictive marker

(D) Inclusionary prognostic marker

Item 143

A 26-year-old woman is interested in genetic testing for *BRCA1* and *BRCA2* gene mutations based on her family history. Her mother was diagnosed with triple-negative breast cancer at age 53 years and died at age 55 years. Her maternal aunt was diagnosed with ovarian cancer at age 48 years and is still alive but is not interested in genetic testing. Her maternal and paternal relatives are of Ashkenazi Jewish descent. The patient is premenopausal and takes no medications.

On physical examination, vital signs are normal. Breast and gynecologic examination findings are normal.

Which of the following is the most appropriate management?

(A) Recommend a direct-to-consumer genetic test

(B) Recommend against genetic testing

(C) Recommend genetic testing for the three *BRCA1* and *BRCA2* mutations most common in patients of Ashkenazi Jewish ethnicity

(D) Refer to a genetic counselor

Item 144

A 28-year-old man is evaluated for a 1-month history of right testicular swelling. His medical history is unremarkable, and he takes no medications.

On physical examination, vital signs are normal. Palpation reveals an enlarged right testicle that is firm and mildly tender.

Scrotal ultrasonography shows a 5-cm right testicular mass.

Which of the following is the most appropriate management?

(A) Measurement of β-human chorionic gonadotropin and α-fetoprotein levels

(B) Needle biopsy

(C) PET-CT scan

(D) Radical inguinal orchiectomy

Item 145

A 40-year-old woman is evaluated in the emergency department for a 2-week history of worsening headache and imbalance. She has metastatic hormone receptor–negative, *HER2*-positive breast cancer with bone metastases and is being treated with paclitaxel, trastuzumab, and pertuzumab with good control of her systemic disease.

On physical examination, the patient is afebrile. Blood pressure is 168/88 mm Hg, pulse rate is 104/min, and respiration rate is normal. She is awake and alert. She has past-pointing on finger-to-nose testing and truncal ataxia. The remainder of the examination is normal.

Head CT scan without contrast in the emergency department shows a 1.5-cm mass in the left cerebellum with surrounding edema and a 1-cm left frontal mass with edema. No midline shift is present.

Which of the following is the most appropriate initial management?

(A) Dexamethasone

(B) Levetiracetam

(C) Mannitol

(D) Urgent neurosurgery

(E) Whole brain radiation

Item 146

A 42-year-old woman is evaluated during a follow-up visit for stage IIA cervical squamous cell cancer. She has completed therapy with pelvic external-beam radiation and concomitant weekly cisplatin chemotherapy, with cervical brachytherapy added during the fourth week of therapy. She has had an excellent response to treatment. She is otherwise well and takes no medications.

On physical examination, vital signs are normal. Pelvic examination reveals no evidence of tumor, and the remainder of the examination is normal.

Which of the following is the most appropriate posttreatment surveillance for this patient?

(A) CT of the pelvis every 6 months

(B) Complete blood count, serum creatinine, and liver chemistry tests every 3 months

(C) History, physical, and gynecologic examination every 3 months

(D) Pelvic ultrasonography every 6 months

Item 147

A 59-year-old woman is evaluated for a 2-month history of shortness of breath and cough. She has a 55-pack-year smoking history. She takes no medications.

On physical examination, vital signs are normal. BMI is 23. Oxygen saturation is normal. Pulmonary examination reveals decreased breath sounds and crackles in the right base posteriorly. Her performance status is good.

CT scan of the chest shows a large, centrally located right lower lobe mass, evidence of mediastinal invasion, bulky mediastinal lymph nodes, and hilar lymphadenopathy.

Bronchoscopy with biopsy of an endobronchial lesion confirms non–small cell lung cancer.

Brain MRI, CT scans of the abdomen and pelvis, and bone scan show no metastatic disease.

Which of the following is the most appropriate management?

(A) Chemotherapy

(B) Combined chemotherapy and radiation

(C) Pembrolizumab

(D) Radiation

(E) Surgical resection of the right lower lobe mass

Item 148

A 48-year-old man is evaluated for increasing dysphagia during the past 2 months. He reports that he first noticed difficulty swallowing solid foods, such as steak, but that this symptom has advanced to occasional difficulty with liquids. He is, however, maintaining adequate hydration and nutrition. He is not currently taking medications.

On physical examination, vital signs are normal. There is a 1.5-cm left supraclavicular node and a liver edge that is palpable below the right costal margin.

A CT scan of the chest and abdomen shows a mass in the lower third of the esophagus just proximal to the gastroesophageal junction. The liver has multiple hypodense lesions consistent with metastases. Endoscopic evaluation reveals a near-obstructing lesion in the distal esophagus. Biopsy shows adenocarcinoma.

Which of the following is the most appropriate diagnostic test to perform next?

(A) Assess tumor tissue for *BRAF* mutation status

(B) Assess tumor tissue for *HER2* amplification

(C) Assess tumor tissue for *RAS* mutation status

(D) Obtain PET/CT scan

(E) Obtain upper gastrointestinal imaging (barium swallow)

Item 149

A 65-year-old man is evaluated after a recent diagnosis of prostate cancer with multiple painful metastases to the lumbar spine. He was treated initially with both bicalutamide and leuprolide for 4 weeks, after which he continued on leuprolide alone with excellent symptomatic relief of bone pain. He started treatment 2 months ago.

On physical examination, vital signs and the remainder of the examination are normal.

Laboratory studies reveal a serum prostate-specific antigen level of 20 ng/mL (20 µg/L), down from 122 ng/mL (122 µg/L) at the time of diagnosis 2 months ago. Complete blood count and liver chemistry test results are normal.

Which of the following is the most appropriate management?

(A) Continue leuprolide alone

(B) Leuprolide plus docetaxel

(C) Radiation to the lumbar spine

(D) Stop leuprolide and start docetaxel

Answers and Critiques

Hematology Answers

Item 1   Answer: B

Educational Objective: Evaluate HIV as a cause of immune thrombocytopenic purpura.

Testing should be performed for HIV. Immune thrombocytopenic purpura (ITP) is caused by autoantibodies directed against glycoproteins on the platelet surface. ITP is diagnosed when thrombocytopenia is found with no alternate cause. ITP can be idiopathic, triggered by medications, or associated with other disorders, such as systemic lupus erythematosus (SLE), chronic lymphocytic leukemia, lymphoma, HIV, hepatitis C, or *Helicobacter pylori* infection. Unless additional cytopenias are discovered or other findings suggest an alternate diagnosis, a bone marrow biopsy in these patients is not necessary. ITP is not uncommon among patients with HIV infection, even early in the disease and in the absence of any other symptoms of immunosuppression or opportunistic infection. ITP is also associated with chronic hepatitis C that may also be asymptomatic. This patient's hepatitis C test was negative, so no further evaluation is needed; however, routine testing for HIV is recommended before starting any immunosuppressive treatment.

Unlike autoimmune hemolytic anemia, no diagnostic test is available for immune-mediated thrombocytopenia. Antiplatelet antibody testing is not recommended because of low sensitivity and specificity, and this test should not be performed in the evaluation of thrombocytopenia.

ITP may be associated with other autoimmune diseases, such as Hashimoto thyroiditis, or with SLE. This patient lacks any history of venous thromboembolism or fetal loss that would suggest an underlying anticardiolipin antibody syndrome and has no other clinical features to suggest SLE; testing for the lupus anticoagulant is unnecessary.

Although vitamin B$_{12}$ and folate deficiency can result in thrombocytopenia, the patient's mean corpuscular volume is normal, so no evidence indicates cobalamin deficiency.

KEY POINT

- Immune thrombocytopenic purpura can be idiopathic, triggered by medications, or associated with other disorders, such as systemic lupus erythematosus, chronic lymphocytic leukemia, lymphoma, HIV, hepatitis C, or *Helicobacter pylori* infection.

Bibliography

Neunert C, Lim W, Crowther M, Cohen A, Solberg L Jr, Crowther MA; American Society of Hematology. The American Society of Hematology 2011 evidence-based practice guideline for immune thrombocytopenia. Blood. 2011;117:4190-207. [PMID: 21325604] doi:10.1182/blood-2010-08-302984

Item 2   Answer: D

Educational Objective: Evaluate for acquired platelet dysfunction.

Patients who present with symptoms of mucocutaneous bleeding and a normal platelet count should be evaluated for acquired platelet dysfunction using the Platelet Function Analyzer-100 (PFA-100). Selective serotonin reuptake inhibitors (SSRIs) such as citalopram decrease serotonin uptake from platelets and have a reported association with gastrointestinal bleeding, especially in older adults. Herbal supplements like ginkgo biloba have been reported to increase platelet dysfunction in patients taking antiplatelet agents and may interact with this patient's SSRI. The PFA-100 provides a rapid screening test of platelet function and has replaced the bleeding time test. Anticoagulated whole blood is passed through small membranes coated with collagen and epinephrine or collagen and adenosine diphosphate. Platelets adhere to the membrane and close a small aperture. A prolonged closure time implies abnormal platelet activity.

Patients with hypofibrinogenemia may have significant bleeding, but it is uncommon as an isolated finding and is much more likely to be seen in patients with liver disease or disseminated intravascular coagulation who also have abnormalities of the prothrombin time (PT), activated partial thromboplastin time (aPTT), and platelet count. Furthermore, the normal thrombin time excludes hypofibrinogenemia.

Rarely, older patients without a personal or family history of bleeding may present with acute new-onset bleeding caused by acquired hemophilia. Such bleeding can be mucocutaneous or intramuscular. The PT is normal, but the aPTT is significantly prolonged, and a 1:1 mixing study of the patient's plasma with normal plasma is unsuccessful at completely correcting the aPTT. This patient's PT and aPTT are normal, and mixing studies will not provide further information.

Although a peripheral blood smear is the first step in evaluating a patient with abnormal platelet counts, all of this patient's cell counts are normal, and a peripheral blood smear review will not help determine the cause of his bleeding.

Serum protein electrophoresis will detect paraprotein, which might cause bleeding by interfering with coagulation factors and prolonging the prothrombin or thrombin times. Because all of this patient's coagulation parameters are normal, looking for a paraprotein is unnecessary at this time.

KEY POINT

- Patients who present with symptoms of mucocutaneous bleeding and a normal platelet count should be evaluated for acquired platelet dysfunction using the Platelet Function Analyzer-100.

Bibliography

Konkle BA. Acquired disorders of platelet function. Hematology Am Soc Hematol Educ Program. 2011;2011:391-6. [PMID: 22160063] doi:10.1182/asheducation-2011.1.391

Item 3   Answer: A

Educational Objective: Treat pulmonary embolism with non–vitamin K antagonist oral anticoagulant monotherapy.

This patient should be treated with apixaban. Patients with pulmonary embolism (PE) were previously hospitalized for anticoagulant therapy. However, admission rates are decreasing because of the recognition that appropriate patients can be safely managed in the outpatient setting. The Outpatient Treatment for Pulmonary Embolism (OTPE) trial was an open-label, randomized, noninferiority trial. A total of 344 patients with acute, symptomatic, objectively confirmed PE were randomly assigned to inpatient or outpatient management. Patients were classified as low risk or high risk of death using the Pulmonary Embolism Severity Index (PESI). Among patients with low-risk PESI scores who were randomly assigned to outpatient or inpatient care, recurrent venous thromboembolism (VTE) occurred within 90 days in 1 of 171 (0.6%) outpatients and zero inpatients, a finding that met the criteria for noninferiority. The PESI stratifies patients into five risk categories for all-cause 30-day mortality based on 11 clinical **parameters**.

TABLE. Pulmonary Embolism Severity Index	
Clinical Parameter	**Score**
Age (in years)	(enter age)
Male sex	10
Current cancer	30
Chronic heart failure	10
Chronic lung disease	10
Pulse rate >110/min	20
Systolic BP <100 mm Hg	30
Respiration rate >30/min	20
Temperature <36 °C (96.8 °F)	20
Disorientation, lethargy, stupor, or coma	60
Oxygen saturation <90%	20

In the appropriate clinical setting, patients with a PESI score less than 65 are very low risk for 30-day mortality (0%), and those with a score less than 85 are low risk for 30-day mortality (1%); patients in these categories can be considered for outpatient management. This patient's PESI score is 59. Therefore, outpatient management can be considered, but the appropriate agent must be selected. The 2016 American College of Chest Physicians guidelines recommend non–vitamin K antagonist oral anticoagulants as first line for patients without cancer with VTE. Dabigatran and

edoxaban require bridging with parenteral anticoagulation, whereas apixaban and rivaroxaban can be used as monotherapy in the treatment of VTE.

Long-term low-molecular-weight heparin is only considered first-line treatment in patients with malignancy. This patient does not have cancer; therefore, apixaban is a more appropriate choice.

KEY POINT

- Patients with a Pulmonary Embolism Severity Index score of less than 65 are at low risk of death and may be managed in the outpatient setting with a non–vitamin K antagonist oral anticoagulant, such as apixaban or rivaroxaban.

Bibliography

Aujesky D, Roy PM, Verschuren F, Righini M, Osterwalder J, Egloff M, et al. Outpatient versus inpatient treatment for patients with acute pulmonary embolism: an international, open-label, randomised, non-inferiority trial. Lancet. 2011;378:41-8. [PMID: 21703676] doi:10.1016/S0140-6736(11)60824-6

Item 4   Answer: D

Educational Objective: Manage inflammatory anemia.

No treatment for anemia is necessary at this time. The patient has findings typical of inflammatory anemia. Inflammatory anemia occurs in response to the inflammatory cytokine IL-6 that leads to hepatic synthesis of hepcidin, which in turn causes proteolysis of the membrane protein ferroportin. As a result, iron absorption from the gut is diminished, as is iron release from macrophages. Patients with chronic infections, such as tuberculosis or osteomyelitis; patients with malignancy; or patients with other chronic inflammatory conditions, such as rheumatologic diseases, can develop inflammatory anemia. Inflammatory anemia is characterized by a hemoglobin level of approximately 10 g/dL (100 g/L) with normocytic or slightly microcytic indices. Characteristically, the serum iron level is low, and the total iron-binding capacity (TIBC) is often low, as well. The serum ferritin level is elevated. In contrast, patients with iron deficiency have a low serum ferritin level and an elevated TIBC. Patients with inflammatory anemia do not require specific therapy.

The use of erythropoiesis-stimulating agents, such as erythropoietin or longer acting darbepoetin, should not be used to treat inflammatory anemia in most patients with cancer because of the lack of benefit and accompanying risks, including hypertension, stroke, and tumor progression. Patients with inflammatory anemia do not respond to oral or parenteral iron supplementation.

KEY POINT

- Inflammatory anemia is usually mild to moderate in severity, characterized by low serum iron levels and total iron-binding capacity and elevated serum ferritin level, and usually requires no specific therapy.

Bibliography
Wang CY, Babitt JL. Hepcidin regulation in the anemia of inflammation. Curr Opin Hematol. 2016;23:189-97. [PMID: 26886082] doi:10.1097/MOH.0000000000000236

Item 5 Answer: D

Educational Objective: Treat a patient with low-risk myelodysplastic syndrome.

This patient with transfusion-dependent myelodysplastic syndrome (MDS) should be treated with lenalidomide. Treatment of MDS has two goals. The first goal is to relieve transfusion dependence; the second is to prevent transformation to acute myeloid leukemia (AML). He has low-risk MDS with chromosome 5q deletion (–5q), and lenalidomide will help with his transfusion-dependent anemia. Patients with infrequent transfusion requirements can be supported with periodic transfusions alone, but in patients requiring frequent transfusions, supplemental treatments to help decrease transfusion requirements should be used to improve quality of life and decrease transfusion-associated iron overload and alloimmunization. In more than 50% of patients with –5q MDS, treatment with low-dose lenalidomide has been shown to achieve transfusion independence and is recommended as first-line therapy. Other second-line treatments for low-risk MDS with –5q include recombinant erythropoietin and the hypomethylating agents azacitidine and decitabine. Hypomethylating agents can reduce transfusion requirements and delay transformation to AML. However, both also worsen blood counts initially and may take up to 6 months to show an effect. Finally, this patient is not at high risk for AML transformation.

Allogeneic hematopoietic stem cell transplantation is usually performed in young patients with high-risk MDS. In patients with low-risk disease, early transplantation is not recommended and can be associated with worse survival.

Immunosuppression with antithymocyte globulin and cyclosporine, similar to that used for aplastic anemia, has been shown to decrease transfusion requirements in younger patients (age <65 years) and those with hypoplastic bone marrow. However, in this 74-year-old patient with –5q mutation, immunosuppression is not effective and has significant adverse effects.

Imatinib is a tyrosine kinase inhibitor that is effective in treating patients with chronic myeloid leukemia and dysregulated tyrosine kinase as a result of the BCR-ABL fusion gene. It is not effective in MDS.

KEY POINT

- In patients with myelodysplastic syndrome requiring frequent transfusions, supplemental treatments to help decrease transfusion requirements, such as lenalidomide, should be used to improve quality of life and decrease transfusion-associated iron overload and alloimmunization.

Bibliography
Giagounidis A, Mufti GJ, Mittelman M, Sanz G, Platzbecker U, Muus P, et al. Outcomes in RBC transfusion-dependent patients with low-/intermediate-1-risk myelodysplastic syndromes with isolated deletion 5q treated with lenalidomide: a subset analysis from the MDS-004 study. Eur J Haematol. 2014;93:429-38. [PMID: 24813620] doi:10.1111/ejh.12380

Item 6 Answer: A

Educational Objective: Evaluate eosinophilia.

This patient should be evaluated for hypereosinophilic syndrome (HES), beginning with an evaluation for helminth infection. He has sustained moderate eosinophilia and end-organ damage (restrictive cardiomyopathy), which are characteristic of HES. Organ involvement is more common when the peripheral eosinophil count is greater than 1500/µL (1.5×10^9/L) as in this patient. The numerous neoplastic and nonneoplastic causes of eosinophilia can be recalled using the mnemonic CHINA (Collagen vascular disease, Helminthic infection, Idiopathic, Neoplasia, Allergy/Atopy/Asthma). Helminth infection is a common cause of eosinophilia and should be evaluated and ruled out in all patients. Eosinophilia of any cause can be associated with end-organ damage, and evaluation for organ involvement is indicated. Organs commonly involved are the skin (eczema, erythroderma, urticaria, and angioedema), lungs (parenchymal infiltrates, pleural effusion, lymphadenopathy, and pulmonary emboli), gastrointestinal tract (eosinophilic gastritis, enteritis, colitis, chronic active hepatitis, focal hepatic lesions, eosinophilic cholangitis, Budd-Chiari syndrome), and heart (mitral or tricuspid regurgitation, cardiomegaly, restrictive cardiomyopathy).

Fat pad biopsy is performed during evaluation for systemic amyloidosis. Amyloidosis involving the heart can cause restrictive heart disease. However, in this patient with sustained elevation of the eosinophil count, HES is more likely the underlying condition.

Prednisone initiation in clinically stable patients with HES without evaluation for the underlying cause of the illness is not recommended because patients with infectious causes of eosinophilia (such as *Strongyloides*) can experience significant symptom flare. In unstable patients, empiric treatment with glucocorticoids must be initiated emergently with ivermectin if risk factors for exposure to strongyloides are present. Patients with negative infectious evaluations should be evaluated for allergic, immunologic, and neoplastic causes of hypereosinophilia, including myeloproliferative disorders, lymphomas, and solid tumors.

Although repeat testing of the eosinophil count is recommended in all patients, at least 1 month apart to confirm sustained elevation, this patient already has two measurements showing sustained hypereosinophilia as well as symptoms of cardiac involvement. Therefore, repeat testing of the eosinophil count in 3 months is not appropriate.

- Hypereosinophilic syndrome is characterized by moderate eosinophilia and end-organ damage commonly involving the skin, lungs, gastrointestinal tract, and heart; secondary causes of eosinophilia should be excluded.

Bibliography

Klion AD. How I treat hypereosinophilic syndromes. Blood. 2015;126:1069-77. [PMID: 25964669] doi:10.1182/blood-2014-11-551614

Item 7   Answer: D

Educational Objective: Manage hereditary spherocytosis during an acute aplastic crisis.

The most appropriate management for this patient is clinical observation. He has hereditary spherocytosis (HS) characterized by a mild lifelong anemia in association with symptomatic cholelithiasis at an early age. The presence of spherocytes is supported by an elevated mean corpuscular hemoglobin concentration frequently seen in this disorder. HS is caused by mutations in several scaffolding proteins that make these cells less distensible and more susceptible to osmotic stress and hemolysis. Patients with this disorder may have mild anemia, an elevated reticulocyte response, and few or no symptoms. The development of pigmented gallstones resulting from excess bilirubin production may result in symptomatic cholelithiasis. Symptoms of anemia may arise when the bone marrow is suppressed, most commonly by an acute infection. In this situation, the reticulocyte count falls, and the patient rapidly develops symptomatic anemia. Parvovirus is most classically linked with bone marrow suppression, but many other viral and infectious agents can have a similar effect. The bone marrow suppression following acute infections is self-limited, but some patients may become symptomatic to the point of requiring blood transfusion.

A subset of patients with HS has chronic hemolytic anemia that is much more severe. These patients will benefit from splenectomy. The spleen is the major site of erythrocyte destruction; after splenectomy, the membrane defect remains unchanged, but erythrocyte survival will be significantly prolonged. Splenectomy is not needed in managing an acute, self-limited aplastic crisis.

Prednisone would be indicated to treat warm antibody autoimmune hemolytic anemia (WAIHA). Spherocytes are also seen in patients with WAIHA, but the direct antiglobulin test result would be positive. WAIHA would not explain the lifelong anemia in this patient.

Erythropoietin deficiency plays no role in the pathogenesis of HS. Endogenous erythropoietin levels are apt to be markedly elevated in this patient, and no evidence indicates that therapy with exogenous erythropoiesis-stimulating agents has any beneficial role.

KEY POINT

- Acute viral infections may trigger a transient aplastic crisis in patients with hereditary spherocytosis.

Bibliography

Perrotta S, Gallagher PG, Mohandas N. Hereditary spherocytosis. Lancet. 2008;372:1411-26. [PMID: 18940465] doi:10.1016/S0140-6736(08)61588-3

Item 8   Answer: B

Educational Objective: Treat a patient with malignancy-associated pulmonary embolism.

The most appropriate treatment for this patient is enoxaparin. Approximately 20% of all venous thromboembolisms (VTEs) occur in patients with cancer. The risk for VTE is determined by general risk factors (age, obesity, personal or family history of VTE, coexisting medical conditions, inherited and acquired thrombophilias) and cancer-specific risk factors (cancer type, cancer stage, chemotherapy type, hormonal therapy, surgery, central venous catheters). Active cancer or cancer actively being treated with chemotherapy or radiation therapy increases the VTE risk approximately five- to sixfold, but a history of cancer, or cancer that has undergone curative therapy without evidence of residual disease, does not. He has been diagnosed with metastatic colon cancer and developed a pulmonary embolism. In patients with active malignancy, studies such as the CLOT trial have shown that low-molecular-weight heparin (LMWH), such as enoxaparin, is the anticoagulant of choice. In the CLOT trial, LMWH was compared with warfarin in patients with malignancy and thrombosis. LMWH was associated with a statistically significant reduction in the rate of recurrent VTE, making it a preferable choice to warfarin. Extended therapy with LMWH is recommended while the cancer remains active. Extended anticoagulation should be weighed against the risk of bleeding, cost of therapy, quality of life, life expectancy, and patient preference. The decision to continue extended therapy requires frequent reassessments of risk and benefit.

Efficacy and safety data are insufficient to recommend either fondaparinux or the non–vitamin K antagonist oral anticoagulants (NOACs) for the treatment of malignancy-associated VTE. Although clinical trials are under way to assess the role of NOACs in patients with cancer, guidelines do not exist at this time, and their use has not been standardized in these patients. Few patients with cancer were included in the original clinical trials of these anticoagulants, and LMWH is still considered standard of care for VTE in these patients.

KEY POINT

- Low-molecular-weight heparin is the anticoagulant of choice for patients with active cancer and a venous thromboembolism.

Bibliography

Lee AY, Levine MN, Baker RI, Bowden C, Kakkar AK, Prins M, et al; Randomized Comparison of Low-Molecular-Weight Heparin versus Oral Anticoagulant Therapy for the Prevention of Recurrent Venous Thromboembolism in Patients with Cancer (CLOT) Investigators.

Low-molecular-weight heparin versus a coumarin for the prevention of recurrent venous thromboembolism in patients with cancer. N Engl J Med. 2003;349:146-53. [PMID: 12853587]

Item 9 Answer: E

Educational Objective: Diagnose pulmonary embolism in a pregnant patient.

A ventilation-perfusion (V/Q) lung scan should be performed next. Pregnant patients with pulmonary embolism (PE) present with symptoms (like dyspnea) that may overlap with symptoms of pregnancy, so a high index of suspicion is needed. New-onset cough is the presenting finding in 24% of pregnant women with PE. Doppler studies may be negative if the primary clot is in the pelvic veins; if results are negative, evaluation for venous thromboembolism requires imaging of the lung. V/Q scanning should be the initial study in pregnant patients. If the V/Q scan is normal, PE can be reliably excluded. If the V/Q scan is strongly positive, showing perfusion defects without matched ventilation abnormalities in this patient with no asthma or underlying lung disease, PE can be reliably diagnosed and therapy initiated.

CT angiography, the gold standard in the diagnosis of PE in most patients, should not be the initial study in pregnant patients because of radiation exposure to both the mother and the fetus. CT angiography should be reserved for instances when the V/Q scan is equivocal.

D-dimer assays are used to guide venous thromboembolism diagnosis in nonpregnant patients with low probability of disease, but D-dimer levels are elevated during pregnancy, with assays only 73% sensitive and 15% specific in this population. Additionally, D-dimer level should be determined only in patients with a low theoretical suspicion for PE. This patient has a moderate or high presumed likelihood.

Magnetic resonance pulmonary angiography has not been evaluated in pregnant patients, but in nonpregnant patients, the sensitivity for PE is only 85% (although the specificity is 98%). In addition, the long-term effects of gadolinium on the fetus are unknown.

Pulmonary function testing would be helpful to rule out bronchospastic disease as a cause for the patient's cough, but it should be done only after the more life-threatening diagnosis of PE is ruled out.

KEY POINT

- In the presence of normal Doppler studies of the lower extremities, ventilation-perfusion lung scanning is the initial lung imaging study to evaluate for pulmonary embolism in pregnant patients; D-dimer testing has no diagnostic role.

Bibliography
Leung AN, Bull TM, Jaeschke R, Lockwood CJ, Boiselle PM, Hurwitz LM, et al; ATS/STR Committee on Pulmonary Embolism in Pregnancy. An official American Thoracic Society/Society of Thoracic Radiology clinical practice guideline: evaluation of suspected pulmonary embolism in pregnancy. Am J Respir Crit Care Med. 2011;184:1200-8. [PMID: 22086989] doi:10.1164/rccm.201108-1575ST

Item 10 Answer: B

Educational Objective: Evaluate preoperative anemia.

Iron studies should be performed next. Preoperative anemia is associated with increased perioperative mortality in patients with cardiovascular disease; it is also a significant predictor for perioperative blood transfusion, which itself is associated with postoperative morbidity. The common causes for preoperative anemia are iron deficiency, vitamin B_{12} deficiency, chronic inflammatory disease, and chronic kidney disease. The hemoglobin level should be measured in the setting of signs or symptoms of anemia or surgery with a large expected blood loss at least 4 weeks before the surgery date. If anemia is identified, laboratory testing should begin with an assessment of iron status. Transferrin saturation less than 15% (or serum ferritin level less than 15 ng/mL [15 µg/L]) is consistent with iron deficiency anemia and should be treated with oral iron. If the response to oral iron is suboptimal because of patient adherence and surgical scheduling, intravenous iron should be used. Iron deficiency in this patient could be attributable to menstrual blood loss, occult gastrointestinal blood loss from NSAID-induced gastritis, or colon cancer. Evaluation and correction of the cause of iron deficiency anemia should take place before elective surgery.

Hemoglobin electrophoresis is useful to detect genetic hemoglobinopathies such as sickle cell disease or thalassemia, which are associated with lifelong anemia unlikely to present for the first time at this patient's age. These conditions could be suspected with examination of a peripheral blood smear.

Vitamin B_{12} deficiency is less common than iron deficiency in most patients scheduled to undergo orthopedic surgery, and it is typically associated with macrocytic anemia, which is not present in this patient.

Ignoring this patient's anemia is not appropriate, considering the increased risk of perioperative allogeneic transfusion, which carries its own risks and is avoidable if the anemia is treated beforehand.

KEY POINT

- Patients scheduled for elective surgery who have anemia should be evaluated for iron deficiency; preoperative management of iron deficiency anemia includes oral iron replacement and evaluation to determine the source of blood loss.

Bibliography
Goodnough LT, Maniatis A, Earnshaw P, Benoni G, Beris P, Bisbe E, et al. Detection, evaluation, and management of preoperative anaemia in the elective orthopaedic surgical patient: NATA guidelines. Br J Anaesth. 2011;106:13-22. [PMID: 21148637] doi:10.1093/bja/aeq361

Item 11 Answer: B

Educational Objective: Reverse warfarin anticoagulation with four-factor prothrombin complex concentrate.

This patient should be given four-factor prothrombin complex concentrate (4f-PCC). Patients who receive anticoagulation

CONT.

with a vitamin K antagonist have an increased risk for major gastrointestinal and central nervous system bleeding and an increased risk for periprocedural bleeding. Although vitamin K alone can be effective in reversing the effect of warfarin, its hemostatic effect can take several hours, and, in urgent situations, simultaneous replacement of the vitamin K–dependent coagulation factors is necessary. 4f-PCC contains factors II, VII, IX, and X as a lyophilized powder and can be administered quickly in a small reconstituted volume. It provides effective hemostasis 90% of the time and is the preferred option for most patients who require urgent warfarin reversal. Thromboembolism is a potential adverse effect. 4f-PCC should be avoided in patients with a history of heparin-induced thrombocytopenia because it contains residual heparin.

Cryoprecipitate would be indicated to treat severe hypofibrinogenemia, usually arising as a consequence of disseminated intravascular coagulation (DIC) or severe liver disease. There is no reason to anticipate DIC in this patient, and he has no history of liver disease.

Plasma transfusion is more time consuming (preparation and administration) and is associated with a much higher risk of fluid overload from the volume needed to replace the coagulation factors. It is no longer the best option to reverse warfarin with the availability of 4f-PCC.

Idarucizumab is a monoclonal antibody that binds the non–vitamin K antagonist oral anticoagulant dabigatran and causes a rapid reduction in available dabigatran in the body for up to 24 hours. Idarucizumab will not reverse warfarin anticoagulation.

KEY POINT

- Four-factor prothrombin complex concentrate should be used to reverse the effects of warfarin anticoagulation in patients experiencing severe bleeding and those requiring urgent surgery.

Bibliography

Goldstein JN, Refaai MA, Milling TJ Jr, Lewis B, Goldberg-Alberts R, Hug BA, et al. Four-factor prothrombin complex concentrate versus plasma for rapid vitamin K antagonist reversal in patients needing urgent surgical or invasive interventions: a phase 3b, open-label, non-inferiority, randomised trial. Lancet. 2015;385:2077-87. [PMID: 25728933] doi:10.1016/S0140-6736(14)61685-8

Item 12   Answer: D

Educational Objective: Evaluate a patient with deep venous thrombosis for occult malignancy.

This patient requires no additional testing. Cancer is eventually found in approximately 10% of patients with an unprovoked venous thromboembolism (VTE) within 1 year of VTE occurrence. Cancers of the ovary, pancreas, and liver are most often found. Testing for cancer in patients with idiopathic VTE leads to diagnosis of cancer at an earlier stage of the disease. However, a recent systematic review concluded that evidence is insufficient to draw definitive conclusions about the effectiveness of extensive testing for undiagnosed cancer in patients with a first episode of unprovoked VTE in reducing

cancer and VTE-related morbidity and mortality. The results are imprecise and could be consistent with either harm or benefit. The authors concluded that further good-quality, large-scale, randomized controlled trials are required before firm conclusions can be made. Furthermore, extensive cancer screening can cause significant economic and psychological burden. A recent economic analysis concluded that addition of a comprehensive CT of the abdomen-pelvis for the screening of occult cancer in patients with unprovoked VTE is not cost effective; it is both more costly and not more effective in detecting occult cancer. Therefore, age-appropriate malignancy screening is advised along with symptom-based assessment. Based on this patient's age and sex, she is up to date on her cancer screening tests, and no further testing is required.

Because the patient has no pulmonary symptoms and has no history of smoking, CT of the chest or abdomen is not necessary at this time.

Although the patient has some persistent lower extremity edema, this can occur during treatment and may persist despite thrombosis resolution. Because the edema seems to be slowly improving and her course of treatment was initiated only 6 weeks ago, repeat Doppler ultrasonography would not be necessary at this time.

KEY POINT

- In approximately 10% of patients in whom an unprovoked venous thromboembolism is diagnosed, cancer will be found within 1 year, so an age-appropriate screening test should be performed.

Bibliography

Carrier M, Lazo-Langner A, Shivakumar S, Tagalakis V, Zarychanski R, Solymoss S, et al; SOME Investigators. Screening for occult cancer in unprovoked venous thromboembolism. N Engl J Med. 2015;373:697-704. [PMID: 26095467] doi:10.1056/NEJMoa1506623

Item 13   Answer: A

Educational Objective: Diagnose acute promyelocytic leukemia.

This patient has pancytopenia, immature leukocytes with morphologic features consistent with promyelocytes, and laboratory features of disseminated intravascular coagulation (DIC), all of which are consistent with acute promyelocytic leukemia (APML). Acute leukemia can present with a leukocyte count within or below the normal range. It can include bleeding, as in this patient, from thrombocytopenia that may be accompanied by coagulopathy. APML is a subset of acute myeloid leukemia that often presents with bleeding and coagulopathy; this coagulopathy contributes to early mortality and morbidity. Features of DIC should prompt transfusion with fresh frozen plasma and cryoprecipitate (for hypofibrinogenemia) in addition to platelet transfusion for thrombocytopenia. A bone marrow aspirate and biopsy should be performed urgently to confirm the diagnosis because the coagulopathy of APML responds to therapy

CONT.

with all-*trans* retinoic acid, which targets the underlying defect in cellular differentiation.

Pancytopenia is expected in patients with aplastic anemia, but those patients would not have the atypical cells seen in the peripheral blood of this patient and would not present with DIC.

Although immature leukocytes, including myelocytes and promyelocytes, may be seen in the peripheral blood in patients with chronic granulocytic leukemia, these patients have leukocytosis, not leukopenia, and most of the increase comes from mature polymorphonuclear leukocytes.

Although severe thrombocytopenia and bleeding are typical of the acute presentation of immune thrombocytopenic purpura, this patient's pancytopenia, coagulopathy, and abnormal leukocytes are inconsistent with this diagnosis.

KEY POINT

- Acute promyelocytic leukemia may present with a reduced total leukocyte count and features of disseminated intravascular coagulation.

Bibliography

Döhner H, Weisdorf DJ, Bloomfield CD. Acute myeloid leukemia. N Engl J Med. 2015;373:1136-52. [PMID: 26376137] doi:10.1056/NEJMra1406184

Item 14   Answer: C

Educational Objective: Evaluate monoclonal gammopathy of undetermined significance.

This patient should have laboratory studies repeated in 6 months. She has incidentally found low-risk monoclonal gammopathy of undetermined significance (MGUS); follow-up in 6 months to 1 year with repeat serum protein electrophoresis, hemoglobin and calcium levels, and kidney function is appropriate. At that time, if the MGUS is stable, the interval for follow-up could be extended further. The risk of progression of MGUS to multiple myeloma or other lymphoproliferative disorders is determined by various risk factors. In this patient with IgG MGUS, an M spike of less than 1.5 g/dL, and normal serum free light chain assay findings, the risk of progression is low at 5% over 20 years. Patients with low-risk MGUS with no other concerning clinical features do not require bone marrow biopsy to evaluate the plasma cell burden. MGUS is seen in 3% of the population older than 50 years, and most of them do not progress, so extensive evaluation is not recommended unless other concerning features are present.

Although kidney injury attributed to multiple myeloma has long been recognized, recent evidence suggests that a portion of patients with MGUS who do not meet criteria for myeloma will, nonetheless, have kidney disease without any other contributing cause beyond the monoclonal protein. These patients have monoclonal gammopathy of renal significance and have characteristic findings on a kidney biopsy specimen. But in this patient with normal

kidney function and no proteinuria, kidney biopsy is not indicated.

In this patient with low-risk MGUS and no symptoms, MRI of the spine is not appropriate. An MRI or CT is more sensitive at detecting bone lesions than plain radiography and should be considered when used to risk stratify patients with smoldering multiple myeloma. MRI or CT may be important to assess spinal cord compression in patients with multiple myeloma and back pain. A skeletal survey is adequate in this low-risk patient.

Measurement of the β_2-microglobulin I level is a part of the risk stratification strategy for patients with multiple myeloma but not for those with MGUS.

KEY POINT

- In patients with IgG monoclonal gammopathy of undetermined significance, an M spike of less than 1.5 g/dL, and normal findings on serum free light chain assay and urine protein electrophoresis, the risk of progression is low, so extensive evaluation is not recommended.

Bibliography

van de Donk NW, Palumbo A, Johnsen HE, Engelhardt M, Gay F, Gregersen H, et al; European Myeloma Network. The clinical relevance and management of monoclonal gammopathy of undetermined significance and related disorders: recommendations from the European Myeloma Network. Haematologica. 2014;99:984-96. [PMID: 24658815] doi:10.3324/haematol.2013.100552

Item 15   Answer: D

Educational Objective: Treat symptomatic secondary hypogammaglobulinemia.

This patient should be given intravenous immune globulin (IVIG). She has acquired hypogammaglobulinemia with recurrent sinus infections. Patients with multiple myeloma are at risk for acquired hypogammaglobulinemia from a decrease in normal plasma cells and the effects of treatment. Patients with acquired hypogammaglobulinemia without recurrent infections should not be offered IVIG replacement. Prophylactic antibiotics are also an option in some patients who have recurrent infections with susceptible organisms. In addition to the cost of infusion, IVIG has numerous adverse effects, including anaphylaxis, serum sickness, kidney failure, hypertension, and headache. In patients with recurrent infections, IVIG provides protection from infection by providing passive immunity; the product is collected from healthy donors who likely have antibodies against the causative organisms. In this patient with recurrent sinus infections, a trial of IVIG should be given. Although efficacy is uncertain, vaccination against influenza, pneumococcus, and *Haemophilus influenzae* is also recommended.

Prophylactic acyclovir is often recommended for patients receiving bortezomib therapy (increased risk for herpes zoster) after autologous stem cell transplantation and for patients with recurrent herpetic infections. It is not provided routinely to patients with multiple myeloma to prevent infection and is unlikely to be of benefit in this patient with recurrent bacterial sinusitis.

Granulocyte colony-stimulating factor is used in conjunction with certain myelotoxic chemotherapies as infection prophylaxis and in some patients with severe neutropenia, such as severe congenital neutropenia. It is not appropriate in this patient with mild neutropenia.

Patients with myeloma are at increased risk for bacterial infection owing to impaired lymphocyte and plasma cell function and hypogammaglobulinemia. The most commonly encountered organisms are *Streptococcus pneumoniae*, *Haemophilus influenzae*, and *Escherichia coli* presenting as sinusitis, pneumonia, and urinary tract infections. Routine prophylaxis against fungal infection with fluconazole is not beneficial.

KEY POINT

- In patients with multiple myeloma, hypogammaglobulinemia, and recurrent infections, intravenous immune globulin should be given to provide passive immunity against causative organisms.

Bibliography

Friman V, Winqvist O, Blimark C, Langerbeins P, Chapel H, Dhalla F. Secondary immunodeficiency in lymphoproliferative malignancies. Hematol Oncol. 2016;34:121-32. [PMID: 27402426] doi:10.1002/hon.2323

Item 16   Answer: A

Educational Objective: Diagnose a delayed hemolytic transfusion reaction.

A direct antiglobulin (Coombs) test (DAT) should be ordered for this patient who is likely experiencing a delayed hemolytic transfusion reaction (DHTR), which is an anamnestic antibody response to previous erythrocyte antigen (non-ABO) sensitization that typically occurs 7 to 14 days after the index transfusion. The primary alloimmunization event is usually a remote transfusion or pregnancy. At the time of the index transfusion, the antibody level is usually lower than the detectable threshold determined by routine blood bank screening. A DHTR is associated with jaundice, low-grade fever, and an otherwise unexplained decrease in the hemoglobin concentration; it is sometimes accompanied by hemoglobinuria, which is confirmed by urinalysis and this patient's presenting symptom of tea-colored urine. Laboratory testing in these patients shows indirect hyperbilirubinemia. The DAT will be positive, whereas the indirect antiglobulin test, which is invariably negative before transfusion, may remain negative or show an unexpected alloantibody. For patients known to have received a recent transfusion, obtaining a transfusion history from the outside blood bank may be helpful.

Flow cytometry will assist in the diagnosis of paroxysmal nocturnal hemoglobinuria (PNH), an acquired clonal stem cell disorder that should be considered in patients presenting with hemolytic anemia, pancytopenia, or unprovoked atypical thrombosis. Hemolytic anemia occurring within days of a transfusion in a previously sensitized individual is more likely to represent DHTR than PNH.

Patients thought to have obscure gastrointestinal bleeding should be considered for repeat upper endoscopy, colonoscopy, or both. Up to 50% of lesions can be identified using this strategy. However, this patient's decrease in hemoglobin level, hemoglobinuria, and elevated total bilirubin level suggest hemolysis, not gastrointestinal bleeding.

Patients who are well compensated for their degree of anemia do not require immediate transfusion.

KEY POINT

- A positive direct antiglobulin (Coombs) test will confirm a delayed hemolytic transfusion reaction, a diagnosis that should be considered in a patient with low-grade fever and features of hemolytic anemia after recent transfusion.

Bibliography

Delaney M, Wendel S, Bercovitz RS, Cid J, Cohn C, Dunbar NM, et al; Biomedical Excellence for Safer Transfusion (BEST) Collaborative. Transfusion reactions: prevention, diagnosis, and treatment. Lancet. 2016;388:2825-2836. [PMID: 27083327] doi:10.1016/S0140-6736(15)01313-6

Item 17   Answer: C

Educational Objective: Treat disseminated intravascular coagulation with cryoprecipitate transfusion.

The most appropriate management for this patient is to transfuse 10 units of pooled cryoprecipitate. Cryoprecipitate is appropriate as adjunctive therapy if bleeding and hypofibrinogenemia persist in disseminated intravascular coagulation (DIC). This patient's clinical presentation of thrombocytopenia, abnormally prolonged clotting times, and low fibrinogen level are consistent with DIC, which is associated with placental abruption and other obstetric emergencies and severe inflammatory immune response syndrome with multiorgan dysfunction. The hemostatic defect in DIC is multifactorial, ultimately involving the consumption of coagulation factors and platelets. Bleeding in DIC typically responds to treatment of the underlying cause and should resolve in this patient with appropriate obstetric management of the placental abruption. However, transfusion support may still be required to address the coagulopathy. Cryoprecipitate is manufactured from fresh frozen plasma and contains fibrinogen in a more concentrated form. The appropriate amount requires pooling 8 to 10 units of cryoprecipitate, each unit being derived from 1 pint of whole blood.

Twenty-five percent albumin is fractionated from large pools of donated plasma and does not contain any coagulation proteins. It is hyperoncotic and used to treat hypotension, commonly in the postoperative setting and after large-volume paracentesis. This patient's blood pressure has stabilized, so she needs definitive management of the coagulopathy. Twenty-five percent albumin would not be appropriate therapy.

Cryo-poor plasma is derived from fresh frozen plasma in which the cryoprecipitate has been separated. Its use is limited to refractory thrombotic thrombocytopenic purpura, although any advantage over fresh frozen plasma in this disorder has not been proven. It is not appropriate for treatment of most coagulopathies.

Although the patient does have thrombocytopenia, a platelet count exceeding 50,000/µL (50×10^9/L) is generally acceptable to manage postsurgical bleeding (with a count of approximately 100,000/µL [100×10^9/L] preferred for intracranial bleeding); therefore, a platelet transfusion is not the most immediate need.

KEY POINT

- Cryoprecipitate is the treatment of choice for patients with bleeding and hypofibrinogenemia secondary to disseminated intravascular coagulation.

Bibliography

Levy JH, Goodnough LT. How I use fibrinogen replacement therapy in acquired bleeding. Blood. 2015;125:1387-93. [PMID: 25519751] doi: 10.1182/blood-2014-08-552000

Item 18   Answer: D

Educational Objective: Diagnose parvovirus B19 infection in a patient with sickle cell disease.

This patient has parvovirus B19 infection presenting with pure red cell aplasia (PRCA). Patients with sickle cell anemia have chronic hemolysis and depend on increased erythrocyte production to maintain the hemoglobin level. Parvovirus B19 infection preferentially affects erythrocyte precursors in the bone marrow, causing transient PRCA. This patient's very low reticulocyte count is consistent with the decreased erythrocyte production seen in PRCA. Infection with parvovirus B19 in children can present as erythema infectiosum with fever and rash. Although adults can have flu-like illness and arthralgia, most are asymptomatic. However, in patients with hemolytic anemia, it can present with transient aplastic crisis. Supportive transfusions are usually required to treat symptoms from severe anemia.

Aplastic anemia (AA) is a condition characterized by pancytopenia with associated neutropenia, anemia, and thrombocytopenia and a severely hypocellular bone marrow. Isolated cytopenias are uncommon despite the designation of anemia. AA is usually acquired and is caused by toxic, viral, or autoimmune mechanisms. The lack of other cytopenias makes AA an unlikely diagnosis.

In some patients with sickle cell disease, a rare condition known as hyperhemolysis is thought to be responsible for an acute hemolytic anemia and reticulocytosis. Episodes have sometimes been associated with delayed transfusion reactions and acute vasoocclusive events. Hyperhemolysis syndrome would be associated with an elevated reticulocyte count, not a reduced count.

Myelodysplastic syndrome (MDS) ranges in severity from an asymptomatic disease characterized by mild normocytic or macrocytic anemia to a transfusion-dependent anemia. The incidence of MDS increases with age. Abnormal erythrocyte forms with basophilic stippling or Howell-Jolly bodies and dysplastic neutrophils with decreased nuclear segmentation and granulation may be present. MDS is unlikely to cause a symptomatic anemia developing over a few days in a young patient with sickle cell disease.

KEY POINT

- Parvovirus B19 infection preferentially affects erythrocyte precursors in the bone marrow, causing transient pure red cell aplasia in patients with sickle cell anemia.

Bibliography

Yawn BP, Buchanan GR, Afenyi-Annan AN, Ballas SK, Hassell KL, James AH, et al. Management of sickle cell disease: summary of the 2014 evidence-based report by expert panel members. JAMA. 2014;312:1033-48. [PMID: 25203083] doi:10.1001/jama.2014.10517

Item 19   Answer: B

Educational Objective: Treat essential thrombocythemia.

The patient has essential thrombocythemia (ET) and should be treated with hydroxyurea. The first step in evaluating thrombocytosis is to rule out a secondary elevation. Chronic infection, collagen vascular disease, malignancy, ongoing bleeding, and iron deficiency can all cause a reactive thrombocytosis. *JAK2* mutation testing is positive in only about 60% of patients with ET, but other clonal mutations involving calreticulin and *MPL* genes have been identified in some patients with *JAK2*-negative ET. Approximately 10% to 15% of patients with ET have negative results for all three mutations (termed triple-negative patients). A bone marrow biopsy specimen showing hypercellularity with increased numbers of enlarged megakaryocytes is required to make the diagnosis in the few patients with ET who do not have any of the three mutations listed previously.

The most significant complications that may occur during follow-up of ET are thrombosis (10%-15% 15-year cumulative risk; arterial is more common than venous), hemorrhage (8.6% 15-year cumulative risk), progression to myelofibrosis (10% 15-year cumulative risk), and transformation to acute leukemia (3% 15-year cumulative risk). The patient's age (older than 60 years) and previous thromboembolic event place her at particularly high risk for subsequent thromboembolic complications. Platelet-lowering therapy is indicated for any patient at high risk. Hydroxyurea is well tolerated in older adult patients and is considered first-line therapy for nonpregnant patients. For that reason, she should be treated with aspirin and hydroxyurea.

Patients with high-risk ET, such as this patient who has a history of stroke, require antiplatelet therapy and platelet-lowering therapy with agents such as hydroxyurea. Changing antiplatelet therapy from aspirin to clopidogrel would not address this patient's need for platelet-lowering therapy nor would adding a second antiplatelet medication, such as clopidogrel, to the aspirin.

Plateletpheresis may be indicated in the emergent management of patients with ET who have markedly elevated platelet counts, usually greater than 1,000,000/µL (1000 × 10^9/L), and acute hemorrhage. Plateletpheresis would not be indicated in this patient.

KEY POINT

- Patients with essential thrombocythemia who are older than 60 years or who have had previous thromboembolic complications should be treated with aspirin and hydroxyurea.

Bibliography

Nangalia J, Massie CE, Baxter EJ, Nice FL, Gundem G, Wedge DC, et al. Somatic CALR mutations in myeloproliferative neoplasms with nonmutated JAK2. N Engl J Med. 2013;369:2391-405. [PMID: 24325359] doi:10.1056/NEJMoa1312542

Item 20   Answer: B

Educational Objective: Diagnose benign ethnic neutropenia.

This patient most likely has benign ethnic neutropenia. Isolated neutropenia usually has a hereditary, toxic, or immune cause. Isolated mild neutropenia (1000-1500/µL [1-1.5 × 10^9/L]) found on routine testing in asymptomatic black patients, or occasionally in other ethnic groups (Sephardic Jews, West Indians, Arabs of the Middle East), likely has a benign ethnic cause. An absolute neutrophil count less than 500/µL (0.5 × 10^9/L) is less likely to be a normal variant and more likely to be associated with increased risk for bacterial and fungal infections. Patients with benign ethnic neutropenia usually have good bone marrow reserve and are not prone to developing infections. A detailed evaluation for other causes of neutropenia is usually not required in these patients. Having a previous history of mild neutropenia supports the diagnosis but is not required.

Autoimmune neutropenia is caused by destruction of the neutrophils by autoantibodies. It is more commonly seen in conjunction with other autoimmune disorders, such as systemic lupus erythematosus or Felty syndrome. Felty syndrome is a triad of rheumatoid arthritis, splenomegaly, and neutropenia. This patient has no signs or symptoms of an autoimmune disorder. Although idiopathic autoimmune neutropenia without an underlying systemic disorder can occur, benign ethnic neutropenia would be a much more likely diagnosis in this asymptomatic black patient with mild neutropenia.

Cyclical neutropenia is a rare congenital disorder in which the neutrophil count nadirs every 2 to 5 weeks with recurrent infections. Diagnosis requires twice-weekly complete blood counts for 6 to 8 weeks. This patient's clinical history does not indicate recurrent infections or other typical findings of cyclical neutropenia.

Drug-induced neutropenia occurs in patients taking medications such as chemotherapy, NSAIDs, carbamazepine, phenytoin, propylthiouracil, cephalosporins, trimethoprim-sulfamethoxazole, or psychotropic drugs. Omeprazole has not been commonly implicated in causing neutropenia. Drug-induced neutropenia is diagnosed by temporal relationship of the neutropenia with starting the medication and improvement with stopping the offending medication. It is important to note that improvement in neutropenia may lag behind by many weeks after stopping the medication.

KEY POINT

- Benign ethnic neutropenia typically appears as an isolated, mild neutropenia (1000-1500/µL [1-1.5 × 10^9/L]) found on routine testing in asymptomatic black persons or certain other ethnic groups.

Bibliography

Gibson C, Berliner N. How we evaluate and treat neutropenia in adults. Blood. 2014;124:1251-8; quiz 1378. [PMID: 24869938] doi:10.1182/blood-2014-02-482612

Item 21   Answer: C

Educational Objective: Manage glucose-6-phosphate dehydrogenase deficiency.

The most appropriate management for this patient is to discontinue dapsone. He most likely has glucose-6-phosphate dehydrogenase (G6PD) deficiency as a result of his dapsone therapy. He developed an acute hemolytic anemia, indicated by an acute reduction in the hemoglobin and haptoglobin levels and reticulocytosis, and the bite cells seen on the peripheral blood smear also suggest G6PD deficiency. A drug reaction should always be suspected in such settings. Dapsone is one of the most commonly encountered drugs leading to G6PD-mediated hemolysis, so this drug should be promptly discontinued. G6PD deficiency is X linked, so it is much more common in men, especially in those of African descent. G6PD levels should not be checked during an acute hemolytic event because they are normal in newly produced erythrocytes but decrease up to 75% as the cells age. As a result, during an acute hemolytic event, the older, more deficient erythrocytes are preferentially destroyed, leaving the newer less deficient cells to circulate. This leads to falsely normal G6PD levels, so G6PD measurement should be delayed for several weeks after a hemolytic event.

Warm antibody autoimmune hemolytic anemia would be appropriately treated with glucocorticoids, such as prednisone, but this disease is unlikely with the negative direct antiglobulin test result and the absence of spherocytes in the peripheral blood.

Rituximab would be indicated to treat cold agglutinin autoimmune hemolytic anemia. However, no agglutinated cells are seen on the peripheral blood smear, and the direct antiglobulin test result would be positive, indicating complement on the erythrocyte surface in this disease.

This patient's platelet count is normal, and no fragmented erythrocytes or schistocytes are seen on the peripheral blood smear, so thrombotic thrombocytopenia purpura, which would be confirmed by a reduction in ADAMTS13 activity, is not likely.

KEY POINT

- Testing for glucose-6-phosphate dehydrogenase activity is reliable in men who are not experiencing an acute hemolytic episode but is less useful during acute episodes because reticulocytes produce higher levels of enzyme, resulting in a falsely normal test result.

Bibliography

Luzzatto L, Seneca E. G6PD deficiency: a classic example of pharmacogenetics with on-going clinical implications. Br J Haematol. 2014;164:469-80. [PMID: 24372186] doi:10.1111/bjh.12665

Item 22   Answer: A

Educational Objective: Diagnose the anemia of kidney disease.

This patient most likely has anemia resulting from erythropoietin deficiency. Normocytic anemia with unremarkable erythrocyte morphology and a low reticulocyte count in a patient with underlying chronic kidney disease is usually caused by erythropoietin deficiency. Measuring erythropoietin levels may be useful in making the diagnosis of the anemia of kidney disease, and low erythropoietin measurements can distinguish these patients from those with other causes of anemia. The modest absolute increase in serum creatinine level underestimates the severity of kidney injury in this frail, older adult patient with reduced muscle mass. Administration of erythropoiesis-stimulating agents will correct the anemia of kidney disease.

The anemia of inflammation is caused by inhibition of iron transport and suppression of erythropoietin by hepcidin and other inflammatory cytokines. Although it is classically seen in patients with chronic infection, cancer, or autoimmune-inflammatory disease, the anemia of inflammation may also occur in patients with diabetes and heart failure and, on occasion, in patients without any overt underlying disease. This patient lacks characteristic laboratory features, including a low total iron-binding capacity and serum iron level and normal or elevated ferritin level.

Iron deficiency is not uncommon in patients with chronic kidney disease because they are at risk for gastrointestinal bleeding from angiodysplasia or ulcer disease, but these patients typically have microcytic erythrocytes, low serum iron and ferritin levels, and elevated total iron-binding capacity.

Patients with myelodysplastic syndrome often have pancytopenia; although early stages and forms of this syndrome with a better prognosis may have isolated anemia, the presence of macrocytosis, which is absent in this patient, is characteristic.

KEY POINT

- Normocytic anemia with a low reticulocyte count and normal erythrocyte morphology in a patient with underlying chronic kidney disease is usually caused by erythropoietin deficiency and will respond to therapy with an erythropoiesis-stimulating agent; however, normalization of the blood count is not advised.

Bibliography

Chapter 1: Diagnosis and evaluation of anemia in CKD. Kidney Int Suppl (2011). 2012;2:288-291. [PMID: 25018948]

Item 23   Answer: A

Educational Objective: Diagnose amyloidosis.

The most appropriate test to perform next is an abdominal fat pad biopsy. This patient has cardiomyopathy, nephrotic syndrome, autonomic dysfunction, and macroglossia, which are likely caused by amyloidosis. Amyloid deposition can occur in one or more organs and cause symptoms related to the sites of deposition. Sites commonly involved are the kidneys, the gastrointestinal tract, and the cardiac, neurologic, coagulation, and musculoskeletal systems. In this patient, nephrotic-range proteinuria, cardiomyopathy, orthostatic hypotension, and macroglossia all suggest amyloidosis. The finding of an IgG λ monoclonal gammopathy can also be associated with amyloidosis. Diagnosis requires biopsy of the affected organ and demonstration of characteristic apple-green birefringence with Congo red staining. Fat pad biopsy is sometimes performed when multiorgan involvement is suspected because it is less invasive; however, if findings are unrevealing, biopsy of the organ(s) involved, such as the kidney, may be required. Because different proteins can be involved in amyloid deposition, protein typing with tests such as mass spectrometry is done after amyloidosis is diagnosed. Proper identification of the amyloid type is critical and guides appropriate therapy.

Cardiac catheterization to evaluate for coronary artery disease is not the best test to perform in this patient with multisystem involvement and no symptoms or signs of acute ischemia. However, cardiac biopsy is sometimes required in patients with suspected isolated cardiac involvement with amyloidosis.

Tilt table testing may be helpful in patients with reflex syncope triggered by standing, patients in high-risk settings with a single unexplained episode of syncope, or patients with recurrent episodes in the absence of organic heart disease. This patient does not have syncope but rather a multiplicity of findings suggesting a systemic disease not likely to be elucidated with tilt table testing.

KEY POINT

- Diagnosis of amyloidosis requires biopsy of the affected organ and demonstration of characteristic apple-green birefringence with Congo red staining; fat pad biopsy is sometimes performed because it is less invasive.

Bibliography

Gillmore JD, Wechalekar A, Bird J, Cavenagh J, Hawkins S, Kazmi M, et al; BCSH Committee. Guidelines on the diagnosis and investigation of AL amyloidosis. Br J Haematol. 2015;168:207-18. [PMID: 25312307] doi:10.1111/bjh.13156

Item 24   Answer: A

Educational Objective: Treat iron deficiency due to malabsorption.

The most appropriate treatment is parenteral iron therapy. This patient has severe iron deficiency and inflammatory bowel disease, which impairs iron absorption in the duodenum and proximal jejunum and commonly leads to increased gastrointestinal blood loss. Several parenteral iron preparations are available, including iron sucrose, ferric gluconate, ferumoxytol, and iron carboxymaltose. These preparations are better absorbed and have a better side effect profile than previous parenteral preparations, such as iron dextran.

Liquid preparations of iron are useful in pediatric populations or to provide an even lower dose of iron than would be present in a single tablet, but no evidence suggests that the liquid form is better absorbed.

Increasing the frequency of oral iron therapy will not address the basic problem of this patient's malabsorption. Additionally, recent information indicates that patients with iron deficiency with normal intestinal function have a paradoxical decrease in iron absorption when supplements are administered multiple times per day compared with once daily, perhaps owing to hepcidin stimulation. Hepcidin, a peptide hormone produced in the liver, is a main regulator of iron homeostasis. It decreases intestinal iron absorption and release of iron stores by down-regulating the ferroportin-mediated release of iron from enterocytes, hepatocytes, and macrophages. Hepcidin is produced by hepatocytes when iron is abundant and in inflammatory anemia; it is suppressed in iron deficiency anemia.

Sustained-release iron preparations should never be used because much of the iron in these preparations is released distal to the jejunal site of absorption.

KEY POINT

- Patients with inflammatory bowel disease have difficulty absorbing oral iron to balance their increased iron loss from bleeding, so parenteral iron is an appropriate alternative for restoring iron stores.

Bibliography

Auerbach M, Adamson JW. How we diagnose and treat iron deficiency anemia. Am J Hematol. 2016;91:31-8. [PMID: 26408108] doi:10.1002/ajh.24201

Item 25   Answer: A

Educational Objective: Diagnose Waldenström macroglobulinemia.

A bone marrow biopsy is the most appropriate diagnostic test to perform in this patient. He has hepatosplenomegaly, anemia, and night sweats along with an IgM spike on laboratory testing, indicating he most likely has Waldenström macroglobulinemia (WM). WM is an indolent B-cell lymphoma with clonal lymphoplasmacytic infiltration of the bone marrow that secretes IgM in the blood. Patients with WM can present with classic "B symptoms" of drenching night sweats, fever, weight loss, and anemia. Tissue infiltration of the lymphoma can cause hepatosplenomegaly and lymphadenopathy. Bone marrow biopsy to document lymphoplasmacytic infiltrate will confirm the diagnosis.

For patients suspected of having a lymphoma, excisional biopsy of a lymph node is preferred to needle biopsy because it provides better architectural detail for distinguishing malignant from benign causes and for classifying the nature of the malignancy. In patients with WM, bone marrow biopsy is predictably diagnostic and a much less invasive option than is para-aortic lymph node excision.

Increased IgM protein in the blood can cause hyperviscosity, with symptoms such as altered vision, headache, hearing loss, tinnitus, dizziness, nystagmus, altered mental status, and nasal and oropharyngeal bleeding. Funduscopic evaluation may show hyperviscosity-related findings, including dilated retinal veins, papilledema, and flame hemorrhages. This patient has no signs or symptoms of hyperviscosity and has an M protein level of less than 400 mg/dL (4 g/L), so serum viscosity testing is not indicated.

KEY POINT

- Waldenström macroglobulinemia is an indolent B-cell lymphoma with clonal lymphoplasmacytic infiltration of the bone marrow that secretes IgM in the blood, and a bone marrow biopsy will confirm the diagnosis.

Bibliography

Castillo JJ, Garcia-Sanz R, Hatjiharissi E, Kyle RA, Leleu X, McMaster M, et al. Recommendations for the diagnosis and initial evaluation of patients with Waldenström Macroglobulinaemia: a task force from the 8th International Workshop on Waldenström Macroglobulinaemia. Br J Haematol. 2016;175:77-86. [PMID: 27378193] doi:10.1111/bjh.14196

Item 26   Answer: D

Educational Objective: Diagnose hereditary hemochromatosis.

The most appropriate test to perform next is transferrin saturation and serum ferritin level. Historically, patients with hereditary hemochromatosis presented with signs of cirrhosis, diabetes mellitus, and skin pigmentation. Because of earlier recognition, fatigue, arthralgias, and loss of libido are more common presenting symptoms. Patients with hemochromatosis have rheumatic symptoms that typically involve the small joints of the hand, especially the second and third metacarpophalangeal (MCP) joints associated with characteristic radiographic findings, including hook-like osteophytes. Guidelines support initial testing with transferrin saturation to diagnosis iron overload. A transferrin saturation greater than 45% is often chosen as the cutoff to warrant additional testing, although this threshold has lower specificity and positive predictive value compared with higher cutoff values. A normal serum ferritin level and transferrin saturation less than 45% have a negative predictive value of 97% to exclude iron overload.

Symmetrical involvement of MCP joints suggests the possibility of rheumatoid arthritis (RA), but hook-like osteophytes on the metacarpal heads is a disease-specific finding for hemochromatosis. For these reasons, RA is an unlikely diagnosis, and it is unnecessary to perform rheumatoid factor and anti–cyclic citrullinated peptide antibody testing. The MCP involvement and radiographic changes also make primary osteoarthritis an unlikely diagnosis.

HFE genotyping is reserved for patients in whom the serum ferritin level is elevated, a high transferrin saturation is noted, or both. It would not be the appropriate initial test to perform in this patient who has had no other testing. C282Y homozygosity accounts for 80% to 85% of typical patients with hereditary hemochromatosis; C282Y/H63D and C282Y/S65C compound heterozygosity are the next most prevalent genotypes.

Since the advent of *HFE* mutational analysis, the role of liver biopsy has diminished. Liver biopsy is generally reserved to stage liver disease in patients known to be C282Y homozygous or compound heterozygous when the serum ferritin level is greater than 1000 ng/mL (1000 µg/L) with or without elevated liver enzyme levels. Liver biopsy may also be useful when other pathogens, including alcohol and chronic hepatitis, might be causing liver injury.

KEY POINT

- Atypical presentations of rheumatoid arthritis and osteoarthritis, particularly with hook-like osteophytes of the second and third metacarpophalangeal joints, suggest the possibility of hemochromatosis; evaluating the transferrin saturation and serum ferritin level should be considered.

Bibliography

Bacon BR, Adams PC, Kowdley KV, Powell LW, Tavill AS; American Association for the Study of Liver Diseases. Diagnosis and management of hemochromatosis: 2011 practice guideline by the American Association for the Study of Liver Diseases. Hepatology. 2011;54:328-43. [PMID: 21452290] doi:10.1002/hep.24330

Item 27   Answer: A

Educational Objective: Treat massive lower extremity deep venous thrombosis.

Thrombolytic therapy with alteplase is the most appropriate management for this patient. He has signs and symptoms of extensive proximal deep venous thrombosis (DVT) leading to progressive edema of the leg, compromising arterial blood flow and causing acute ischemic injury. He is at risk for amputation of the leg and increased risk of death. Results of a systematic review of thrombolytic therapy showed greater improvement in venous patency, increased complete clot lysis, and reduced postthrombotic syndrome compared with anticoagulant therapy alone. Thrombolytic therapy was not associated with significant differences in mortality, stroke or intracerebral hemorrhage, pulmonary embolism, or leg ulceration; however, there were few events overall and with wide confidence intervals, and the review could not rule out clinically relevant differences. Bleeding risk with thrombolytic therapy is slightly greater than that associated with anticoagulant therapy, and strict eligibility criteria to reduce the risk of bleeding complications limit the applicability of this

treatment. Thrombolytic agents include tissue plasminogen activator, streptokinase, and urokinase. Derivatives of tissue plasminogen activator, such as alteplase, are most commonly used in the setting of thrombosis because they more selectively activate fibrin-bound plasminogen.

The parenteral direct thrombin inhibitors argatroban and lepirudin are reserved for the treatment of heparin-induced thrombocytopenia. Argatroban and lepirudin are not thrombolytic.

Rivaroxaban, a non–vitamin K antagonist oral anticoagulant, is an accepted monotherapy for DVT (heparin not required). However, rivaroxaban has no immediate effect on thrombus dissolution.

Unfractionated heparin potentiates the natural anticoagulant activity of antithrombin and acts as a nonspecific anticoagulant, mostly against thrombin and activated factor X. Heparin will prevent propagation of the thrombus but does not provide an immediate decrease in the size of an existing thrombus; therefore, it will not reverse tissue ischemia.

The role of an inferior vena cava filter in a patient with massive proximal DVT is uncertain. Although it might decrease the short-term risk of pulmonary embolism, it will predispose to subsequent DVT and increase the risk of postphlebitic syndrome. If a filter were used, it should be inserted after thrombolytic therapy.

KEY POINT

- Thrombolysis should be considered as the initial therapy for patients with iliofemoral deep venous thrombosis with acute limb ischemia.

Bibliography

Watson L, Broderick C, Armon MP. Thrombolysis for acute deep vein thrombosis. Cochrane Database Syst Rev. 2014 Jan 23;(1):CD002783. doi:n10.1002/14651858.CD002783.pub3. Review. Update in: Cochrane Database Syst Rev. 2016 Nov 10;11:CD002783. [PMID: 24452314]

Item 28   Answer: C

Educational Objective: Treat autoimmune hemolytic anemia with transfusion of crossmatch-incompatible blood.

The most appropriate management is to transfuse with crossmatch-incompatible blood. Although the goal of pretransfusion testing is to ensure the provision of ABO and Rh crossmatch-compatible blood, compatibility might not be achievable in autoimmune hemolytic anemia. Autoimmune hemolytic anemia is caused by the production of autoreactive antibodies against the patient's own erythrocytes. The direct antiglobulin test detects the presence of IgG or complement coating the patient's erythrocytes. In many patients who have IgG autoantibodies, the autoantibodies are of sufficient concentration in the serum or plasma to cause an incompatible crossmatch with donor erythrocytes because the autoantibody is directed against a core antigen on erythrocytes that is present not only on the patient's erythrocytes but also on all donor cells. Although the autoantibody will shorten the

CONT.

survival of transfused cells, they will still survive for days or even weeks and should provide effective therapy for problems related to acute anemia until immunosuppressive therapy becomes effective. A response to immunosuppressive therapy takes 1 to 2 weeks. The major risk in these patients is the failure to identify any additional alloantibody that may be present and could lead to more fulminant acute hemolytic transfusion reactions. In the absence of pregnancy or previous transfusion, the likelihood of non-ABO erythrocyte alloantibody development is extremely low. Therefore, a unit that is ABO and Rh matched is appropriate, even if crossmatch incompatible.

It is not appropriate to withhold transfusion when a patient has severe anemia-related symptoms.

Plasma exchange therapy is not effective for removing IgG antibodies because of a large extravascular space for IgG distribution that equilibrates back into the vascular pool as plasma is removed.

Using "universal" group O–negative or group O–positive blood provides no advantage. It would still be crossmatch incompatible because of the underlying autoantibody. Uncrossmatched blood is reserved for situations of exsanguination in which blood transfusion is urgently required before "type and cross" can be completed.

KEY POINT

- In patients with severe symptomatic autoimmune hemolytic anemia, the autoantibody typically reacts against all erythrocytes, and a completely crossmatch-compatible unit may be impossible to find; these patients should receive ABO and Rh-matched blood even if it is not crossmatch compatible.

Bibliography
Lechner K, Jäger U. How I treat autoimmune hemolytic anemias in adults. Blood. 2010;116:1831-8. [PMID: 20548093] doi:10.1182/blood-2010-03-259325

Item 29   Answer: B

Educational Objective: Identify an increased risk of infection after autologous hematopoietic stem cell transplantation.

This patient is at increased risk of infection. The most common indications for autologous hematopoietic stem cell transplantation (HSCT) are multiple myeloma and relapsed non-Hodgkin lymphoma. With appropriate supportive care, many older patients are eligible for autologous HSCT. Fatigue, altered taste, diminished appetite, and persistent mild diarrhea are common adverse effects of high-dose chemotherapy, an integral part of HSCT. The most common concern in patients who have undergone HSCT is the increased risk of infection, which persists for 6 to 12 months after HSCT. This risk is attributed to compromised function of neutrophils and lymphocytes and is sometimes associated with mild neutropenia and lymphopenia. For this reason, patients should be counseled to report warning symptoms, such as fever and

respiratory or other localizing symptoms of infection, early in the course.

Graft-versus-host disease (GVHD) is a major risk of allogeneic HSCT. Acute GVHD occurs when graft T cells recognize the patient's normal gut, skin, and liver sinusoids as foreign. Severe GVHD is life threatening and is treated with high-dose glucocorticoids. Anti–T-lymphocyte immune globulin as part of the myeloablative conditioning regimen can markedly reduce the prevalence of chronic GVHD 2 years after allogeneic HSCT in HLA-matched siblings. GVHD is not a complication of autologous HSCT.

Hematopoietic clonal disorders, including myelodysplasia, leukemia, and lymphoma, can occur decades after completion of therapy. Typical agents associated with therapy-related myelodysplasia include alkylators, anthracyclines, and topoisomerase II inhibitors. Likewise, leukemia and lymphoma can develop as a late consequence of exposure to chemotherapy and radiation. But these disorders would not occur in the months immediately following uncomplicated autologous HSCT.

KEY POINT

- Immediately following hematopoietic stem cell transplantation, patients are at increased risk of infection because of compromised function of lymphocytes and neutrophils.

Bibliography
Hashmi SK. Basics of hematopoietic cell transplantation for primary care physicians and internists. Prim Care. 2016;43:693-701. [PMID: 27866586] doi:10.1016/j.pop.2016.07.003

Item 30   Answer: C

Educational Objective: Evaluate smoldering multiple myeloma with whole body MRI.

Whole body MRI is the most appropriate next diagnostic test for this patient. Smoldering multiple myeloma (MM) is characterized by a serum M protein level of 3 g/dL or greater (or ≥500 mg/24 hr of urinary monoclonal free light chains) or bone marrow plasma clonal cells of 10% or greater and no evidence of myeloma-related signs or symptoms requiring therapy. All patients with MM should be assessed for skeletal lesions at diagnosis, periodically thereafter, and when any new symptoms occur. Skeletal survey with plain radiography is commonly used to assess for lytic lesions in patients with monoclonal gammopathy. However, MRI has recently been found to be more sensitive at identifying myeloma bone lesions and soft tissue lesions from plasmacytoma. The International Myeloma Working Group recommends that all patients with smoldering MM undergo whole body MRI (or spine and pelvic MRI if whole body MRI is not available). Whole body MRI is considered the gold standard for imaging of the axial skeleton, for the evaluation of painful lesions, and for distinguishing benign versus malignant osteoporotic vertebral fractures. If a patient is discovered to have more than one lesion greater than 5 mm, the patient

Answers and Critiques

should be considered symptomatic and requires consideration for treatment. With equivocal small lesions, a second MRI should be performed after 3 to 6 months; if the MRI shows progression, the patient should be treated as having symptomatic myeloma. In this patient with smoldering MM, negative findings on plain radiographs do not reliably rule out a skeletal lesion, and MRI is needed for further evaluation.

Although bone scans are useful in detecting bone metastases from underlying cancer, the bone lesions in MM are often purely lytic and lack the enhanced osteoblastic activity that is shown by bone scan imaging. Bone scans should not be used to assess bone involvement in myeloma.

CT is more sensitive than plain radiography in detecting bone lesions but is less sensitive than MRI in detecting small lesions. Additionally, patients with MM are at high risk for contrast nephropathy from CT contrast.

No further testing is inappropriate because the detection of asymptomatic focal lesions on whole body MRI determines the plan of care for patients with smoldering MM.

KEY POINT

- The International Myeloma Working Group recommends that all patients with smoldering multiple myeloma undergo whole body MRI to assess for lytic lesions.

Bibliography

Dimopoulos MA, Hillengass J, Usmani S, Zamagni E, Lentzsch S, Davies FE, et al. Role of magnetic resonance imaging in the management of patients with multiple myeloma: a consensus statement. J Clin Oncol. 2015; 33:657-64. [PMID: 25605835] doi:10.1200/JCO.2014.57.9961

Item 31   Answer: C

Educational Objective: Treat warfarin-associated bleeding.

The most appropriate treatment for this patient is vitamin K and prothrombin complex concentrates (PCCs), specifically, four-factor PCC. Four-factor PCC is a combination of inactivated factors II, VII, IX, and X. Treatment recommendations for over-anticoagulation with warfarin are based on the degree of over-anticoagulation as measured by the INR and clinical manifestations of bleeding. The first step in all cases of over-anticoagulation is withholding warfarin. For patients with an INR of 4.5 to 10 and with no evidence of bleeding, routine use of vitamin K is not recommended. For patients with an INR greater than 10 and with no evidence of bleeding, oral vitamin K is recommended. For patients with major bleeding, such as this patient with an intracerebral hemorrhage, rapid reversal of anticoagulation is recommended with four-factor PCC rather than fresh frozen plasma (FFP). These patients are also likely to benefit from the addition of vitamin K by slow intravenous injection rather than using coagulation factors alone. Clinical trials have shown four-factor PCC to be noninferior to FFP in reversing

warfarin anticoagulation. However, four-factor PCC is preferred because of its rapid reversal of the INR, rapid infusion and administration, and no risk of volume overload as is sometimes seen with plasma infusions. Additionally, four-factor PCC does not require thawing or typing.

Although FFP contains the appropriate clotting factors, it requires thawing and large volumes to correct the INR. This patient also has heart failure, making infusion of FFP problematic because of the volume needed.

Idarucizumab is a monoclonal antibody approved for reversal of the anticoagulant effects of dabigatran. It is not used to reverse the effects of vitamin K–antagonist anticoagulants.

Recombinant activated factor VII has been found to reduce the INR in warfarin-associated bleeding, but its overall effect on outcome has been unclear, with a varied rate of thromboembolic events. It is not recommended for acute warfarin reversal.

KEY POINT

- In patients with INR elevation and bleeding associated with warfarin administration, urgent reversal of anticoagulation should be accomplished using vitamin K and prothrombin complex concentrates.

Bibliography

Sarode R, Milling TJ Jr, Refaai MA, Mangione A, Schneider A, Durn BL, et al. Efficacy and safety of a 4-factor prothrombin complex concentrate in patients on vitamin K antagonists presenting with major bleeding: a randomized, plasma-controlled, phase IIIb study. Circulation. 2013;128:1234-43. [PMID: 23935011] doi:10.1161/CIRCULATIONAHA.113.002283

Item 32   Answer: A

Educational Objective: Treat secondary iron overload.

This patient should begin deferasirox for treatment of secondary iron overload. In most cases, secondary iron overload occurs in patients with severe anemia who require chronic transfusion therapy. Because iron excretion has no regulated mechanism, multiple transfusions (for anemias not stemming from blood loss or iron deficiency) lead to iron overload, with subsequent secondary organ damage. If these anemias resolve (either from hematopoietic stem cell transplantation or remission of leukemias), phlebotomy should be initiated. When anemia is ongoing, such as in this patient, iron chelation is required, for which deferoxamine or deferasirox may be used. These agents are relatively toxic, leading to potential kidney and liver damage, agranulocytosis, or ocular and ophthalmic disorders; therefore, careful monitoring is required. Serum ferritin level correlates with iron burden in patients receiving chronic transfusion, and levels greater than 1000 ng/mL (1000 µg/L) are generally considered an indication for therapy. Deferoxamine is only available for parenteral administration, which is much less convenient in the long-term outpatient setting than oral iron chelation. The availability of oral iron chelation with deferasirox has increased medication adherence for patients who develop secondary iron overload from chronic transfusions for hemoglobinopathies or myelodysplastic syndrome. Deferasirox commonly causes gastrointestinal side effects. The medication is often better tolerated in the evening, before the evening meal.

Succimer is used to chelate lead and enhance excretion in patients with chronic lead intoxication. It would not be used to treat iron overload.

Therapeutic phlebotomy is the management of choice for hereditary (primary) hemochromatosis. It effectively removes 200 mg of iron with each pint of blood removed. However, therapeutic phlebotomy is not suitable for patients with symptomatic anemia who require chronic transfusion, as is the case with this patient.

Withholding transfusion is not appropriate because of this patient's age and her symptomatic anemia.

> **KEY POINT**
>
> - Secondary iron overload from chronic transfusions can be effectively treated with oral chelation agents, such as deferasirox.

Bibliography

Nolte F, Angelucci E, Breccia M, Gattermann N, Santini V, Vey N, et al. Updated recommendations on the management of gastrointestinal disturbances during iron chelation therapy with deferasirox in transfusion dependent patients with myelodysplastic syndrome - emphasis on optimized dosing schedules and new formulations. Leuk Res. 2015;39:1028-33. [PMID: 26293555] doi:10.1016/j.leukres.2015.06.008

Item 33   Answer: A

Educational Objective: Treat the anemia of chronic kidney disease with an erythropoiesis-stimulating agent.

Darbepoetin should be administered to achieve a hemoglobin level of 11 to 12 g/dL (110-120 g/L). Erythropoiesis-stimulating agents (ESAs) such as erythropoietin and darbepoetin have dramatically reduced the need for transfusion in patients with the anemia of chronic kidney disease (CKD) but have little impact on quality of life or mortality. This patient has symptomatic anemia of CKD, which is determined by ruling out other causes of anemia in patients with reduced kidney function. Although symptomatic anemia occurs commonly in patients with advanced CKD who are receiving hemodialysis, it may also occur in patients with stages III and IV CKD. Regardless of stage, patients with symptomatic anemia of CKD will benefit from ESAs by reducing their transfusion requirements. However, a "normal" hemoglobin threshold is not the preferred target level for patients taking ESAs. Numerous studies have shown that ESAs increase adverse cardiovascular outcomes when the hemoglobin level exceeds 11 to 12 g/dL (110-120 g/L). Additionally, ESAs can cause hypertension and thrombosis.

Iron stores must be normal for ESAs to be effective. Patients undergoing dialysis are often treated with additional parenteral iron along with ESAs even if they are not overtly iron deficient. Although supplemental iron with darbepoetin may be required in this patient, iron therapy alone, either by oral or parenteral routes of administration, will not correct anemia in this patient who has no laboratory findings to support the diagnosis of iron deficiency.

> **KEY POINT**
>
> - Patients with symptomatic anemia of chronic kidney disease may be treated with erythropoiesis-stimulating agents to reduce transfusion requirements with a target hemoglobin level of 11 to 12 g/dL (110-120 g/L) to avoid increased risk of adverse cardiovascular events.

Bibliography

Palmer SC, Saglimbene V, Craig JC, Navaneethan SD, Strippoli GF. Darbepoetin for the anaemia of chronic kidney disease. Cochrane Database Syst Rev. 2014:CD009297. [PMID: 24683046] doi:10.1002/14651858.CD009297.pub2

Item 34   Answer: E

Educational Objective: Manage minor bleeding in a patient taking a non–vitamin K antagonist oral anticoagulant.

Observation is most appropriate in this patient at this time. She has no major or clinically relevant bleeding; therefore, a conservative treatment approach is reasonable. Her hemoglobin level is normal, she is hemodynamically stable, and she has no other signs of bleeding. The elimination half-life of dabigatran is 12 hours with anticoagulant effect for 24 hours in patients with normal kidney function. Dabigatran should be withheld for 24 hours or longer in this patient pending evaluation of her urinary tract. She has nonglomerular hematuria (no proteinuria, casts, or dysmorphic erythrocytes) and requires an evaluation of the upper and lower urinary tract for a cause of the hematuria. The necessity to fully evaluate hematuria is not influenced by the use of anticoagulant therapy.

Fresh frozen plasma has been used in patients experiencing major bleeding while taking a non–vitamin K antagonist oral anticoagulant, but it is not typically adequate monotherapy in patients experiencing severe bleeding; it is often combined with four-factor prothrombin complex concentrate (4f-PCC). However, neither fresh frozen plasma nor 4f-PCC would be necessary in this patient because she is hemodynamically stable, the bleeding is not life threatening, and the anticoagulant effect of dabigatran will dissipate in 24 hours.

Idarucizumab is a humanized monoclonal antibody fragment with a very high affinity for dabigatran. It is approved for dabigatran reversal for emergency surgery, for urgent procedures, or in patients experiencing life-threatening or uncontrolled bleeding. Severe adverse effects may include thromboembolic events and possible hypersensitivity reactions, such as bronchospasm and pruritus. Because this patient does not have life-threatening bleeding, idarucizumab is not indicated.

Vitamin K administration has no effect on bleeding caused by non–vitamin K antagonist oral anticoagulants such as dabigatran. Vitamin K can be used to reverse over-anticoagulation with warfarin.

KEY POINT

- Minor bleeding in patients taking a non–vitamin K antagonist oral anticoagulant can be managed by discontinuation of the anticoagulant alone without additional therapy.

Bibliography

Pollack CV Jr, Reilly PA, Eikelboom J, Glund S, Verhamme P, Bernstein RA, et al. Idarucizumab for dabigatran reversal. N Engl J Med. 2015;373:511-20. [PMID: 26095746] doi:10.1056/NEJMoa1502000

Item 35   Answer: C

Educational Objective: Manage preoperative transfusion in sickle cell anemia.

The patient should receive preoperative simple transfusion to achieve a hemoglobin level of 10 g/dL (100 g/L). Transfusions may have significant adverse effects, including infection, alloimmunization, and cumulative risk of iron overload. Therefore, persons with sickle cell disease (SCD) should not receive transfusions unless they have significant symptoms or signs of end-organ failure from their anemia or are preparing for surgery. Patients with SCD are at increased risk for perioperative pulmonary, infectious, and thrombotic complications. In 1994, a landmark study was published showing that simple transfusion to a target hemoglobin level of 10 g/dL (100 g/L) was equivalent to exchange transfusion in low- to medium-risk surgeries (low-risk surgeries include adenoidectomy and inguinal-hernia repair; medium-risk surgeries include cholecystectomy and joint replacement) in reducing surgical complications in patients with SCD with less risk, reduced cost, and increased convenience. More recently, guidelines have been published on the care of patients with SCD that strongly recommend simple transfusion to a target hemoglobin level of 10 g/dL (100 g/L) in patients requiring general anesthesia. In addition to transfusion, the use of incentive spirometry has also been shown in a randomized trial to improve surgical outcomes in patients with SCD. Overtransfusion should be avoided in these patients because of complications arising from increased blood viscosity. Typically, hemoglobin levels are kept at or below 10 g/dL (100 g/L).

Exchange transfusion is used for acute stroke or retinal artery occlusion or in patients with severe acute chest syndrome. When indicated, the target hemoglobin S level should be less than 30%.

KEY POINT

- Simple transfusion to achieve a hemoglobin level of 10 g/dL (100 g/L) in patients having low- to moderate-risk surgery reduces surgical complications equivalent to exchange transfusion with less risk and cost.

Bibliography

Yawn BP, Buchanan GR, Afenyi-Annan AN, Ballas SK, Hassell KL, James AH, et al. Management of sickle cell disease: summary of the 2014 evidence-based report by expert panel members. JAMA. 2014;312:1033-48. [PMID: 25203083] doi:10.1001/jama.2014.10517

Item 36   Answer: C

Educational Objective: Diagnose protein C deficiency.

The most likely diagnosis is protein C deficiency. The patient's skin condition is most likely retiform purpura. The term "retiform" describes the angulated or netlike configuration that reflects the vascular structure in the skin. The color is often a dark brick-red or purple. Retiform purpura is caused by local skin ischemia caused by occlusion or breakdown of vascular integrity that may lead to necrosis, which may become life-threatening if not aggressively treated. Various conditions can cause retiform purpura, many of which disrupt arterial blood flow. Thrombotic and embolic causes should be considered first. Thrombotic causes include alterations to the coagulation cascade such as disseminated intravascular coagulation, thrombotic thrombocytopenic purpura, and drug-induced thrombosis (warfarin or heparin).The patient's clinical presentation is consistent with warfarin-induced skin necrosis, which is a rare complication of warfarin therapy. The pathophysiology is thought to be caused by a transient hypercoagulable state resulting from protein C deficiency, which can be inherited or acquired. A family history of pulmonary embolism suggests the possibility of inherited protein C deficiency. Congenital protein C deficiency is an autosomal dominant inherited thrombophilia associated with an increased risk of venous thromboembolism. When protein C is activated, it inactivates the activated coagulation factors V and VIII, which are needed for factor X activation. When warfarin is initiated, an initial reduction in protein C activity of 50% occurs, which leads to a transient hypercoagulable state. If the patient is receiving heparin and warfarin therapy, the lesions may appear when the heparin is discontinued, which likely accounts for the appearance of the rash on day 3 of her hospitalization. Treatment involves the discontinuation of warfarin, continuation of alternate anticoagulation (such as a non–vitamin K antagonist oral anticoagulant), vitamin K for warfarin reversal, and fresh frozen plasma in an attempt to improve decreased protein C levels.

Warfarin-induced skin necrosis is not associated with factor V Leiden mutation, plasminogen activator inhibitor 1 deficiency, or prothrombin gene mutation.

KEY POINT

- Protein C or S deficiency is associated with warfarin-associated skin necrosis.

Bibliography

Thornsberry LA, LoSicco KI, English JC 3rd. The skin and hypercoagulable states. J Am Acad Dermatol. 2013 Sep;69(3):450-62. doi:10.1016/j.jaad.2013.01.043. [PMID: 23582572]

Item 37   Answer: D

Educational Objective: Evaluate a patient with dyspnea using the Pulmonary Embolism Rule-Out Criteria.

The patient requires no further testing for pulmonary embolism. Many patients present to the emergency department with shortness of breath or chest pain. Inappropriate use of D-dimer testing and CT angiography led to the development of new American College of Physicians guidelines regarding the evaluation of patients with possible pulmonary embolism (PE). These guidelines use clinical decision tools (such as the Pulmonary Embolism Rule-Out Criteria [PERC]) to help risk stratify patients who present with shortness of breath or chest pain.

The PERC are defined as

- Age younger than 50 years
- Heart rate less than 100/min
- Oxygen saturation 95% or greater
- No hemoptysis
- No estrogen use
- No previous deep venous thrombosis or PE
- No unilateral leg swelling
- No surgery or trauma requiring hospitalization in the last 4 weeks

To avoid unnecessary testing, patients with a low pretest probability using a validated prediction tool such as the Wells Criteria for Pulmonary Embolism and negative PERC should undergo no further evaluation. In patients with intermediate pretest probability or positive PERC, the D-dimer level should be obtained. Patients with a high pretest probability should proceed directly to imaging, without D-dimer testing.

Because this patient has a low pretest probability and the PERC are negative, neither D-dimer testing nor CT angiography of the chest should be performed. A study of multiorgan ultrasonography was shown to be helpful in the diagnosis of PE in adults with a Wells score of 4 or greater or a positive D-dimer test. A positive test was defined by any one of the following: one or more pulmonary subpleural infarctions on lung ultrasonography; right ventricular dilatation or thrombi on heart ultrasonography; or deep venous thrombosis on lower extremity ultrasonography. Multiorgan ultrasonography was found to be 90% sensitive and 86% specific compared with CT angiography. Multiorgan ultrasonography was significantly more sensitive than individual ultrasonographic examinations of the lungs, heart, or lower extremities.

Echocardiography is unlikely to be helpful in this patient because her pretest probability of pulmonary embolism was very low, and echocardiography alone is an insensitive test.

KEY POINT

- Patients identified as low risk and meeting the Pulmonary Embolism Rule-Out Criteria do not require D-dimer testing to eliminate the need for further diagnostic imaging.

Bibliography

Kline JA, Courtney DM, Kabrhel C, Moore CL, Smithline HA, Plewa MC, et al. Prospective multicenter evaluation of the pulmonary embolism rule-out criteria. J Thromb Haemost. 2008;6:772-80. [PMID: 18318689] doi:10.1111/j.1538-7836.2008.02944.x

Item 38   Answer: C

Educational Objective: **Treat chronic myeloid leukemia with an oral tyrosine kinase inhibitor.**

This patient should be treated with imatinib, a tyrosine kinase inhibitor (TKI); he has chronic myeloid leukemia (CML) presenting in the chronic phase and requires therapy targeting the BCR-ABL fusion gene. Translocation of the long arm of chromosomes 9 and 22 leads to the fusion gene of BCR-ABL, which is characteristic of CML. CML is divided into the chronic phase, accelerated phase, or blast crisis depending on clinical and pathologic characteristics. Approximately 90% of patients with CML present in the chronic phase with less than 10% blasts in the blood and bone marrow. TKIs are effective in the treatment of the chronic phase of CML and are usually first-line treatment. The three TKIs approved for initial treatment of CML are imatinib, dasatinib, and nilotinib. Other newer generation TKIs are approved for patients who are intolerant of these first three TKIs or who have CML resistant to them. Although TKIs have some unique adverse effects and drug interactions, they are well tolerated compared with chemotherapy and transplantation.

Bone marrow transplantation for CML in the chronic phase is reserved for patients with resistant disease or who are intolerant of TKIs.

Chemotherapy with idarubicin and cytarabine is used for patients with CML in blast crisis with more than 20% blasts and is not intended for the chronic phase as in this patient. This therapy is similar to the treatment of acute myeloid leukemia.

Part of the differential diagnosis for extreme granulocytic leukocytosis (leukocyte count >50,000/μL [50 × 10^9/L]) is the leukemoid reaction. When sepsis occurs, the bone marrow responds by releasing early cells into circulation, and a leukemoid reaction may be difficult to distinguish from CML in an acutely ill patient. However, few patients with typical sepsis, even gram-negative bacillary bacteremia, develop such counts. Blasts and basophils are much less likely with a leukemoid reaction. This patient has been chronically, not acutely, ill, and CML is a much more likely explanation of the leukocytosis than is sepsis; therefore, antibiotics are not needed.

KEY POINT

- Tyrosine kinase inhibitors such as imatinib are effective for initial treatment of chronic myeloid leukemia in the chronic phase.

Bibliography

Cortes J, Kantarjian H. How I treat newly diagnosed chronic phase CML. Blood. 2012;120:1390-7. [PMID: 22613793] doi:10.1182/blood-2012-03-378919

Item 39   Answer: B

Educational Objective: **Diagnose paroxysmal nocturnal hemoglobinuria.**

Flow cytometry is the most appropriate test to perform next. This patient has pancytopenia with significant intravascular hemolysis and hemoglobinuria, most likely caused by paroxysmal nocturnal hemoglobinuria (PNH). Patients with PNH commonly note fatigue and nonspecific abdominal pain, which worsens during times of increased hemolysis. These patients have a mutation in the gene that regulates production of glycophosphatidylinositol-anchoring proteins. Flow cytometry will demonstrate the absence of glycophosphatidylinositol-linked proteins, such as CD55 and CD59, on leukocytes; these proteins normally prevent complement activation on the erythrocyte surface. Bone marrow aplasia and corresponding pancytopenia in these patients are common, and they have an increased risk of evolving to a myelodysplastic syndrome or acute leukemia. Patients with PNH also have an increased risk for thrombotic complications, including thrombi in unusual sites, such as the portal venous system or sagittal veins in the central nervous system.

Hereditary angioedema is caused by the unregulated activation of the complement cascade owing to lack of or ineffective function of C1 esterase inhibitor, leading to increased vascular permeability. C1 esterase inhibitor deficiency has no role in the pathogenesis of PNH.

While complement-mediated hemolysis is a core feature of PNH, the complement system functions normally. Neither excess of complement nor IgG antibodies are noted on the erythrocyte surface that would be revealed by a direct antiglobulin test.

Vitamin B_{12} deficiency can cause pancytopenia and is commonly associated with some features of intramedullary hemolysis resulting from ineffective erythropoiesis. However, vitamin B_{12} deficiency is associated with macrocytic anemia, which is not present in this patient. Hemoglobinuria is present in PNH but not seen in vitamin B_{12} deficiency. The first step in diagnosing vitamin B_{12} deficiency is a cobalamin measurement. Methylmalonic acid and homocysteine measurements may be helpful in cases of diagnostic uncertainty because they are elevated in 98% of patients with cobalamin deficiency. Methylmalonic acid measurement is unnecessary in this patient.

KEY POINT

- Diagnosis of paroxysmal nocturnal hemoglobinuria is based on flow cytometry results, which can detect CD55 and CD59 deficiency on the surface of peripheral erythrocytes or leukocytes.

Bibliography

Sutherland DR, Illingworth A, Keeney M, Richards SJ. High-sensitivity detection of PNH red blood cells, red cell precursors, and white blood cells. Curr Protoc Cytom. 2015;72:6.37.1-30. [PMID: 25827482] doi:10.1002/0471142956.cy0637s72

Item 40   Answer: C

Educational Objective: Treat coagulopathy of liver disease.

This patient should receive a transfusion with cryoprecipitate. He has the coagulopathy of liver disease, characterized by thrombocytopenia, prolonged activated partial thromboplastin time (aPTT) and prothrombin time (PT), elevated D-dimer level, and hypofibrinogenemia. The patient's hemodynamic instability is addressed with fluids and erythrocyte transfusion. Vitamin K will help correct the PT, but he may also need fresh frozen plasma (FFP). Thrombocytopenia is addressed with platelet transfusion. Fibrinogen levels less than 100 mg/dL (1 g/L) associated with active bleeding should be corrected. Cryoprecipitate contains more fibrinogen than FFP and is the blood component of choice for treating this patient. It is often difficult to distinguish between disseminated intravascular coagulation (DIC) and the coagulopathy of liver disease, but a normal or increased factor VIII level points to liver disease instead of DIC. Somewhat paradoxically, factor VIII levels are supranormal in the coagulopathy of liver disease because it is produced in extrahepatic endothelial cells, and a hepatically synthesized factor is required for factor VIII clearance. The management of these coagulopathies is often the same.

Recombinant activated factor VII is preferred for treating patients with acquired hemophilia associated with high titers of antibody directed against factor VIII. It may be used to treat uncontrolled bleeding in patients with liver disease unresponsive to replacement of platelets, FFP, vitamin K, and cryoprecipitate.

ε-Aminocaproic acid (EACA), an inhibitor of fibrinolysis, has been shown to reduce blood loss after cardiac and orthopedic surgery. Accelerated fibrinolysis plays some role in the coagulopathy of bleeding in liver disease, and EACA may reduce bleeding in some of these patients. No laboratory test correlates fibrinolysis with bleeding risk, and EACA should not be used before treating more objective measures of coagulopathy, such as low fibrinogen levels.

Four-factor prothrombin complex concentrate is used to treat patients with warfarin toxicity and life-threatening bleeding. It should not be used more routinely to treat patients with the coagulopathy of liver disease and bleeding until conventional component support proves ineffective.

KEY POINT

- Patients with coagulopathy of liver disease and low fibrinogen levels who are experiencing bleeding should receive immediate cryoprecipitate transfusion.

Bibliography

Tripodi A, Mannucci PM. The coagulopathy of chronic liver disease. N Engl J Med. 2011;365:147-56. [PMID: 21751907] doi:10.1056/NEJMra1011170

Item 41   Answer: B

Educational Objective: Prevent venous thromboembolism in a hospitalized patient with cancer.

This patient should receive prophylactic enoxaparin. Venous thromboembolism (VTE) is a major contributor to morbidity and mortality in patients with cancer. It is the second leading cause of death after the cancer itself. Hospitalized patients with cancer have an even greater thrombotic risk. The Prophylaxis in Medical Patients with Enoxaparin (MEDENOX)

CONT.

trial enrolled 1102 medically ill patients who were randomly assigned to receive one of three subcutaneous regimens: enoxaparin sodium, 20 mg/d; enoxaparin sodium, 40 mg/d; or placebo. The frequency of VTE was reduced in a statistically significant manner in patients receiving enoxaparin sodium, 40 mg/d. For hospitalized patients with cancer and acute illness, pharmacologic prophylaxis should be used unless a clear contraindication exists.

Although aspirin has a role for prevention of recurrent VTE in patients without cancer, it does not have a place in primary prophylaxis.

The American College of Physicians guideline on VTE prophylaxis in hospitalized patients recommends against the use of graduated compression stockings because of the lack of difference in risk for mortality or symptomatic VTE. However, risk for lower-extremity skin damage was increased among patients treated with compression stockings.

The American College of Physicians guideline also noted that in patients at high risk for bleeding events or in whom heparin is contraindicated for other reasons, intermittent pneumatic compression may be a reasonable option because evidence suggests it is beneficial in surgical patients. However, intermittent pneumatic compression has not been sufficiently evaluated as a stand-alone intervention in medical patients to reliably estimate benefits and harms.

Warfarin is typically not used as VTE prophylaxis in hospitalized patients with cancer because of its delayed onset of antithrombotic action and the need for dose adjustment. Although low-molecular-weight heparin is more effective than warfarin for treatment of cancer-associated VTE, no randomized trials have compared the benefit of prophylactic heparin with warfarin in hospitalized medical patients.

KEY POINT

- In patients with cancer who are hospitalized, prophylactic anticoagulation with low-molecular-weight heparin should be provided to reduce the risk of venous thromboembolism.

Bibliography

Samama MM, Cohen AT, Darmon JY, Desjardins L, Eldor A, Janbon C, et al. A comparison of enoxaparin with placebo for the prevention of venous thromboembolism in acutely ill medical patients. Prophylaxis in Medical Patients with Enoxaparin Study Group. N Engl J Med. 1999;341:793-800. [PMID: 10477777]

Item 42   Answer: E

Educational Objective: Manage sickle cell disease in an uncomplicated pregnancy.

This patient requires no treatment other than expectant care. She should be closely monitored and treatment should be withheld until symptoms appear or some measurable parameter changes. Sickle cell disease (SCD) is associated with maternal morbidity and mortality from stroke, vaso-occlusive crisis, and acute chest syndrome. Furthermore, the risk of eclampsia is higher in pregnant women with SCD. Fetal complications are also more common in patients with SCD, including low birth weight, spontaneous abortion, early delivery, and growth retardation. No routine interventions have been proven to decrease these complications, so close follow-up by hematologic and obstetric specialists and prompt management of evolving problems is important. Pregnancy outcomes are difficult to predict in pregnant patients with SCD, but one of the best indicators is the outcome from a previous pregnancy, which is encouraging in this patient.

Antiplatelet drugs, such as clopidogrel, have been associated with increased risk of bleeding and ablatio placenta without any clear benefit in pregnant patients with SCD.

Although the role of transfusion in the management of pregnant patients with SCD lacks consensus, no clear benefit has been seen with either simple or exchange transfusion in patients with uncomplicated disease or pregnancy. However, pregnant patients with SCD who have worsening symptomatic anemia should undergo transfusion. Those with past or new severe obstetric or fetal complications, those with twins, or those with chronic organ dysfunction may also benefit from transfusion. The decision to transfuse must be balanced against the risks of transfusion, including alloimmunization and delayed transfusion reaction, as well as iron and volume overload. Because this patient has an uncomplicated pregnancy, exchange or simple transfusion is not indicated.

Hydroxyurea therapy results in decreased mortality in SCD and is indicated in patients with recurrent painful episodes, acute chest syndrome, and symptomatic anemia. However, because of its potential teratogenicity, hydroxyurea should not be administered during pregnancy. Proper contraception before hydroxyurea initiation should be discussed with the nonpregnant patient. This patient has no indication for hydroxyurea treatment.

KEY POINT

- Patients with sickle cell disease and uncomplicated pregnancy should be closely monitored and treatment withheld until symptoms appear or some measurable parameter changes.

Bibliography

Boga C, Ozdogu H. Pregnancy and sickle cell disease: a review of the current literature. Crit Rev Oncol Hematol. 2016;98:364-74. [PMID: 26672916] doi:10.1016/j.critrevonc.2015.11.018

Item 43   Answer: D

Educational Objective: Diagnose α-thalassemia trait.

The most likely diagnosis is α-thalassemia trait. This patient has a chronic microcytic anemia. Patients with α-thalassemia trait have inadequate production of two copies of the α gene on chromosome 16 (α-/α- or --/αα). Such patients have a chronic microcytic anemia with hemoglobin levels of approximately 10 g/dL (100 g/L). Hemoglobin A levels, although reduced in quantity, are otherwise normal in these patients and will migrate in a normal pattern on electrophoresis. Furthermore, there is no increase in the minor hemoglobin components, hemoglobin A_2 and hemoglobin F. It is possible to identify specific chromosomal abnormalities that establish the diagnosis of α-thalassemia, but physicians typically make a clinical diagnosis based on family history, complete blood count, peripheral blood smear, and hemoglobin electrophoresis and by ruling out other causes of microcytic anemia. Patients with thalassemia should receive supplemental folate but should not receive iron supplementation; they are not iron deficient and they have an increased ability to absorb iron, which can lead to iron overload. Genetic counseling may be indicated in reproductive planning.

This patient's iron study results are normal, and her serum ferritin level is greater than 100 ng/mL (100 µg/L), essentially ruling out iron deficiency.

Inflammatory anemia, also known as anemia of chronic disease, is characterized by a low serum iron level and often a concomitant reduction in iron-binding capacity in the absence of iron deficiency. The iron studies in this patient are inconsistent with that diagnosis. Mild microcytosis may be seen in the anemia of inflammation but not as severely as in this patient.

Patients who are silent carriers for α-thalassemia have a defect in production of a single α gene. These patients have a normal hemoglobin level and no microcytosis. They are clinically healthy.

Patients with β-thalassemia minor also have a chronic microcytic anemia and a normal electrophoretic pattern for hemoglobin A. But in β-thalassemia, the excess α chains link with δ and γ chains to produce increased amounts of hemoglobin A_2 and hemoglobin F, respectively.

KEY POINT

- Patients with α-thalassemia trait have chronic microcytic anemia with hemoglobin levels of approximately 10 g/dL (100 g/L) and a normal hemoglobin electrophoresis pattern.

Bibliography

Brancaleoni V, Di Pierro E, Motta I, Cappellini MD. Laboratory diagnosis of thalassemia. Int J Lab Hematol. 2016;38 Suppl 1:32-40. [PMID: 27183541] doi:10.1111/ijlh.12527

Item 44   Answer: D

Educational Objective: Manage an elevated INR.

The patient's warfarin therapy should be withheld, and her INR should be remeasured in 2 days. Warfarin acts by inhibiting the synthesis of vitamin K–dependent clotting factors, which include factors II, VII, IX, and X. Variations in INR can occur with dietary changes. Other factors associated with prolonged elevation of INR include age 80 years or older, lower maintenance dose of warfarin, decompensated heart failure, active cancer, and use of medications known to potentiate the effect of warfarin. The 30-day risk of major bleeding is less than 1% with an INR between 5 and 9.

Accordingly, warfarin should be withheld in patients with elevated INRs between 4.5 and 10 who are not bleeding and have no major risk factors for bleeding. Approximately one third of patients with an INR greater than 6 will still have an abnormal INR after withholding warfarin for two consecutive doses. Warfarin can be reinstituted when the INR returns to a therapeutic level.

The patient is asymptomatic, with no evidence of bleeding. Therefore, neither vitamin K nor fresh frozen plasma should be given. Patients who are not bleeding, are not at high risk for bleeding, and have an INR less than 10 can be managed simply by withholding warfarin. For patients with an INR greater than 10, oral vitamin K, 2.5 mg, should be given. Oral vitamin K and intravenous vitamin K appear equally effective and more effective than subcutaneous vitamin K or placebo for reversing excessive warfarin-induced anticoagulation.

The American Society of Hematology recommends against administering plasma or prothrombin complex concentrates for nonemergent reversal of vitamin K antagonists (including situations other than major bleeding, intracranial hemorrhage, or anticipated emergent surgery). However, the 30-day mortality is approximately 13% in patients with major bleeding during treatment with warfarin. In these patients with acute major bleeding as a result of warfarin therapy, in addition to vitamin K, prothrombin complex concentrates are preferred to fresh frozen plasma. Prothrombin complex concentrate is more effective than fresh frozen plasma for reducing 30-day all-cause mortality and the INR in patients with major bleeding or requiring surgical or invasive procedures.

KEY POINT

- Patients with asymptomatic INR elevation between 4.5 and 10 are managed by simply withholding warfarin.

Bibliography

Lee A, Crowther M. Practical issues with vitamin K antagonists: elevated INRs, low time-in-therapeutic range, and warfarin failure. J Thromb Thrombolysis. 2011;31:249-58. [PMID: 21274594] doi:10.1007/s11239-011-0555-z

Item 45   Answer: B

Educational Objective: Manage pre-eclampsia in a pregnant woman with thrombocytopenia.

The most appropriate management of this patient is emergency delivery of the fetus. Several disorders are characterized by microangiopathic hemolytic anemia (MAHA) and thrombocytopenia during pregnancy. Pre-eclampsia, HELLP (Hemolysis, Elevated Liver enzymes, and Low Platelets) syndrome, and thrombotic thrombocytopenic purpura–hemolytic uremic syndrome (TTP-HUS) have different clinical features but with significant overlap. Pre-eclampsia typically presents with hypertension, peripheral edema, and proteinuria, most commonly in the third trimester of pregnancy. TTP-HUS is characterized by MAHA and thrombocytopenia developing in the first or second trimester. Additionally, neurologic findings and fever are more common in TTP-HUS than in the other syndromes. HELLP syndrome is characterized by right upper quadrant pain and elevated liver enzyme levels. Disseminated intravascular coagulation parameters may be found in patients with pre-eclampsia and HELLP syndrome but should be absent in those with TTP-HUS. This patient has pre-eclampsia, defined as hypertension (systolic blood pressure >140 mm Hg or diastolic blood pressure >90 mm Hg) after the 20th week of gestation with edema and proteinuria, which requires immediate delivery. Symptoms usually resolve with delivery. HELLP syndrome is similarly treated.

Eculizumab is used to treat atypical hemolytic uremic syndrome (HUS), which is the most common form of HUS in pregnancy. It is associated with congenital defects in the alternate pathway of the complement system. Although this patient has proteinuria, the normal creatinine level makes this an unlikely diagnosis because marked kidney disease is a hallmark of this disorder.

High-dose glucocorticoids would be useful to treat immune thrombocytopenic purpura (ITP) in pregnancy, especially toward the end of the third trimester. ITP is diagnosed when an isolated thrombocytopenia is discovered, but it is not associated with hypertension, proteinuria, or schistocytes on the peripheral blood smear.

Although she has thrombocytopenia, fragmented erythrocytes, and headache, her elevated blood pressure, edema, and proteinuria point to pre-eclampsia as a more likely diagnosis than TTP. Therefore, plasma exchange would not be appropriate.

KEY POINT

- Pre-eclampsia, HELLP (Hemolysis, Elevated Liver enzymes, and Low Platelets) syndrome, and thrombotic thrombocytopenic purpura–hemolytic uremic syndrome can all present with microangiopathic hemolytic anemia and thrombocytopenia during pregnancy; pre-eclampsia is defined by hypertension, edema, and proteinuria after the 12th week of gestation.

Bibliography

Shatzel JJ, Taylor JA. Syndromes of thrombotic microangiopathy. Med Clin North Am. 2017;101:395-415. [PMID: 28189178] doi:10.1016/j.mcna.2016.09.010

Item 46   Answer: D

Educational Objective: Diagnose von Willebrand disease.

Von Willebrand disease (vWD) is the most common inherited hemostatic defect. Quantitative or qualitative abnormalities in the portion of the factor VIII molecule that facilitates binding of platelets to injured endothelium lead to bleeding. Often the hemostatic defect is mild, characterized as mucosal

or endometrial bleeding, and requires an additional hemostatic insult, such as surgery, menstruation, or platelet injury from NSAIDs, to provoke bleeding. The patient's bleeding history and normal prothrombin time (PT), activated partial thromboplastin time (aPTT), and platelet count, along with an abnormal screening of platelet function, support the diagnosis of vWD. This diagnosis can be confirmed by finding a quantitative reduction in von Willebrand antigen and a qualitative reduction in von Willebrand ristocetin cofactor activity.

Congenital hemophilia A is an X-linked hereditary disorder of factor VIII deficiency. Although women may be carriers, they rarely have symptomatic bleeding. Laboratory features in inherited hemophilia would include a prolonged aPTT that corrects with mixing studies and a normal PT. Assay of individual factor levels would confirm factor VIII deficiency. Platelet function should be normal. These features are not present in this patient, making this diagnosis unlikely.

Factor XI deficiency is expressed in a clinically heterogeneous manner. Many patients are asymptomatic, even when stressed with major surgery, but some might have a bleeding history similar to this patient's. The diagnosis is more prevalent in patients of Jewish descent, and the aPTT should be prolonged and should correct with mixing. This patient's normal aPTT and platelet dysfunction make this an unlikely diagnosis.

The lupus anticoagulant is an acquired autoantibody to phospholipids that behaves like an inhibitor in the test tube. Typically, the aPTT is prolonged and does not correct when mixed with normal plasma. Despite the prolonged aPTT, lupus anticoagulants are associated with thrombosis, not bleeding. The patient's normal aPTT and abnormal Platelet Function Analyzer-100 result are not compatible with the presence of a lupus anticoagulant.

KEY POINT

- A history of mucosal or endometrial bleeding, normal prothrombin and activated partial thromboplastin times, and normal platelet count with evidence of a qualitative platelet defect suggest the diagnosis of von Willebrand disease.

Bibliography

Tcherniantchouk O, Laposata M, Marques MB. The isolated prolonged PTT. Am J Hematol. 2013;88:82-5. [PMID: 22811044] doi:10.1002/ajh.23285

Item 47   Answer: B

Educational Objective: Diagnose hemoglobin S β-thalassemia.

This patient most likely has hemoglobin S β-thalassemia (Sβ-thalassemia). Patients with Sβ-thalassemia generally have milder disease than those homozygous for hemoglobin S (HbS). However, patients with Sβ-thalassemia can have painful crises of varied frequency and intensity. Some of the variability in presentation depends on the relative expression of the β-globin gene (from β^+ to β^0), which in turn determines the relative amount of hemoglobin A (HbA). Most black persons with Sβ-thalassemia are β^+ and have between 5% and 30% HbA; the more HbA present, the less severe the symptoms and fewer the complications. Occasionally, with a milder disease course, patients do not present until adolescence or early adulthood. Hemoglobin electrophoresis is essential in making a specific diagnosis of a sickling disorder. Patients with Sβ-thalassemia have a slightly reduced hemoglobin level and microcytic erythrocytes. Characteristically, their HbS levels are about 60%. In contrast, patients with sickle cell trait have HbS levels well below 50%, typically closer to 30%, and proportionally more HbA. More notably, patients with sickle cell trait do not experience painful crises and have normal hemoglobin levels.

Patients with hemoglobin SS disease (sickle cell anemia) have greater than 90% HbS and no HbA. The clinical expression and severity of sickle cell anemia may be quite variable, and some patients may have few acute pain events and no other major complications, so that the diagnosis may not be suspected until later in life. The level of hemoglobin F detected in these patients may also vary, with increased hemoglobin F levels correlating with milder disease, but Hb A should be undetectable and no microcytosis should be seen.

Hemoglobin E disease results from a point mutation in the β-globin gene that causes decreased production of β-globin and results in a thalassemia-like syndrome. Hemoglobin E migrates in a different pattern than HbA and would be revealed on hemoglobin electrophoresis, in addition to increased levels of HbA2, as with other β-thalassemias. Although patients with hemoglobin E disease will have mild anemia, they do not experience acute pain events.

KEY POINT

- Patients who coinherit hemoglobin S and β-thalassemia genes typically have lifelong mild hemolytic anemia with microcytosis and detectable hemoglobin A on electrophoresis; the amount of hemoglobin A is inversely related to the severity of the symptoms and risk of complications.

Bibliography

Benites BD, Bastos SO, Baldanzi G, Dos Santos AO, Ramos CD, Costa FF, et al. Sickle cell/β-thalassemia: Comparison of Sβ(0) and Sβ(+) Brazilian patients followed at a single institution. Hematology. 2016;21:623-629. [PMID: 27237196]

Item 48   Answer: A

Educational Objective: Manage acute upper gastrointestinal bleeding with a restrictive transfusion strategy.

This patient should continue to receive crystalloid resuscitation. In the absence of symptoms of anemia, hemodynamic instability, or massive bleeding, a patient such as this one does not require a blood transfusion. A randomized controlled trial of 900 patients with acute upper gastrointestinal bleeding and a hemoglobin level less than 12 g/dL (120 g/L) compared a restrictive transfusion strategy (hemoglobin transfusion threshold of 7 g/dL [70 g/L]) to a liberal strategy (hemoglobin transfusion threshold of 9 g/dL [90 g/L]). Half of the patients had peptic ulcer disease as the source of bleeding. Mortality was lower in the restrictive group compared with the liberal transfusion group (5% versus 9%). Half of the patients in the restrictive group did not receive transfusion at all. Therefore, crystalloid volume resuscitation is appropriate and erythrocyte transfusion unnecessary in this patient.

Plasma transfusion is not indicated in the absence of coagulopathy. Fresh frozen plasma (FFP) contains all of the coagulation factors. FFP use is excessive in the United States and other countries despite published guidelines regarding its use. FFP is ineffective at treating mild coagulopathies. Indications for the use of FFP and other plasma-based products include treatment or prevention of coagulopathy from massive transfusion, bleeding associated with multiple acquired clotting factor deficiencies (liver disease, disseminated intravascular coagulation), and major warfarin-associated hemorrhage when a four-factor prothrombin complex concentrate is not available. There is no reason to suspect that this patient has a coagulopathy requiring replacement of clotting factors.

Platelet counts greater than 50,000/μL (50 × 10⁹/L) do not warrant platelet transfusion in most situations when thrombocytopenia is the only hemostatic defect. The exception is neurosurgical patients, in whom platelet counts of approximately 100,000/μL (100 × 10⁹/L) should be maintained.

KEY POINT

- A hemoglobin transfusion threshold of less than 7 g/dL (70 g/L) for hemodynamically stable patients is associated with less blood use and lower mortality compared with a more liberal hemoglobin transfusion threshold of 9 g/dL (90 g/L).

Bibliography

Villanueva C, Colomo A, Bosch A, Concepción M, Hernandez-Gea V, Aracil C, et al. Transfusion strategies for acute upper gastrointestinal bleeding. N Engl J Med. 2013;368:11-21. [PMID: 23281973] doi:10.1056/NEJMoa1211801

Item 49   Answer: B

Educational Objective: Prevent complications of sickle cell disease with hydroxyurea.

The most appropriate management for this patient is to begin hydroxyurea therapy. The benefits of hydroxyurea in reducing painful crises and complications of sickle cell disease (SCD) were discovered 20 years ago. Hydroxyurea acts as a nitric oxide donor and can decrease vascular and platelet activity. It also increases levels of hemoglobin F, which, in turn, enhances hemoglobin oxygen avidity and decreases the likelihood of sickling. Hydroxyurea therapy is indicated for patients who experience frequent painful episodes or have a history of acute chest syndrome, severe vaso-occlusive events, or severe symptomatic anemia. It has been shown to decrease vaso-occlusive episodes and acute chest syndrome, to decrease transfusion requirements and hospitalizations, and to prolong overall survival. Unfortunately, hydroxyurea remains underused.

As in other hemolytic anemias, folate is consumed during active hemolysis, which could lead to a megaloblastic anemia. Folic acid supplementation, 1 mg/d, is recommended for most patients with chronic hemolytic anemia. This patient has an elevated mean corpuscular volume related to the reticulocytosis, so additional folate is not needed.

Incentive spirometry is useful in preventing acute chest syndrome in patients hospitalized with an acute pain event and chest symptoms, but it is unnecessary to continue treatment after the patient is pain free.

Although simple or exchange transfusion may be indicated in the therapy of acute chest syndrome, no evidence supports continuing transfusion therapy after the patient has recovered. Additionally, persons with SCD should not receive transfusions unless they have significant symptoms from their anemia (dizziness, shortness of breath, chest pain that is significantly worse than their typical vaso-occlusive symptoms) or they have signs of end-organ damage (such as acute neurologic symptoms, acute chest syndrome, multiorgan failure). Transfusions for simple vaso-occlusive pain are generally not indicated.

KEY POINT

- In patients with sickle cell disease, hydroxyurea therapy has been shown to decrease vaso-occlusive episodes and acute chest syndrome, to decrease transfusion requirements and hospitalizations, and to prolong overall survival.

Bibliography

Kato GJ. New insights into sickle cell disease: mechanisms and investigational therapies. Curr Opin Hematol. 2016;23:224-32. [PMID: 27055046] doi:10.1097/MOH.0000000000000241

Item 50   Answer: B
Educational Objective: Diagnose polycythemia vera.

The most appropriate diagnostic test to perform is for the *JAK2 V617F* mutation. Polycythemia vera (PV) is a disorder of the myeloid and erythroid stem cells that causes erythropoietin-independent proliferation of erythrocytes. This older adult patient has an elevated hematocrit level, a low erythropoietin level, and splenomegaly, indicating a likely diagnosis of PV. More than 97% of patients with PV have the *JAK2* mutation. The 2016 World Health Organization major criteria for PV include increased hemoglobin level

(>16.5 g/dL [165 g/L] in men and >16 g/dL [160 g/L] in women), a bone marrow biopsy specimen showing hypercellularity and increased reticulin and collagen fibrosis, and positive findings for *JAK2* or exon 12 mutation. *JAK2* mutation testing can be done on peripheral blood granulocytes.

Calreticulin mutation has been recently found in *JAK2*-negative myeloproliferative disorders such as essential thrombocythemia and myelofibrosis. Evaluation for the calreticulin mutation would not be indicated in the absence of thrombocytosis or cytopenia.

Translocation of chromosomes 9 and 22, resulting in a *BCR-ABL* fusion gene, is seen in patients with chronic myeloid leukemia (CML). CML can present with elevated leukocyte and platelet counts, but polycythemia is not a typical presentation.

Most causes of secondary erythrocytosis share the mechanism of an elevated erythropoietin level, which is most commonly driven by hypoxemia. Polycythemia can be the presenting symptom of undiagnosed sleep apnea, and all patients with polycythemia should be screened for symptoms and signs of sleep apnea. However, in this patient with no symptoms, a low erythropoietin level, and splenomegaly, PV is much more likely, and *JAK2* mutational analysis should be performed first.

KEY POINT

- *JAK2 V617F* mutation is present in 97% of patients with polycythemia vera, so testing should be performed in patients in whom the disease is suspected.

Bibliography

Arber DA, Orazi A, Hasserjian R, Thiele J, Borowitz MJ, Le Beau MM, et al. The 2016 revision to the World Health Organization classification of myeloid neoplasms and acute leukemia. Blood. 2016;127:2391-405. [PMID: 27069254] doi:10.1182/blood-2016-03-643544

Item 51   Answer: C
Educational Objective: Diagnose thrombotic thrombocytopenic purpura.

The finding of schistocytes on the peripheral blood smear is all that is needed to initiate therapy for presumed thrombotic thrombocytopenic purpura (TTP). This patient's clinical features of fever, change in mental status, thrombocytopenia, and features of hemolytic anemia (low haptoglobin level, elevated lactate dehydrogenase level, elevated reticulocyte count) suggest TTP. The presence of schistocytes on the peripheral blood smear will confirm the diagnosis of a microangiopathic hemolytic anemia (MAHA) and a presumptive diagnosis of TTP and allows for early treatment. Prompt diagnosis is critical because TTP is fatal in 90% of patients without therapy. Patients require emergent treatment with plasma exchange.

The most common cause of TTP results from a deficiency in the protease ADAMTS13, which cleaves the high-molecular-weight multimers of von Willebrand

CONT.

factor (vWF). The decrease in ADAMTS13 activity leads to accumulation of clumps of ultra-large-molecular-weight vWF multimers, which bind to masses of platelets leading to microvascular occlusion and thrombocytopenia. If the peripheral blood smear supports the diagnosis of TTP, testing for ADAMTS13 activity is important to confirm the diagnosis and establish the autoimmune cause. However, the turn-around time for this test result is long, and therapy should not be delayed while awaiting results. This patient's clinical history, laboratory findings, and schistocytes on the peripheral blood smear are sufficient to initiate life-saving treatment.

Coagulation studies are almost always normal in patients with TTP. Tissue ischemia may result in laboratory findings consistent with disseminated intravascular coagulation, but neither normal nor abnormal coagulation studies affect the decision to initiate early therapy.

In a patient with thrombocytopenia, MAHA, and bloody diarrhea, stool cultures and toxin testing for Shiga toxin or Shiga toxin–producing organisms are indicated to differentiate TTP from hemolytic uremic syndrome. Because this patient does not have diarrhea, stool studies are not indicated, and results do not dictate when to initiate therapy.

> **KEY POINT**
>
> - In the proper clinical setting, a peripheral blood smear showing schistocytes in a patient with thrombocytopenia and hemolytic anemia establishes a presumptive diagnosis of thrombotic thrombocytopenic purpura and confirms the need to initiate early, life-saving therapy.

Bibliography
George JN, Nester CM. Syndromes of thrombotic microangiopathy. N Engl J Med. 2014;371:654-66. [PMID: 25119611] doi:10.1056/NEJMra1312353

Item 52   **Answer: D**

Educational Objective: Screen for hyperlipidemia and diabetes in adult survivors of pediatric leukemia.

A lipid profile and fasting blood glucose should be performed. Adult survivors of childhood leukemia (primarily acute lymphoblastic leukemia [ALL]) have health risks largely secondary to the cancer therapy they received. Requesting a treatment summary or referral to a survivor clinic at a comprehensive cancer center is the first step in providing care. Increased risks of cardiovascular disease, the metabolic syndrome, and secondary cancer are the most relevant concerns. Compared with control populations, survivors of ALL are more likely to have features of the metabolic syndrome, including high BMI, truncal obesity, dyslipidemia, insulin resistance, and hypertension. Screening for lipid profile, diabetes, and hypertension is recommended by multiple guidelines for adult survivors of childhood ALL.

Survivors of ALL in continuous remission for more than 20 years have virtually no risk for ALL recurrence, although they are at risk for therapy-associated myelodysplastic syndrome or acute myeloid leukemia up to 15 years after treatment. With normal complete blood count findings, surveillance bone marrow examinations and whole genome sequencing are not indicated.

Leukemia therapy in childhood does not typically compromise ovarian function, and the patient's regular periods attest to the presence of normal ovarian function; obtaining estrogen and progesterone levels is not necessary.

Anthracyclines, such as doxorubicin, are the most common cause of dose-dependent chemotherapy-induced cardiomyocyte damage, leading to late and irreversible chronic heart failure. Exposure to anthracycline chemotherapy during childhood can cause heart failure in adulthood. However, echocardiography, not an exercise stress test, is the appropriate test to evaluate for abnormal myocardial function that may be asymptomatic. Echocardiography before pregnancy may be particularly important in women previously treated with anthracyclines because they are at risk for further deterioration of myocardial function during pregnancy.

> **KEY POINT**
>
> - Survivors of acute lymphoblastic leukemia are at increased risk for the metabolic syndrome, including high BMI, truncal obesity, dyslipidemia, insulin resistance, and hypertension.

Bibliography
Diller L. Clinical practice. Adult primary care after childhood acute lymphoblastic leukemia. N Engl J Med. 2011;365:1417-24. [PMID: 21995389] doi:10.1056/NEJMcp1103645

Item 53   **Answer: C**

Educational Objective: Diagnose transfusion-associated circulatory overload.

The most likely diagnosis is transfusion-associated circulatory overload, which is an underrecognized and underreported transfusion reaction affecting 1% to 8% of transfusion recipients. Risk factors include older age, pre-existing cardiac or kidney disease, receipt of multiple blood components, and rapid administration rate. The definition includes respiratory distress within 6 hours of transfusion, positive fluid balance, elevated central venous pressure, elevated B-type natriuretic peptide, and radiographic findings of pulmonary edema. Management consists of transfusion discontinuation, diuretic therapy, and supportive care. Prevention includes a slower infusion rate (1 mL/kg/hour) and diuretic therapy between transfusions to maintain euvolemia for those at risk.

Intravascular acute hemolytic transfusion reactions are characterized by the immediate destruction of donor erythrocytes by recipient antibodies. Signs and symptoms include

Answers and Critiques

CONT.

fever, chills, dyspnea, red urine, flank pain, kidney injury, disseminated intravascular coagulation, and hypotension or shock; they do not include circulatory overload as seen in this patient.

Anaphylaxis is associated with respiratory distress. Manifestations include the sudden onset of respiratory distress, bronchospasm, angioedema, urticaria, nausea and vomiting, abdominal pain, tachycardia, and hypotension. It is not associated with pulmonary edema.

Transfusion-related acute lung injury (TRALI) is the leading cause of transfusion-related mortality. It is characterized by the development of acute lung injury within 6 hours of transfusion of erythrocytes, platelets, or fresh frozen plasma. TRALI is mediated by initial priming of neutrophils in the recipient's lung parenchyma followed by their activation by anti-HLA and antineutrophil antibodies present in donor plasma. Signs and symptoms escalate quickly and include dyspnea, hypoxia, fever, chills, and hypotension. The chest radiograph shows diffuse bilateral pulmonary infiltrates. The presence of circulatory overload is not consistent with TRALI. Management of TRALI is supportive.

KEY POINT

- Signs of transfusion-associated circulatory overload include respiratory distress within 6 hours of transfusion, positive fluid balance, elevated central venous pressure, elevated B-type natriuretic peptide, and radiographic findings of pulmonary edema.

Bibliography

Delaney M, Wendel S, Bercovitz RS, Cid J, Cohn C, Dunbar NM, et al; Biomedical Excellence for Safer Transfusion (BEST) Collaborative. Transfusion reactions: prevention, diagnosis, and treatment. Lancet. 2016;388:2825-2836. [PMID: 27083327] doi:10.1016/S0140-6736(15)01313-6

Item 54   Answer: B

Educational Objective: Treat acute chest syndrome.

The most appropriate management is to perform immediate exchange transfusion. The patient has acute chest syndrome (ACS), defined clinically by fever, respiratory findings that include tachypnea and hypoxia, and evolving infiltrates on chest radiograph. ACS is one of the most common complications of sickle cell disease and is the most common cause of death. ACS may occur secondary to infection, fat or bone marrow embolism, in situ thrombosis, or any combination of these. ACS remains a clinical diagnosis. Patients should receive supplemental oxygen, incentive spirometry, analgesics if they have concomitant pain, and antibiotics to treat common causes of pneumonia. The severity of ACS determines the need for transfusion and type of transfusion (simple versus exchange transfusion). Mild episodes require no transfusion, moderate episodes are managed with simple or exchange transfusion, and severe episodes require exchange transfusion. The target hemoglobin level is 10 g/dL (100 g/L). Most experts agree that patients

requiring mechanical ventilation or experiencing shock or other signs of multiorgan dysfunction should receive exchange transfusion.

Venous thromboembolism is not a common precipitant of ACS, and filling defects in the pulmonary vasculature are more likely to be caused by bone marrow or fat emboli than by venous thromboembolism. Without evidence for venous thrombosis of the lower extremity or other risk factors, CT pulmonary angiography should not be obtained, and therapeutic anticoagulation with heparin should not be started. Similarly, duplex Doppler imaging of the lower extremities should not be performed in the absence of clinical features such as unilateral leg swelling or edema and dilatation of the venous pattern that suggest acute venous thrombosis.

Acute infection is a common precipitant of ACS, and antibiotics to treat common causes of pneumonia should be routinely administered. Although a broad range of bacterial and viral agents have been linked to ACS, infection with fungal organisms is rare, and amphotericin is not indicated.

KEY POINT

- Patients with sickle cell disease and acute chest syndrome with respiratory distress requiring mechanical ventilation should receive emergent exchange transfusion.

Bibliography

Novelli EM, Gladwin MT. Crises in sickle cell disease. Chest. 2016;149:1082-93. [PMID: 26836899] doi:10.1016/j.chest.2015.12.016

Item 55   Answer: C

Educational Objective: Reverse non–vitamin K antagonist oral anticoagulation before emergent surgery.

The most appropriate management of this patient is to administer idarucizumab. To proceed with urgent procedures or surgery in patients taking anticoagulants, the continued presence of the anticoagulant must be determined, and the anticoagulant effect must be reversed. Idarucizumab is a humanized monoclonal antibody fragment that binds with high affinity to free and thrombin-bound dabigatran. The REVERSE AD study assessed the efficacy and safety of idarucizumab for patients with serious bleeding or requiring urgent procedures. Among the 36 patients in the study who underwent a procedure, normal hemostasis was reported in 92%. The half-life of dabigatran in patients with normal kidney function is 12 to 17 hours. Although the patient's last dose of dabigatran was 16 hours ago, her impaired kidney function (serum creatinine level, 1.7 mg/dL [150 µmol/L]) will likely extend the half-life of the drug. In patients taking dabigatran, prolongation of the activated partial thromboplastin time is a good indication of bleeding risk with emergency surgery. Low levels of dabigatran can be detected by elevation of the dilute thrombin time.

CONT.

Dabigatran is cleared through the kidney, and dialysis has been used in patients experiencing bleeding. However, treatment duration is unclear, and a rebound increase in dabigatran levels after discontinuation of dialysis has been noted; therefore, dialysis would not be the best, or even the most practical, management choice for this patient who requires emergency surgery.

Fresh frozen plasma should not be used in this patient. It would require a large volume to overcome inhibition of factor Xa, putting the patient at great risk for transfusion-associated circulatory overload (TACO). TACO is a common adverse event in which hypervolemia develops toward completion or within several hours of a blood product transfusion.

Although three- and four-factor prothrombin complex concentrates (PCCs) have been used in bleeding associated with non–vitamin K antagonist oral anticoagulants, the benefit of PCCs has not been confirmed in randomized trials and remains unclear. Because idarucizumab is available as a reversal agent for dabigatran, its use would be first line in this setting.

KEY POINT

- Patients taking dabigatran and requiring urgent surgery should be given idarucizumab, a monoclonal antibody fragment that binds free and thrombin-bound dabigatran and neutralizes its activity.

Bibliography

Pollack CV Jr, Reilly PA, Eikelboom J, Glund S, Verhamme P, Bernstein RA, et al. Idarucizumab for dabigatran reversal. N Engl J Med. 2015;373:511-20. [PMID: 26095746] doi:10.1056/NEJMoa1502000

Item 56   Answer: B

Educational Objective: Diagnose folate deficiency.

The most likely diagnosis is folate deficiency. The patient has a macrocytic anemia associated with malnutrition and presumed decreased consumption of folate-rich foods and chronic alcoholism. A major source of folate is grains and green leafy vegetables, but folate absorption is decreased in the presence of chronic alcoholism. This patient is at risk for folate deficiency based on his homelessness, cachetic appearance suggesting malnutrition, and chronic alcoholism. Folate is not efficiently stored, and folate deficiency can develop within weeks of inadequate intake. Measuring the folate level is often of limited utility because of the ease and safety of initiating folate replacement. This patient should receive supplemental folate in addition to mental health and social service support.

Cobalamin deficiency will also produce a macrocytic anemia with hematologic features identical to that seen in folate deficiency. Unlike folate, cobalamin is effectively stored, and dietary inadequacy is not a common cause of deficiency. Alcohol dependence is not a risk factor for cobalamin deficiency. Although cobalamin deficiency is a

conceivable cause of anemia in this patient, folate deficiency is much more likely.

Inflammatory anemia is caused by underlying proinflammatory states, such as infection, cancer, and autoimmune disease, and other conditions not traditionally characterized as proinflammatory, including chronic heart failure and diabetes mellitus. It is associated with a normocytic or microcytic anemia, not with macrocytosis or hypersegmented neutrophils as seen in this patient.

The hallmark of iron deficiency is a microcytic hypochromic anemia. Macrocytosis and hypersegmented neutrophils are not seen, making iron deficiency an unlikely diagnosis in this patient.

KEY POINT

- Folate deficiency should be suspected in patients with macrocytic anemia, malnutrition, and alcohol dependence.

Bibliography

Green R, Dwyre DM. Evaluation of macrocytic anemias. Semin Hematol. 2015;52:279-86. [PMID: 26404440] doi:10.1053/j.seminhematol. 2015.06.001

Item 57   Answer: D

Educational Objective: Diagnose multiple myeloma.

Serum protein electrophoresis (SPEP) and serum free light chain analysis are the most appropriate next diagnostic steps. He has the classic signs and symptoms of multiple myeloma (MM) (hyperCalcemia, Renal failure, Anemia, and Bone lesions [CRAB]; the bone lesions in this instance manifest by a compression fracture). In addition to these features, he has elevated total protein and low serum albumin levels, which indicate an elevated globulin level that can be seen with MM. SPEP and serum free light chain assay are the initial screening tests for MM because they identify most myelomas, which secrete a clonal immunoglobulin, a light chain, or both. Rarely, some patients with MM do not secrete a protein, and bone marrow biopsy is required for diagnosis.

Bone scans are not obtained in MM because myeloma lesions are usually lytic and lack the associated increase in osteoblast activity that leads to positive bone scan findings typical of other forms of metastatic cancer. Plain radiography of the bones (skeletal surveys) is the most common imaging used to assess lytic lesions, but PET scan and MRI are more sensitive than skeletal survey at identifying MM bone lesions.

Prostate cancer with bone metastasis can cause hypercalcemia, bone pain, anemia, and, possibly, kidney failure from obstruction or hypercalcemia. But it would not cause the elevated protein seen in this patient.

Although primary hyperparathyroidism can cause hypercalcemia and decreased bone density leading to increased risk of vertebral body fractures, this patient's anemia and protein elevation do not fit with that diagnosis.

KEY POINT

- Patients with hypercalcemia, renal failure, anemia, and bone disease should have further testing with serum protein electrophoresis and serum free light chain assay to evaluate for multiple myeloma.

Bibliography

Rajkumar SV, Dimopoulos MA, Palumbo A, Blade J, Merlini G, Mateos MV, et al. International Myeloma Working Group updated criteria for the diagnosis of multiple myeloma. Lancet Oncol. 2014;15:e538-48. [PMID: 25439696] doi:10.1016/S1470-2045(14)70442-5

Item 58   Answer: B

Educational Objective: Evaluate megaloblastic anemia.

Serum cobalamin and folate levels should be obtained next. The clinical features, pancytopenia with macrocytic erythrocytes and hypersegmented neutrophils, suggest megaloblastic anemia, and serum levels of cobalamin and folate should be assessed. The patient described also has an elevated indirect bilirubin level and an elevated lactate dehydrogenase (LDH) level, which indicate ineffective erythropoiesis and intramedullary hemolysis seen in megaloblastic anemia. This constellation of findings is consistent with cobalamin deficiency, which often occurs simultaneously with other autoimmune conditions, such as Hashimoto thyroiditis. Similar hematologic findings are seen in folate deficiency, which would be more likely in patients with poor nutrition or alcohol dependence. A reasonable first step in evaluating suspected vitamin B_{12} deficiency is serum cobalamin measurement, with levels greater than 300 pg/mL (221 pmol/L) making deficiency unlikely and levels less than 200 pg/mL (148 pmol/L) strongly suggesting deficiency. If diagnostic uncertainty exists, methylmalonic acid and homocysteine measurement may be helpful. Both are elevated in 98% of patients with cobalamin deficiency, even in patients who have neurologic symptoms without anemia. Methylmalonic acid and total homocysteine levels are helpful in differentiating cobalamin deficiency (both levels are elevated) from folate deficiency (elevated homocysteine level but normal methylmalonic acid level).

Bone marrow biopsy is seldom indicated to diagnose megaloblastic anemia. Although a marrow sample may be useful to diagnose myelodysplasia, which can also present as a macrocytic anemia, a bone marrow biopsy would not be the appropriate next test for this patient without first excluding vitamin B_{12} and folate deficiency.

Flow cytometry would not be helpful in the absence of abnormal leukocytes or other findings that raise suspicion for myelodysplasia or leukemia (for example, immature cells, leukopenia, or leukocytosis).

Patients with glucose-6-phosphate dehydrogenase (G6PD) deficiency do not have a macrocytic anemia or hypersegmented neutrophils. During episodes of hemolysis, peripheral blood smears show typical bite cells and Heinz bodies, which are not present in this patient's peripheral smear. Additionally, G6PD deficiency is an X-linked condition uncommon in women. Furthermore, patients with suspected G6PD deficiency should not have G6PD levels measured during an acute hemolytic event because G6PD levels are relatively preserved in the non-hemolyzed cells remaining in circulation, so false-negative results are common.

KEY POINT

- Patients with pancytopenia, macrocytic erythrocytes, hypersegmented neutrophils, and findings consistent with intramedullary hemolysis should have vitamin B_{12} and folate levels assessed to determine the cause of megaloblastic anemia.

Bibliography

Stabler SP. Clinical practice. Vitamin B12 deficiency. N Engl J Med. 2013;368:149-60. [PMID: 23301732] doi:10.1056/NEJMcp1113996

Item 59   Answer: A

Educational Objective: Diagnose acquired von Willebrand disease.

Acquired von Willebrand disease (vWD) should be suspected in a patient who has previously been well without bleeding symptoms but now has bleeding manifestations and laboratory features consistent with vWD. Acquired vWD typically occurs in patients who develop an autoantibody to von Willebrand factor, analogous to that seen with acquired factor VIII deficiency, and in conditions of high sheer pressure within the vasculature, traditionally in patients with a prosthetic heart valve that has become dislodged but also in patients with prosthetic heart valves that appear normal in function and in those with valvular heart disease who have not had surgery. More recently, this disorder has been linked to left ventricular assist devices (LVADs). This patient has the expected INR elevation associated with therapeutic-dose warfarin routinely prescribed after LVAD implantation. But the relatively abrupt onset of bleeding manifestations is associated with prolongation of the Platelet Function Analyzer-100 test, suggesting a new qualitative platelet defect. Acquired vWD can be confirmed by low levels of von Willebrand antigen or ristocetin cofactor activity.

The liver is responsible for synthesizing all clotting factors as well as anticoagulant and antifibrinolytic factors. Because of this fact, patients with severe liver disease will have significantly prolonged prothrombin and activated partial thromboplastin times (PT and aPTT) resulting from decreased levels of coagulation factors. This patient only has slightly prolonged aPTT and PT and no history or evidence of severe liver disease, making the coagulopathy of liver disease unlikely.

Acquired fibrinogen abnormalities are relatively common, whereas inherited fibrinogen disorders are rare. The most common causes include liver disease (dysfibrinogenemia), disseminated intravascular coagulation (hypofibrinogenemia), and certain medications. This patient has no evidence of liver disease, and his fibrinogen level is normal, which together exclude disseminated intravascular coagulation.

Immune thrombocytopenic purpura is associated with a low platelet count and not with a qualitative platelet abnormality.

> **KEY POINT**
> - High sheer force seen in some patients with prosthetic heart valves, abnormal native valves, and left ventricular assist device placement may cause an acquired von Willebrand disease with clinical bleeding.

Bibliography

Nascimbene A, Neelamegham S, Frazier OH, Moake JL, Dong JF. Acquired von Willebrand syndrome associated with left ventricular assist device. Blood. 2016;127:3133-41. [PMID: 27143258] doi:10.1182/blood-2015-10-636480

Item 60   Answer: B

Educational Objective: Diagnose myelodysplastic syndrome.

This older adult patient should undergo bone marrow biopsy. He has macrocytic anemia likely resulting from myelodysplastic syndrome (MDS), and a bone marrow biopsy will help confirm the diagnosis. The peripheral blood smear shows a dysplastic neutrophil with abnormal segmentation and hypogranularity and a nucleated erythrocyte, which are characteristic in patients with MDS. MDS is an acquired bone marrow failure syndrome with ineffective hematopoiesis and peripheral cytopenias. A bone marrow biopsy specimen showing hypercellular marrow with dysplastic myeloid progenitor cells and lack of orderly maturation is diagnostic. Bone marrow biopsy also helps with risk stratification of MDS, which determines treatment. Other causes of dysplasia, including chronic infections (HIV), vitamin B_{12} deficiency, alcohol use, and medications such as sulfamethoxazole, must be ruled out.

BCR-ABL translocation involving chromosomes 9 and 22 is pathognomonic for chronic myeloid leukemia (CML), a myeloproliferative neoplasm. CML typically presents in the chronic phase with elevated neutrophils or platelets, or both. CML cannot explain this patient's pancytopenia and abnormal peripheral blood smear findings.

Positivity for the *JAK2* mutation is seen in certain other myeloproliferative neoplasms, such as essential thrombocythemia, polycythemia vera, and primary myelofibrosis. Primary myelofibrosis can present with cytopenias, but patients usually have other systemic symptoms, such as fever, night sweats, and malaise; findings of splenomegaly; and a peripheral blood smear showing teardrop erythrocytes and a leukoerythroblastic picture. This patient's clinical presentation with cytopenias and dysplastic neutrophils does not fit that of CML or other myeloproliferative neoplasms, so performing *JAK2* mutation testing or polymerase chain reaction for *BCR-ABL* translocation is not necessary at this time.

Although patients with multiple myeloma may present with pancytopenia, anemia is more likely to be normochromic or normocytic and not megaloblastic as seen in this patient. Furthermore, patients with multiple myeloma do not have dysplastic leukocytes or nucleated erythrocytes in the peripheral blood.

> **KEY POINT**
> - Bone marrow biopsy can help confirm the diagnosis of myelodysplastic syndrome in patients with macrocytic anemia and other cytopenias and a peripheral blood smear showing dysplastic, hypogranular neutrophils and nucleated erythrocytes.

Bibliography

Fenaux P, Haase D, Sanz GF, Santini V, Buske C; ESMO Guidelines Working Group. Myelodysplastic syndromes: ESMO Clinical Practice Guidelines for diagnosis, treatment and follow-up. Ann Oncol. 2014;25 Suppl 3:iii57-69. [PMID: 25185242] doi:10.1093/annonc/mdu180

Item 61   Answer: B

Educational Objective: Diagnose pulmonary hypertension related to sickle cell disease.

Echocardiography is the most appropriate diagnostic test to perform next. The patient's symptoms, cardiac examination, and electrocardiography suggest pulmonary hypertension (PH). PH is associated with significant morbidity and a 30% to 50% mortality rate. Prevalence is approximately 10% in nonpregnant patients but increases in women with sickle cell disease (SCD) who become pregnant. Risk factors for development of PH include severity of anemia, iron overload from transfusions, and history of thromboembolic disease. Although cardiac ultrasonography may underestimate the severity of PH, it remains a useful initial noninvasive screening test even if right heart catheterization is eventually required to more definitively evaluate the hemodynamics.

Cardiac MRI would be useful in evaluating infiltrative cardiomyopathy from iron overload or amyloidosis. Secondary iron overload is seen in SCD but invariably in the setting of multiple blood transfusions over years of time, a history that is lacking in this patient.

Although chest pain could be associated with coronary artery disease and angina, patients with SCD are not especially predisposed to this complication. Exercise stress testing would be contraindicated in those with suspected severe PH and a recent episode of exertion-triggered syncope.

Although pregnancy is a risk factor for dissecting thoracic aortic aneurysm, it is somewhat debated whether additional conditions, such as sustained hypertension, Marfan syndrome, or other connective tissue disorders, are required. This patient's clinical features do not warrant aortography before additional tests are performed, including cardiac ultrasonography.

> **KEY POINT**
> - Pulmonary hypertension, a known complication in sickle cell disease, may worsen during pregnancy and should be initially evaluated by echocardiography.

Bibliography

Gordeuk VR, Castro OL, Machado RF. Pathophysiology and treatment of pulmonary hypertension in sickle cell disease. Blood. 2016;127:820-8. [PMID: 26758918] doi:10.1182/blood-2015-08-618561

Item 62   Answer: D

Educational Objective: Diagnose testosterone supplementation as a secondary cause for polycythemia.

This patient's polycythemia is likely caused by testosterone injections. Polycythemia is a common adverse effect of testosterone (and anabolic steroid) supplementation, and evaluating the hematocrit level at initiation, 3 to 6 months after testosterone initiation, and annually thereafter is recommended by Endocrine Society guidelines. Guidelines also recommend interrupting the testosterone supplementation if the hematocrit value is greater than 54%. Secondary polycythemia can cause symptoms, such as headaches and elevated blood pressure, and increase the risk of thromboembolism. The risk of venous thromboembolic disease is directly related to hematocrit level. In this patient, stopping the testosterone supplementation until his polycythemia improves and restarting at a lower dose is recommended. In patients with severe symptoms, phlebotomy can also be considered. Testosterone supplementation can also exacerbate undiagnosed sleep apnea, and evaluation for an underlying sleep disorder should be performed in these patients with polycythemia.

Anemia rather than erythrocytosis may be seen in patients with both hyperthyroidism and hypothyroidism, and levothyroxine, even if given at inappropriately high or low doses, does not cause polycythemia.

Lisinopril does not cause polycythemia. ACE inhibitors, such as lisinopril, are actually used to treat secondary polycythemia after kidney transplantation. Posttransplant erythrocytosis occurs in up to 15% of patients after kidney transplantation. ACE inhibitors reduce erythrocytosis in 90% of patients in a dose-response manner. The mechanism is unknown, but apoptosis of the erythroid precursors has been suggested as well as renin-angiotensin system inhibition that may decrease erythropoietin production.

Polycythemia vera (PV) is a disorder of the myeloid and erythroid stem cells that causes erythropoietin-independent proliferation of erythrocytes and splenomegaly. PV should be considered in all patients with polycythemia; however, in this patient who is receiving testosterone supplementation, has an elevated erythropoietin level, and does not have splenomegaly, PV is unlikely. If PV is suspected, mutational analysis for *JAK2 V617F* should be performed.

KEY POINT

- Polycythemia is a common adverse effect of testosterone injections, and testosterone supplementation should be interrupted if the hematocrit level exceeds 54%.

Bibliography

Bhasin S, Cunningham GR, Hayes FJ, Matsumoto AM, Snyder PJ, Swerdloff RS, et al; Task Force, Endocrine Society. Testosterone therapy in men with androgen deficiency syndromes: an Endocrine Society clinical practice

guideline. J Clin Endocrinol Metab. 2010;95:2536-59. [PMID: 20525905] doi:10.1210/jc.2009-2354

Item 63   Answer: A

Educational Objective: Treat heparin-induced thrombocytopenia.

The most appropriate management is to discontinue heparin and initiate argatroban. This patient has heparin-induced thrombocytopenia (HIT). He was in the hospital 1 month ago for chronic heart failure and most likely received subcutaneous heparin at that time, so he has a history of heparin exposure. A scoring system for determining the pretest probability of a patient having HIT has been developed (4T score). High probability scores are associated with a 50% decrease in platelet count, onset between days 5 and 10 of heparin exposure, new thrombosis, and no other cause of thrombocytopenia. This patient's platelet count decreased more than 50% from admission 5 days ago, he has a new thrombotic event, and he has no other likely explanation for the thrombocytopenia. HIT can be a life-threatening condition if not addressed rapidly. Heparin must be discontinued and an alternate, immediately effective anticoagulant, such as argatroban, must be initiated. A strongly positive immunoassay for HIT antibody will help confirm the diagnosis. The risk of thrombosis persists after resolution of the thrombocytopenia, so treatment with warfarin should begin when the platelet count normalizes; most experts recommend 3 to 6 months of therapy.

Patients with HIT must have all heparin products stopped. Replacing low-molecular-weight heparin with unfractionated heparin does not mitigate the risk of additional thrombosis. Most experts advise delaying warfarin therapy until the platelet count has normalized.

Placement of an inferior vena cava filter will not prevent additional thrombotic events.

KEY POINT

- Patients with a high probability of heparin-induced thrombocytopenia should have heparin stopped, and therapy with an immediately effective anticoagulant, such as argatroban, should be initiated.

Bibliography

Greinacher A. Clinical practice. Heparin-induced thrombocytopenia. N Engl J Med. 2015;373:252-61. [PMID: 26176382] doi:10.1056/NEJMcp1411910

Item 64   Answer: B

Educational Objective: Diagnose hemolytic uremic syndrome.

This patient most likely has hemolytic uremic syndrome (HUS). HUS is a diarrhea-associated syndrome of microangiopathic hemolytic anemia, thrombocytopenia, and acute kidney injury caused by Shiga toxin–producing *Escherichia coli*, typically with serotypes O157:H7, O104:H4, and, less commonly, *Shigella dysenteriae*. Shiga toxin binds to endothelial cells, triggering thrombosis and resulting in a thrombotic microangiopathy. It also binds to renal mesangial cells, podocytes, and renal tubular cells, causing direct damage. These actions lead to acute kidney injury. Although it is more commonly seen in children, it can also present in adults. Supportive care is a cornerstone of treatment, and fluid management with volume expansion is critical despite any existing oliguria.

Atypical HUS is a congenital syndrome caused by overwhelming complement activation that is not preceded by a diarrheal illness as typical HUS is. The distinction between thrombotic thrombocytopenic purpura and typical and atypical HUS is difficult but important to make because atypical HUS is effectively treated by infusions of eculizumab, a monoclonal antibody directed against the terminal components of the complement cascade.

The combination of an immune-mediated hemolytic anemia, usually warm antibody, IgG mediated, and immune thrombocytopenic purpura is known as Evans syndrome. Although this patient has evidence of a hemolytic anemia and thrombocytopenia, the direct antiglobulin test is negative, and schistocytes, reflecting microangiopathic hemolysis, were noted on the peripheral blood smear. Spherocytes would be expected in IgG-mediated autoimmune hemolytic anemia.

Patients with rapidly progressive glomerulonephritis (RPGN) typically present with the nephritic syndrome and may sometimes be in advanced kidney failure at the time of presentation. Other symptoms and clinical findings related to an underlying cause may also be present, such as systemic signs of vasculitis (arthritis, epistaxis, hemoptysis) or lung hemorrhage (Goodpasture syndrome). The absence of active urinary sediment and the presence of microangiopathic hemolytic anemia make RPGN an unlikely diagnosis.

> **KEY POINT**
>
> - Classic hemolytic uremic syndrome is a diarrhea-associated syndrome of microangiopathic hemolytic anemia, thrombocytopenia, and acute kidney injury caused by Shiga toxin–producing *Escherichia coli* and, less commonly, *Shigella dysenteriae*.

Bibliography

Mele C, Remuzzi G, Noris M. Hemolytic uremic syndrome. Semin Immunopathol. 2014;36:399-420. [PMID: 24526222] doi:10.1007/s00281-014-0416-x

Item 65   Answer: D

Educational Objective: Diagnose valve hemolysis.

This patient most likely has valve hemolysis. She has a persistent mild anemia with laboratory features consistent with intravascular hemolysis (undetectable haptoglobin levels and elevated lactate dehydrogenase levels). The peripheral blood smear shows rare schistocytes, which are fragmented erythrocytes consistent with micro- or macroangiopathic hemolysis. Patients with artificial valves or

those with left ventricular assist devices can develop anemia resulting from erythrocyte fragmentation known as macroangiopathic hemolysis. A normal echocardiographic examination does not exclude mild valve hemolysis; in fact, the peripheral blood smear is more sensitive than echocardiography for detecting valve dysfunction. In addition to the peripheral blood smear, the most sensitive laboratory test is the serum haptoglobin level, but this test lacks specificity. Although the peripheral blood smear is a reliable indicator of the integrity of valve function, it is a less reliable indicator of the degree of hemodynamically significant perivalvular regurgitation. As such, the presence of mild hemolysis may not necessitate valve replacement, and the timing of valve replacement would become a clinical decision based on patient and valve characteristics, pattern and pace of hemolysis, and changes in echocardiographic findings over time.

This patient is taking no medications associated with drug-induced hemolytic anemia (for example, cephalosporins, penicillins, NSAIDs, quinidine, isoniazid). In addition, schistocytes are not present in drug-induced hemolysis, making this a very unlikely diagnosis.

The peripheral blood smear does not show features, such as microcytosis or anisopoikilocytosis, found in iron deficiency from blood loss, making gastrointestinal bleeding unlikely. However, patients with significant intravascular hemolysis and hemoglobinuria may excrete enough iron in the urine to become iron deficient. This patient does not have such severe hemolysis nor does she have any hematologic features of iron deficiency.

This patient lacks the peripheral blood smear findings associated with glucose-6-phosphate dehydrogenase deficiency, including bite cells and Heinz bodies. Similarly, none of the medications prescribed (for example, sulfonamides, some antimalarials, rasburicase) are associated with glucose-6-phosphate dehydrogenase deficiency, an X-linked condition that is uncommon in women.

> **KEY POINT**
>
> - Patients with artificial valves or those with left ventricular assist devices can develop anemia resulting from erythrocyte fragmentation known as macroangiopathic hemolysis.

Bibliography

Beris P, Picard V. Non-immune hemolysis: diagnostic considerations. Semin Hematol. 2015;52:287-303. [PMID: 26404441] doi:10.1053/j.seminhematol.2015.07.005

Item 66   Answer: A

Educational Objective: Treat provoked deep venous thrombosis.

The most appropriate management is to continue anticoagulation for a 3-month course. Decisions on anticoagulation therapy duration depend on the recurrent venous thromboembolism (VTE) risk without anticoagulation, the bleeding risk with anticoagulants, and the patient's preference. In patients with proximal leg deep venous thrombosis (DVT) or pulmonary embolism, the cumulative VTE recurrence risk after discontinuation of anticoagulation is (1) 1% after 1 year and 3% after 5 years for VTE provoked by major surgery; (2) 5% after 1 year and 15% after 5 years for VTE provoked by a nonsurgical reversible risk factor; and (3) 10% after 1 year and 30% after 5 years for unprovoked VTE. This patient experienced a provoked DVT after major surgery. In provoked thrombosis with reversible risk factors, guidelines recommend 3 months of anticoagulation.

Because of the high risk of recurrence with discontinuation of anticoagulant therapy, an unprovoked VTE is a consideration for extended anticoagulant therapy. When extended (long-term) anticoagulation therapy is chosen, the risks, benefits, and burden of long-term therapy must be re-evaluated periodically. This patient's DVT was provoked by surgery; therefore, extended anticoagulation is not a reasonable option.

Identifying an inherited thrombophilia often does not change treatment decisions in a patient with VTE. Recent guidelines recommend against routine thrombophilia testing because identification of inherited abnormalities does not alter the duration of recommended anticoagulation or reliably predict risk of VTE recurrence. Finally, the American Society of Hematology's Choosing Wisely Campaign specifically recommends against thrombophilia testing in adults with VTE that occurs in the setting of a major transient risk factor, such as surgery, prolonged immobility, or trauma.

In patients with unprovoked DVT, a common strategy has been to measure D-dimer levels 2 weeks after discontinuation of a 3-month course of anticoagulant therapy. Patients with elevated D-dimer levels were considered for further anticoagulation. However, although elevated levels of D-dimer can identify persons at risk, this test has low specificity, and a normal D-dimer level cannot safely rule out the possibility of future recurrence, thus limiting the utility of this testing strategy. Furthermore, this patient had a provoked DVT, which is another reason not to perform follow-up D-dimer testing.

KEY POINT

- In provoked deep venous thrombosis with reversible risk factors, 3 months of anticoagulation is recommended.

Bibliography

Kearon C, Akl EA, Ornelas J, Blaivas A, Jimenez D, Bounameaux H, et al. Antithrombotic therapy for VTE disease: CHEST Guideline and Expert Panel Report. Chest. 2016;149:315-52. [PMID: 26867832] doi:10.1016/j.chest.2015.11.026

Item 67   Answer: D

Educational Objective: Diagnose pseudothrombocytopenia.

The most likely diagnosis in this patient is pseudothrombocytopenia. A review of the peripheral blood smear is the first step in evaluating a patient with thrombocytopenia. Platelet clumping, or pseudothrombocytopenia, is caused by antibodies directed against the anticoagulant ethylenediaminetetraacetic acid and is not associated with any medical problem. Additionally, in the absence of platelet clumping, review of the peripheral blood smear might show schistocytes or abnormal leukocytes, suggesting possible diagnoses accounting for true thrombocytopenia. An accurate platelet count would be obtained by drawing a blood sample in a heparinized tube.

Patients with essential thrombocythemia may have large platelets and platelet clumping, but the platelet count would be elevated, not normal as was found with the heparinized blood specimen.

Immune thrombocytopenic purpura is an autoimmune disorder that results in a low platelet count. The peripheral smear typically shows scant large platelets that do not form clumps, and the platelet count would be consistently low, even when drawn in a heparinized tube.

The diagnosis of myelodysplastic syndrome should be suspected in patients with macrocytic anemia or pancytopenia in whom vitamin B_{12} and folate deficiency have been excluded. Abnormal erythrocyte forms with basophilic stippling or Howell-Jolly bodies and dysplastic neutrophils with decreased nuclear segmentation and granulation may be present. Increased myeloblasts can be seen in more advanced disease. This patient's microcytic anemia, thrombocytopenia with platelet clumping, and correction of the thrombocytopenia by using a heparinized tube is not consistent with the diagnosis of myelodysplastic syndrome.

KEY POINT

- Evaluation of the peripheral blood smear to assess platelet clumping should be done in patients with isolated thrombocytopenia; if clumping is detected, the platelet count should be repeated in a heparinized blood specimen.

Bibliography

Lippi G, Plebani M. EDTA-dependent pseudothrombocytopenia: further insights and recommendations for prevention of a clinically threatening artifact [Editorial]. Clin Chem Lab Med. 2012;50:1281-5. [PMID: 22868791] doi:10.1515/cclm-2012-0081

Item 68   Answer: C

Educational Objective: Treat multiple myeloma and skeletal lesions.

All patients with multiple myeloma (MM) requiring therapy should be given intravenous bisphosphonates, such as zoledronic acid or pamidronate, in addition to antimyeloma therapy. Zoledronic acid and pamidronate have been shown to prevent new skeletal-related events in patients with MM, but only zoledronic acid has been shown to improve survival. Close monitoring of kidney function and calcium level should be performed in all patients taking zoledronic acid; monitoring for pain and swelling that may be early signs of osteonecrosis of the jaw is also essential. Calcium and vitamin D supplementation is usually given to patients taking intravenous bisphosphonates unless a contraindication exists. Patients with MM are given intravenous zoledronic acid every 3 to 4 weeks. Experts have not reached a consensus on duration of therapy, but indefinite bisphosphonate therapy is often used. It is reasonable to consider remission status, extent of skeletal disease, kidney function, and patient preference when determining the duration of bisphosphonate therapy. In patients who stop therapy, bisphosphonates should be restarted at disease relapse.

In patients with monoclonal gammopathy of undetermined significance and smoldering MM, dual-energy x-ray absorptiometry (DEXA) is performed to evaluate for osteoporosis or osteopenia in determining bisphosphonate therapy. This patient has MM requiring therapy with lytic lesions. Bone density scanning with DEXA is unnecessary to determine treatment.

With the advent of effective antimyeloma therapy, limited use of radiation is recommended to preserve the bone marrow. Radiation therapy is recommended to control pain or prevent impending pathologic fracture or spinal cord compression. In this patient with adequate pain control, no evidence of spinal cord compression, and no neurologic symptoms, radiation therapy is not appropriate.

Patients with MM requiring therapy are at high risk for recurrent skeletal-related events. Therefore, continuing with antimyeloma therapy alone without specifically addressing the bone disease is not adequate.

KEY POINT

• Zoledronic acid has been shown to prevent new skeletal-related events and improve survival in patients with multiple myeloma requiring therapy.

Bibliography
Terpos E, Morgan G, Dimopoulos MA, Drake MT, Lentzsch S, Raje N, et al. International Myeloma Working Group recommendations for the treatment of multiple myeloma-related bone disease. J Clin Oncol. 2013; 31:2347-57. [PMID: 23690408] doi:10.1200/JCO.2012.47.7901

Item 69   Answer: C
Educational Objective: Treat cold agglutinin disease.

The most appropriate treatment for this patient is rituximab. She has profound anemia and evidence of intravascular (decreased haptoglobin, hemoglobinuria, elevated lactate dehydrogenase) and extravascular (elevated indirect hyperbilirubinemia level) hemolysis. The positive direct antiglobulin test showing C3 on erythrocytes with agglutinated erythrocytes on the peripheral blood smear suggests cold agglutinin autoimmune hemolytic anemia. The improbably high mean corpuscular volume (MCV) calculated by the Coulter counter likely reflects measurement of agglutinated cells, although the reticulocytosis will also elevate the MCV. This disease can be primary, with no other underlying disorders, but may be associated with lymph-

oproliferative disorders, such as Waldenström macroglobulinemia, other B-cell non-Hodgkin lymphomas, and IgM monoclonal gammopathy of undetermined significance. Cold agglutinin disease may also be precipitated by infections, typically *Mycoplasma pneumoniae* or Epstein-Barr virus. In cold agglutinin disease, IgM antibodies are directed against erythrocyte antigens, resulting in complement fixation and intravascular hemolysis as well as clearance of complement-coated erythrocytes by Kupffer cells in the liver. Rituximab, a monoclonal antibody to the B-cell antigen CD20, has shown efficacy in case series of patients with cold agglutinin disease. Additionally, all patients with cold agglutinin disease should be kept warm, and all infusions should be administered at body temperature.

Unlike in patients with warm antibodies, prednisone and intravenous immune globulin do not decrease the hemolytic process in patients with cold agglutinin disease.

Because cold agglutinin disease does not involve splenic clearance of erythrocytes, splenectomy is not effective at reducing this type of hemolysis compared with warm antibody-mediated hemolysis.

KEY POINT

• Cold avoidance and rituximab are effective treatments for cold agglutinin disease; glucocorticoids, splenectomy, and intravenous immune globulin are not helpful.

Bibliography
Barcellini W. Immune hemolysis: diagnosis and treatment recommendations. Semin Hematol. 2015;52:304-12. [PMID: 26404442] doi:10.1053/j.seminhematol.2015.05.001

Item 70   Answer: B

Educational Objective: Diagnose antithrombin deficiency as a cause of heparin resistance.

The most likely diagnosis is antithrombin deficiency (ATD). This patient's clinical presentation is consistent with heparin resistance, which occurs when the activated partial thromboplastin time (aPTT) does not increase into the therapeutic range despite increasing doses of heparin or when unusually high doses of heparin are required to achieve a therapeutic aPTT. Heparin achieves its anticoagulant effect through antithrombin. The heparin-antithrombin complex then inactivates thrombin, activated factor X (fXa), and other activated clotting factors. If the amount of available antithrombin is decreased, a reduced response to heparin is seen. Heparin resistance can also occur with increased clearance of heparin or an increase in acute phase reactant proteins such as factor VIII, which can bind to and neutralize heparin. ATD is diagnosed by assaying antithrombin activity. Acquired causes must be ruled out.

Antiphospholipid antibodies are acquired autoantibodies against phospholipids and phospholipid-binding proteins, such as cardiolipin and β_2-glycoprotein I. In vitro, they can prolong clotting tests, but in vivo, they increase the

CONT. risk of venous and arterial thrombosis. Antiphospholipid syndrome (APS) can be a primary disorder with no underlying comorbidity or a secondary disorder associated with autoimmune diseases, malignancy, or drugs. This patient's clotting test fails to prolong with heparin therapy; this finding is incompatible with APS.

Factor V Leiden mutation is the most common inherited thrombophilia. Factor V Leiden mutation is associated with about 95% of cases of activated protein C (APC) resistance. APC is a naturally occurring anticoagulant; the primary manifestation of APC resistance is venous thromboembolism. Patients with factor V Leiden mutation are not resistant to the effects of heparin.

Protein C is a vitamin K–dependent natural anticoagulant; it is converted during the coagulation process to APC, which inactivates coagulation factors Va and VIIIa. Protein C deficiency is inherited in an autosomal dominant fashion. Protein C deficiency is a risk factor for venous thromboembolism and arterial thromboembolism. Patients with protein C deficiency are not resistant to the effects of heparin.

KEY POINT

- Antithrombin deficiency is a cause of heparin resistance.

Bibliography

Gaman AM, Gaman GD. Deficiency of antithrombin III (AT III) - case report and review of the literature. Curr Health Sci J. 2014;40:141-3. [PMID: 25729597] doi:10.12865/CHSJ.40.02.12

Item 71   Answer: A

Educational Objective: Treat acquired factor VIII deficiency.

The most appropriate management of this patient is to administer activated factor VII. She has an acquired hemophilia A with an autoantibody against factor VIII. An association of this disorder with hematologic malignancies such as chronic lymphocytic leukemia has been recognized. The prolonged activated partial thromboplastin time (aPTT) did not fully correct with mixing, suggesting the presence of an inhibitor. Acquired hemophilia typically presents in adults older than 60 years, and women are affected more often than men. Patients present with ecchymoses and subcutaneous or muscle bleeding. Treatment with factor VIII infusion is not successful because the inhibitor will interfere with factor efficacy, so an activated factor product is required. Recombinant activated factor VII (or activated prothrombin complex concentrate) promotes clotting by bypassing several coagulation steps.

Bleeding associated with a prolonged aPTT should raise concern for disseminated intravascular coagulation (DIC) with hypofibrinogenemia requiring cryoprecipitate; however, severe factor VIII deficiency (1%) is unusual in DIC, and the normal prothrombin time and platelet count also argue against that diagnosis. Finally, the patient has none of the common triggers of DIC, such as sepsis, metastatic cancer, or systemic immune response syndrome.

Desmopressin is used in the treatment of von Willebrand disease (vWD) and causes preformed stores of von Willebrand factor and factor VIII to be released from endothelial cells. However, in patients with vWD, the aPTT would correct in a mixing study. This patient's aPTT did not correct, making the diagnosis of vWD unlikely.

Fresh frozen plasma is used to treat patients with massive bleeding and dilutional coagulopathy and has been used in patients with warfarin toxicity. It would be ineffective in treating hemophilia with acquired factor VIII inhibitor because the inhibitor will interfere with factor efficacy.

KEY POINT

- A prolonged activated partial thromboplastin time that does not fully correct with a mixing study suggests the presence of a factor inhibitor and the diagnosis of acquired hemophilia A; treatment is with activated factor VII.

Bibliography

Franchini M, Mannucci PM. Acquired haemophilia A: a 2013 update. Thromb Haemost. 2013;110:1114-20. [PMID: 24008306] doi:10.1160/TH13-05-0363

Item 72   Answer: A

Educational Objective: Treat vitamin K deficiency.

Administering vitamin K is the most appropriate management at this time. This patient has developed vitamin K deficiency from poor oral intake and a prolonged course of antibiotics combined with diarrhea from concurrent *Clostridium difficile* infection. Although vitamin K is found in many foods, most vitamin K needed for coagulation is derived from saprophytic bacteria in the colon, and antibiotics destroy these bacteria. Diarrhea (from any cause) results in decreased absorption of vitamin K. Vitamin K is needed to activate certain factors (II, VII, IX, and X), and the prothrombin time (PT), which is most sensitive to a decrease in factor VII levels, will be elevated out of proportion to the activated partial thromboplastin time (aPTT), which will be normal or only mildly elevated. Vitamin K deficiency can be managed with oral or parenteral vitamin K, and the coagulopathy will begin to correct within 1 day.

Although atorvastatin can cause an elevation in liver enzyme levels, this patient's coagulopathy is not a result of liver disease, because the factor V level is in the normal range. With the exception of factor VIII, all clotting factors are produced in the liver, and liver disease results in a decrease in all factors with corresponding abnormalities in aPTT and PT.

Discontinuing this patient's low-dose heparin is unnecessary because this heparin formulation will not prolong the PT.

Although fresh frozen plasma will correct the underlying vitamin K deficiency, it is not the safest or most cost-effective treatment option, and the duration of effect is limited by the short half-life of factor VII. Vitamin K is a safer, more cost-effective intervention and will last much longer.

Bibliography

Brenner B, Kuperman AA, Watzka M, Oldenburg J. Vitamin K–dependent coagulation factors deficiency. Semin Thromb Hemost. 2009;35:439-46. [PMID: 19598072] doi:10.1055/s-0029-1225766

Item 73   Answer: D

Educational Objective: Determine when a thrombophilia evaluation should be performed.

The ideal testing strategy is to temporarily stop rivaroxaban in 1 year and test 2 weeks later. Long-term anticoagulation is indicated in the setting of idiopathic thrombosis. Because of the unprovoked nature of this patient's thrombotic event, his thrombotic risk remains high even after 3 months of anticoagulation. Therefore, it is safer to continue anticoagulation for 1 year before testing. Testing for inherited thrombophilia remains controversial. Guidelines and systematic reviews recommend against routine population screening or screening in most adults with idiopathic venous thromboembolism (VTE) and in asymptomatic family members of patients with VTE and known factor V Leiden or prothrombin *G20210A* gene mutation. Most experts agree that thrombophilia evaluation can be considered in select populations, such as patients with thromboses at unusual sites or recurrent idiopathic thrombosis, patients younger than 45 years with unprovoked thrombosis, patients with VTE and a clear family history of thrombosis in one or more first-degree relatives, and patients with warfarin-induced skin necrosis. After an informed discussion of the risks and benefits of testing, patients who desire evaluation should receive genetic counseling before testing. Testing typically focuses on factor V Leiden mutation; prothrombin *G20210A* mutation; protein C, protein S, and antithrombin deficiencies; and antiphospholipid antibody syndrome. However, the thrombophilia evaluation should not be performed during an acute episode of thrombosis. Additionally, although genetic tests such as factor V Leiden and prothrombin gene mutation can be performed at any time, the other assays can be variably affected by the presence of an acute thrombosis, heparin, and other anticoagulants. For example, during the acute phase of thrombosis, plasma levels of antithrombin and occasionally proteins C and S may transiently decrease, and fibrinogen and factor VIII levels may increase. Depending on the assay used, dabigatran therapy may result in increased measurements of antithrombin and protein S and C levels, whereas the factor Xa inhibitors (for example, rivaroxaban and apixaban) may result only in increased measurements of antithrombin. Warfarin therapy reduces vitamin K–dependent factors, including proteins C and S, which do not resolve for 4 to 6 weeks after discontinuation. Most experts agree that with the exception of testing for genetic mutations, testing should not be done in the acute setting or while receiving anticoagulant therapy and should be delayed at least 2 weeks after discontinuation of anticoagulant therapy to minimize diagnostic error.

KEY POINT

- With the exception of testing for genetic mutations, thrombophilia testing should not be performed in the acute setting or while receiving anticoagulant therapy and should be delayed at least 2 weeks after discontinuation of anticoagulant therapy to minimize diagnostic error.

Bibliography

Meyer MR, Witt DM, Delate T, Johnson SG, Fang M, Go A, et al. Thrombophilia testing patterns amongst patients with acute venous thromboembolism. Thromb Res. 2015;136:1160-4. [PMID: 26477821] doi:10.1016/j.thromres.2015.10.019

Item 74   Answer: D

Educational Objective: Diagnose a myeloproliferative neoplasm in a patient with hepatic vein thrombosis.

This patient should be evaluated for the *JAK2 V617F* gene mutation. This mutation is present in more than 95% of patients with polycythemia rubra vera and 50% of patients with essential thrombocytosis, even without the presence of erythrocytosis or thrombocytosis. Thromboses, including abdominal vein thromboses, are a major cause of morbidity and mortality in patients with myeloproliferative neoplasms (MPNs). Approximately 50% of cases of Budd-Chiari syndrome and 25% of cases of portal vein thrombosis are the result of an MPN, and *JAK2 V617F* gene mutations should be evaluated even in the absence of erythrocytosis or thrombocytosis. Portal hypertension and splenomegaly are often found, which may account for the relatively normal blood counts seen in some patients.

Although hepatocellular carcinoma, which could possibly be diagnosed by α-fetoprotein, can be associated with the development of abdominal thrombosis, this diagnosis is unlikely in this patient, considering her viral studies are negative and she has no evidence of cirrhosis or malignancy on imaging.

Factor VIII testing is not considered a standard component of a thrombophilia evaluation because of its mixed results regarding long-term implications. It would be inappropriate to evaluate the patient's factor VIII level at this time.

Paroxysmal nocturnal hemoglobinuria is also associated with abdominal vein thrombosis, but her normal haptoglobin level and absence of indirect hyperbilirubinemia indicate no evidence of hemolysis. Performing flow cytometry to evaluate for loss of CD 55/59 would not be appropriate.

KEY POINT

- Patients with abdominal thrombosis, splenomegaly, and portal hypertension should be evaluated for the presence of a myeloproliferative neoplasm, specifically the *JAK2 V617F* gene mutation, even in the absence of erythrocytosis or thrombocytosis.

Bibliography

Smalberg JH, Arends LR, Valla DC, Kiladjian JJ, Janssen HL, Leebeek FW. Myeloproliferative neoplasms in Budd-Chiari syndrome and portal vein thrombosis: a meta-analysis. Blood. 2012;120:4921-8. [PMID: 23043069] doi:10.1182/blood-2011-09-376517

Item 75   Answer: B

Educational Objective: Diagnose drug-induced autoimmune hemolytic anemia.

This patient most likely has drug-induced hemolysis. She has an acute anemia in association with ceftriaxone treatment for Lyme-related meningoencephalitis. Acute anemia in hospitalized patients should raise the suspicion for blood loss (including from laboratory testing) or hemolysis. An elevated lactate dehydrogenase level along with the positive direct antiglobulin test (DAT) and spherocytes on the peripheral blood smear should further raise suspicion for hemolysis from an IgG autoantibody. Many drugs are associated with drug-induced hemolytic anemia, and antibiotics are the most frequently encountered cause of this condition, with ceftriaxone being one of the most common. It is believed that ceftriaxone may become affixed to the erythrocyte membrane, leading to an immune reaction resulting in erythrocyte hemolysis. Treatment of drug-induced hemolysis involves stopping the offending drug. Importantly, Lyme disease itself is not associated with hemolysis.

Although warm antibody hemolysis can cause a hemolytic anemia that is DAT positive for IgG, cold agglutinin disease is DAT positive for C3. The peripheral blood smear would show agglutinated cells, and spherocytes would not be present. Furthermore, cold agglutinin disease is not associated with Lyme disease. Cold agglutinin disease can be primary or associated with lymphoproliferative disorders and certain infections, typically *Mycoplasma pneumoniae* or Epstein-Barr virus.

Glucose-6-phosphate dehydrogenase (G6PD) deficiency can cause acute hemolysis with certain medications (for example, sulfonamides, some antimalarials, rasburicase), but ceftriaxone is not a drug associated with G6PD deficiency-induced hemolysis. Also, G6PD-mediated hemolysis is an X-linked disease and is uncommon in women. Finally, the positive DAT and presence of spherocytes on the peripheral blood smear are inconsistent with G6PD deficiency; bite cells and Heinz bodies, which are denatured oxidized hemoglobin visualized as intranuclear inclusions seen on supravital stain, are the expected finding.

KEY POINT

- Many drugs are associated with drug-induced hemolytic anemia, and antibiotics are the most frequently encountered cause of this condition, with ceftriaxone being one of the most common causative agents.

Bibliography

Mayer B, Bartolmäs T, Yürek S, Salama A. Variability of findings in drug-induced immune haemolytic anaemia: experience over 20 years in a single centre. Transfus Med Hemother. 2015;42:333-9. [PMID: 26696803] doi:10.1159/000440673

Item 76   Answer: A

Educational Objective: Diagnose transfusion-transmitted babesiosis.

The patient most likely has transfusion-transmitted babesiosis. This tickborne disease, caused primarily by *Babesia microti* in the United States, can be transmitted through transfusion but is not routinely screened for in blood donors. *Babesia* is endemic in New England and regions of the upper Midwest. Although blood donors who report a history of babesiosis are excluded from donating, 80% of infected persons are asymptomatic and may be parasitemic for months. The incubation period for transfusion-related babesiosis ranges from 11 to 176 days. Risk factors for severe disease include older age, splenectomy, or compromised immune function. Symptoms include fatigue, malaise, fever, nausea, anorexia, myalgia, abdominal pain, and diarrhea. Hemolytic anemia, thrombocytopenia, and elevated serum aminotransferase and alkaline phosphatase levels are common. The first clue often comes on the blood smear examination from the unexpected detection of the protozoal ring forms within erythrocytes; babesiosis is then confirmed by polymerase chain reaction.

Bacterial contamination in blood components is much less common in erythrocytes compared with platelets, and symptoms and signs, such as fever and hypotension, begin during or within hours of the transfusion. This patient's illness, beginning 3 weeks after transfusion, would not be consistent with bacterial contamination.

The transmission of cytomegalovirus is associated with a generally benign mononucleosis-like syndrome in immunocompetent patients. Patients typically have lymphocytosis and atypical lymphocytosis but would not have hemolytic anemia or erythrocyte inclusions.

West Nile virus infection has an incubation period of only 2 weeks or less and is associated with fever and headaches. Zika virus may be transmitted through transfusion, but the incubation period is 2 weeks or less. Symptoms typically include rash and arthralgia. Neither West Nile virus nor Zika virus would be associated with hemolytic anemia, elevated liver chemistry test results, or erythrocyte inclusions.

KEY POINT

- *Babesia microti* is a transfusion-transmissible pathogen that can be responsible for malaria-like symptoms, hemolytic anemia, thrombocytopenia, and abnormal liver chemistry study results.

Bibliography

Manian FA, Barshak MB, Lowry KP, Basnet KM, Stowell CP. Case records of the Massachusetts General Hospital. Case 27-2016. N Engl J Med. 2016;375:981-91. [PMID: 27602671] doi:10.1056/NEJMcpc1607091

Item 77   Answer: D

Educational Objective: Treat chronic immune thrombocytopenic purpura during pregnancy.

No management beyond monitoring her platelet count and treating her urinary tract infection is needed for this patient.

Women with immune thrombocytopenic purpura (ITP) can be safely monitored during their pregnancy without intervention as long as they are asymptomatic and the platelet count remains greater than 30,000/µL (30 × 10⁹/L). If the platelet count drops unexpectedly, other diagnoses, in addition to worsening ITP, must be considered, such as pre-eclampsia, HELLP syndrome (Hemolysis, Elevated Liver enzymes, and Low Platelets), thrombotic thrombocytopenic purpura (TTP), or hemolytic uremic syndrome (HUS). This patient's normal blood pressure, absence of proteinuria, and normal liver chemistry tests make pre-eclampsia and HELLP syndrome unlikely. The absence of schistocytes on her peripheral blood smear excludes TTP, HUS, and HELLP syndrome. Her currently decreased platelet count is probably related to her intercurrent infection. However, her platelet count should be monitored closely because it is close to the cut-off for treatment.

Intravenous immune globulin is a first-line therapy option in treating ITP in pregancy, but treatment is unnecessary when the platelet count is greater than 30,000/µL (30 × 10⁹/L).

This patient does not require therapy at this time. If treatment is needed, prednisone is another first-line option in ITP. Orofacial abnormalities have been reported in neonates when used in the first trimester, but prednisone is safe to use after the 12th week of gestation. However, this patient is only at 10 weeks' gestation, so prednisone would not be preferred if treatment were needed.

Patients with ITP should not receive platelet transfusions because autoantibodies will cross-react with the transfused platelets, interfering with any potential improvement in platelet counts. However, their use in patients with severe bleeding is not disputed.

> **KEY POINT**
>
> - Pregnant women with immune thrombocytopenic purpura can be safely monitored during their pregnancy without intervention as long as they are asymptomatic and the platelet count remains greater than 30,000/µL (30 × 10⁹/L).

Bibliography

Gernsheimer T, James AH, Stasi R. How I treat thrombocytopenia in pregnancy. Blood. 2013;121:38-47. [PMID: 23149846] doi:10.1182/blood-2012-08-448944

Oncology Answers

Item 78   Answer: C

Educational Objective: Treat limited small cell lung cancer with combined chemotherapy and radiation.

The most appropriate treatment is combined chemotherapy and radiation. This patient has limited small cell lung cancer. Limited disease is defined as nonmetastatic disease that can be encompassed within a single radiation portal. Because this patient's cancer is confined to the left chest and is not metastatic, it meets this definition. Although surgery can be considered for patients with small isolated tumors, this cancer most commonly presents with large centrally located tumors that are not amenable to resection, as it did in this patient. For these patients, standard management is combined chemotherapy and radiation, which can result in cure for about 20% to 30% of patients. Chemotherapy consists of a cisplatin-based combination (usually cisplatin and etoposide) and is started at the same time as radiation. It is important to integrate radiation early in the course of chemotherapy, as delaying radiotherapy has been shown to result in inferior outcomes. Chemotherapy typically continues for a total of four to six cycles.

Chemotherapy alone does not sufficiently control local disease and is also not curative in small cell lung cancer, even in the limited-stage setting.

There is no proven role for chemotherapy followed by radiation. Studies of the use of sequential versus concurrent chemotherapy and radiation have found that concurrent treatment seems to be more effective than sequential treatment. Although in the one reported randomized trial the improvement in survival did not reach statistical significance, the preponderance of available evidence suggests that concurrent treatment is superior to sequential treatment. Therefore, it remains standard care for this patient population.

Radiation alone is not effective and does not result in cure. Small cell lung cancer has a high predilection for metastatic spread, which cannot be prevented by radiation therapy.

> **KEY POINT**
>
> - For patients with small cell lung cancer who have large centrally located tumors that are not amenable to resection, standard management is combined chemotherapy and radiation, which can result in cure for about 20% to 30% of patients.

Bibliography

Tam K, Daly M, Kelly K. Treatment of locally advanced non-small cell lung cancer. Hematol Oncol Clin North Am. 2017 Feb;31(1):45-57. doi:10.1016/j.hoc.2016.08.009. [PMID: 27912833]

Item 79   Answer: C

Educational Objective: Treat high-risk prostate cancer with a gonadotropin-releasing hormone agonist plus radiation.

The most appropriate treatment is a gonadotropin-releasing hormone (GnRH) agonist plus radiation. High-risk prostate cancer is defined as a prostate-specific antigen (PSA) level greater than 20 ng/mL (20 µg/L), a Gleason score of 8 to 10, or evidence of extraprostatic extension of the cancer. Imaging studies, such as pelvic CT or MRI, can be used to assess regional lymph node enlargement in selected patients. Imaging is reserved for patients with a PSA level greater 20 ng/mL (20 µg/L), a Gleason score 8 or greater, and other factors. Patients with high-risk prostate cancer have a significant risk of eventually developing metastatic disease, and they all require treatment unless significant medical comorbidity precludes treatment. In this patient population, there is significant risk of both local recurrence and distant metastatic disease. Studies have shown that the addition of androgen deprivation therapy (most commonly with a GnRH agonist, such as leuprolide) to radiation results in an improvement in 10-year disease-free and overall survival compared with radiation alone in men with high-risk prostate cancer. Based on this data, the combination of radiation with a GnRH agonist for up to 2 to 3 years is the standard care for this patient population.

Brachytherapy is not indicated in patients with high-risk prostate cancer because no evidence supports the efficacy of brachytherapy in this setting. Brachytherapy is typically only recommended for men with low-risk and limited-volume cancer.

Use of a GnRH agonist alone has no role in the treatment of nonmetastatic prostate cancer. In this patient, local treatment (with either radiation or surgery) is definitively indicated, and treatment with a GnRH agonist alone provides no local treatment.

Radiation alone is not recommended given the survival advantage associated with combined GnRH agonist and radiation treatment in men with high-risk and very-high-risk prostate cancer.

KEY POINT

- Combination therapy with radiation and a gonadotropin-releasing hormone agonist for up to 2 to 3 years results in an improvement in 10-year disease-free and overall survival and is the standard care for patients with high-risk and very-high-risk prostate cancer.

Bibliography

Bolla M, Van Tienhoven G, Warde P, et al. External irradiation with or without long-term androgen suppression for prostate cancer with high metastatic risk: 10-year results of an EORTC randomized study. Lancet Oncol. 2010 Nov;11(11):1066-73. [PMID: 20933466]

Item 80   Answer: B

Educational Objective: Treat locally advanced head and neck cancer.

The most appropriate treatment is cetuximab plus radiation. Several options exist for treatment of locally advanced head and neck cancer. However, in many cases, surgery is not recommended as first-line treatment. In addition, significant morbidity is expected with open surgery to resect large, locally advanced cancers. For these reasons, nonsurgical treatment is often recommended in this setting. The standard treatment of such patients is a combination of radiation with systemic therapy, most commonly either cisplatin or cetuximab. Randomized trials have clearly demonstrated improved survival in patients treated with either cisplatin or cetuximab plus radiation compared with those treated with radiation alone. For example, 3-year survival in a pivotal randomized trial was 55% in patients receiving cetuximab and radiation compared with 45% in patients treated with radiation alone.

No study to date has determined whether cetuximab or cisplatin is preferred in this setting. However, because of long-term experience with cisplatin and the significantly higher cost of cetuximab, cisplatin is preferred unless there is a contraindication to use of this agent. For this patient, who has chronic kidney disease with a baseline creatinine level of 1.8, cisplatin is clearly contraindicated and, therefore, cetuximab combined with radiotherapy is the most appropriate treatment.

There is no evidence to support a role for bevacizumab, a monoclonal antibody directed against vascular endothelial growth factor, in the treatment of locally advanced head and neck cancer.

Although radiation alone can be used for treatment of very-early-stage disease, this patient has locally advanced disease, and radiation alone is not sufficient treatment based on data clearly identifying an improvement in survival with combined radiation and systemic therapy, as discussed above.

KEY POINT

- The standard treatment for locally advanced head and neck cancer is a combination of radiation with systemic therapy, most commonly cisplatin or cetuximab.

Bibliography

Bonner JA, Harari PM, Giralt J, et al. Radiotherapy plus cetuximab for squamous-cell carcinoma of the head and neck. N Engl J Med. 2006 Feb 9;354(6):567-78. [PMID: 16467544]

Item 81   Answer: A

Educational Objective: Manage early-stage cervical cancer while maintaining fertility.

The most appropriate management for this patient with early-stage cervical cancer and concerns about future fertility is conization, which consists of excision of a cone-shaped portion of the cervix. Discussion of the impact of treatment options on fertility is important for reproductive-age patients with cancer and especially relevant for women with cervical cancer, almost half of whom are younger than 45 years of age. Patients with early-stage cervical cancer, which includes stage IA (microscopic disease without visible tumor), and stage IB1 (visible tumor less than 4 cm in size confined to the cervix) who desire future childbearing are candidates for fertility-sparing surgery. Conization is an option limited to stage IA disease without vascular invasion.

Patients with stage IA1 disease with vascular invasion and patients with stage IA2 or IB1 disease are candidates for radical trachelectomy. Vaginal radical trachelectomy is a fertility preservation surgery that involves removal of the cervix with conservation of the uterus. A permanent cerclage is placed in the uterine isthmus. In one study of patients who underwent vaginal radical trachelectomy, the 5-year recurrence-free survival was 95.8%. Fifty-eight of 125 women conceived a total of 106 pregnancies, with 75% of the pregnancies carried to term.

Neoadjuvant chemotherapy in women with early-stage cervical cancer is not needed; its use in more advanced-stage disease has not been well studied.

Radiation therapy can be used for early-stage cervical cancer, particularly in patients with poor performance status who are not candidates for surgery, but radiation would result in infertility and is thus not the best option in this patient.

Similarly, in early-stage cervical cancer, there is no difference in the rate of recurrence or mortality with more limited surgery that allows future child-bearing compared to radical or simple hysterectomy.

KEY POINT

- Conization, or excision of a cone-shaped portion of the cervix, is a fertility preservation surgery for patients who have stage IA cervical cancer, defined as microscopic disease without visible tumor.

Bibliography

Qian Q, Yang J, Cao D, You Y, Chen J, Shen K. Analysis of treatment modalities and prognosis on microinvasive cervical cancer: a 10-year cohort study in China. J Gynecol Oncol. 2014;25:293-300. [PMID: 25142622] doi:10.3802/jgo.2014.25.4.293

Item 82   Answer: A

Educational Objective: Treat early-stage hormone receptor–positive breast cancer with tamoxifen in a premenopausal patient.

The most appropriate management for this patient with early-stage hormone receptor–positive breast cancer is to continue tamoxifen for 5 more years. Two large randomized controlled studies have confirmed the benefit of extending tamoxifen to 10 years in decreasing breast cancer recurrence and breast cancer mortality. Ten years of tamoxifen compared with 5 years reduces breast cancer mortality by one third in the first 10 years and by one half after 10 years. The major adverse event with 5 additional years of tamoxifen use was a small increase in the risk for endometrial cancers with no increase in endometrial cancer deaths. There were no increases in fatal pulmonary emboli, stroke, or ischemic heart disease.

In postmenopausal women, estrogen is no longer made in the ovaries but rather in other tissues, such as fat and muscle, through the aromatase enzymes. Use of aromatase inhibitors alone, therefore, is an ineffective strategy in premenopausal women who still have ovarian estrogen production. Because this patient is still having periods, anastrozole will be ineffective; aromatase inhibitors should be used in postmenopausal women only.

Ovarian suppression with leuprolide or other gonadotropin-releasing hormone agonists combined with aromatase inhibitors has been shown to decrease the risk for breast cancer recurrence in premenopausal patients with early hormone receptor–positive breast cancer who receive chemotherapy for higher-risk cancers. Based on recent large randomized controlled trials, ovarian suppression does not improve disease-free or overall survival in patients with lower-risk cancers who did not receive initial chemotherapy.

KEY POINT

- In patients with low-risk, early-stage hormone receptor–positive breast cancer, use of tamoxifen for 10 years has been shown to decrease the risk for breast cancer recurrence and breast cancer mortality.

Bibliography

Burstein HJ, Temin S, Anderson H, et al. Adjuvant endocrine therapy for women with hormone receptor–positive breast cancer: American Society of Clinical Oncology clinical practice guideline focused update. J Clin Oncol. 2014 Jul 20;32(21):2255-69. [PMID: 24868023]

Item 83   Answer: B

Educational Objective: Treat classic Hodgkin lymphoma.

The most appropriate management for this young man with Hodgkin lymphoma is chemotherapy. Hodgkin lymphoma encompasses four classic histologic subtypes (nodular sclerosing, mixed cellularity, lymphocyte predominant, and lymphocyte depleted) and one nonclassic subtype (nodular lymphocyte-predominant subtype expressing the CD20 cell surface antigen). The presentation is consistent among subtypes and is characterized by palpable, firm lymph nodes and, in some patients, B symptoms (fever, night sweats, weight loss). Other physical examination findings include splenomegaly (30%) and hepatomegaly (5%). Hodgkin lymphoma is a highly curable disease, and the best outcomes are achieved with systemic therapy, sometimes in combination with radiation therapy. In the United States, doxorubicin, bleomycin, vinblastine, and dacarbazine is the most commonly used chemotherapy regimen for classic Hodgkin lymphoma. The need for radiation after chemotherapy for early-stage disease depends on the initial bulk of disease, the response to treatment, and patient and institutional preference.

Bone marrow biopsy, in the absence of unexplained blood abnormalities, is not indicated in the evaluation of patients with Hodgkin lymphoma. Staging no longer includes routine bone marrow biopsy, lymphangiography, or staging laparotomy and splenectomy. High-resolution CT, PET, and the routine use of systemic therapy in even early-stage disease have obviated the need for these staging modalities. Patients with extensive lymph node involvement above the diaphragm are now typically treated with chemotherapy; therefore, there is no need for staging laparotomy and splenectomy to determine the presence of microscopic disease below the diaphragm as the treatment would be no different. With this approach, the short-term morbidity of the staging surgery and long-term risk of overwhelming sepsis from asplenia can be avoided.

Radiation therapy may have a role in this patient's management; however, it is given after completion of chemotherapy for consolidation. Although radiation therapy alone may have a high cure rate for classic Hodgkin lymphoma, the cure rate is higher and toxicity is reduced when chemotherapy is used as the primary treatment modality.

KEY POINT

- All patients with classic Hodgkin lymphoma, regardless of stage, receive chemotherapy, usually the doxorubicin, bleomycin, vinblastine, and dacarbazine regimen, obviating the need for staging laparotomy and splenectomy.

Bibliography

Ansell SM. Hodgkin lymphoma: diagnosis and treatment. Mayo Clin Proc. 2015;90:1574-83. [PMID: 26541251] doi:10.1016/j.mayocp.2015.07.005

Item 84   Answer: B

Educational Objective: Treat advanced ovarian cancer with germline *BRCA1* and *BRCA2* mutations using olaparib.

The most appropriate treatment is an oral poly (adenosine diphosphate [ADP]-ribose) polymerase (PARP) inhibitor. Olaparib is an oral PARP inhibitor that is FDA-approved monotherapy for patients with germline *BRCA*-mutated advanced ovarian cancer previously treated with three or more lines of chemotherapy. PARP inhibition leads to the formation of double-stranded DNA breaks that in *BRCA*-competent tumors are repaired by homologous recombination. Tumors with germline *BRCA* mutations are unable to repair these defects, leading to cell death (referred to as synthetic lethality). A study of 298 patients with germline *BRCA1*- or *BRCA2*-associated cancers showed responses in ovarian, breast, pancreatic, and prostate cancers, with a 31% response rate and median duration of response of 7 months in platinum-resistant ovarian cancers. The most common side effects of olaparib were fatigue, nausea, vomiting, and anemia. In addition to the 15% of ovarian cancers with germline *BRCA1* and *BRCA2* mutations, up to 50% of high-grade serous ovarian cancers may be deficient in homologous recombination repair due to somatically acquired *BRCA1* and *BRCA2* mutations, epigenetic inactivation of *BRCA1*, or other defects in the homologous recombination pathway. These ovarian cancers with a "BRCAness" phenotype are also responsive to PARP inhibitors.

High-dose chemotherapy with hematopoietic stem cell transplantation is not recommended for the treatment of ovarian cancer, neither as initial treatment nor after recurrence.

Intraperitoneal chemotherapy is not effective in patients with recurrent ovarian cancer.

Given the activity of olaparib in the setting of a germline *BRCA1* mutation and this patient's good performance status, it is reasonable to recommend continuing cancer-directed therapy at this time. In patients who did not benefit from previous treatment and with poor performance status (Eastern Cooperative Oncology Group performance status, 3-4) or in those with bowel obstruction in the setting of refractory ovarian cancer, changing to supportive care would be appropriate.

KEY POINT

- Olaparib is FDA approved as monotherapy for patients with germline *BRCA*-mutated advanced ovarian cancer previously treated with three or more lines of chemotherapy.

Bibliography

Kaufman B, Shapira-Frommer R, Schmultzer RK, et al. Olaparib monotherapy in patients with advanced cancer and a germline BRCA1/2 mutation. J Clin Oncol. 2015 Jan 20;33(3):244-50. [PMID: 25366685]

Item 85   Answer: C

Educational Objective: Manage fertility in a female patient with cancer.

The most appropriate option for this patient is to meet with a fertility specialist. Young women with cancer who may wish to bear children after cancer treatment can be seen emergently and counseled about their options. An established fertility preservation option for a woman with a partner is in vitro fertilization with embryo freezing. Newer options include freezing of unfertilized eggs and ovarian cryopreservation with future reimplantation. Delaying initiation of chemotherapy for a brief time in a stable patient so she can be assessed and eggs or embryos harvested if appropriate is acceptable. Premenopausal women with breast cancer who do not wish to become pregnant should use a nonhormonal method of birth control.

Although a hormone receptor–negative, *HER2*-positive cancer is potentially aggressive and initiation of her neoadjuvant treatment should not be unnecessarily delayed, it is not an emergency and there is time for her to meet with a fertility specialist. With the use of chemotherapy and anti-*HER2* therapy in combination with appropriate local therapy, she should have a reasonably high likelihood of cure. Restricting her therapy to only local therapy with surgery and radiation decreases her chance for cure and is not the best option.

There is no evidence that women who become pregnant after a diagnosis of breast cancer have a higher rate of recurrence than similarly staged patients who do not become pregnant. Therefore, there is no reason to counsel this patient against future pregnancies.

KEY POINT

- For women who desire future childbearing who are medically stable, initiation of chemotherapy can be delayed for a brief time to allow assessment by a fertility specialist.

Bibliography

Lambertini M, Del Mastro L, Pescio MC, et al. Cancer and fertility preservation: international recommendations from an expert meeting. BMC Med. 2016 Jan 4;14:1.doi: 10.1186/s12916-015-0545-7. [PMID: 26728489]

Item 86   Answer: C

Educational Objective: Evaluate a woman with ovarian cancer with *BRCA1* and *BRCA2* genetic testing.

This patient should be referred to a genetic counselor for genetic testing for *BRCA1* and *BRCA2* mutations. Current guidelines recommend *BRCA1* and *BRCA2* genetic testing for all women with epithelial ovarian cancer, regardless of age of onset, family history, or ancestry. Of women with ovarian cancer, 10% to 15% carry a mutation in one of these genes. Approximately 75% of epithelial ovarian cancers are serous histology–the type most likely to be associated with a *BRCA1* or *BRCA2* mutation. This patient has a family history of breast cancer in a paternal aunt who was age 52 years, but even with no family history of breast or ovarian cancer, *BRCA1* and *BRCA2* genetic testing would still be recommended. Although she had her ovaries removed, positive test results for a *BRCA1* or *BRCA2* mutation would have implications for breast cancer risk and screening, with annual mammography and breast MRI recommended. She may also consider prophylactic mastectomies. If she carries a *BRCA1* or *BRCA2* mutation, her siblings and children have a 50% chance of inheriting the same mutation. Genetic testing is best performed by a genetic counselor, with appropriate pre- and post-test counseling.

Routine surveillance imaging studies are not recommended for monitoring patients in clinical remission after initial treatment; therefore, neither annual chest radiography nor an abdominal-pelvic CT scan in 3 months would be recommended unless the patient develops signs or symptoms suggestive of recurrent disease.

Hereditary nonpolyposis colon cancer (HNPCC), also known as Lynch syndrome, is an autosomal dominant disorder caused by a germline mutation in one of the DNA mismatch repair genes. Patients with Lynch syndrome have a 3% to 14% lifetime risk of ovarian cancer, and the possibility of HNPCC mutation testing should be considered in patients with ovarian cancer. However, testing for HNPCC mutations is usually only offered to patients who have a personal or family history, or both, of additional HNPCC-related cancers, particularly colorectal, small bowel or endometrial cancers, or transitional cell cancers of the renal pelvis or ureters. This patient has no personal or family history of these cancers and would not usually be offered HNPCC testing based on her history of ovarian cancer alone. Models such as PREMM$_{1,2,6}$ can be used to determine if a patient is eligible for HNPCC testing.

KEY POINT

- Current guidelines recommend *BRCA1* and *BRCA2* genetic testing for all women with epithelial ovarian cancer, regardless of age of onset, family history, or ancestry.

Bibliography

Alsop K, Fereday S, Meldrum C, et al. BRCA mutation frequency and patterns of treatment response in BRCA mutation-positive women with ovarian cancer: a report from the Australian Ovarian Cancer Study Group. J Clin Oncol. 2012 Jul 20;30(21);2654-63. Erratum in: J Clin Oncol. 2012 Nov 20;30(33):4180. [PMID: 22711857]

Item 87   Answer: D

Educational Objective: Treat gastric MALT lymphoma associated with *Helicobacter pylori* infection.

The appropriate treatment for this patient with gastric mucosa-associated lymphoid tissue (MALT) lymphoma associated with *Helicobacter pylori* infection is proton pump inhibitor

and dual antibiotic therapy, such as clarithromycin and amoxicillin, for 7 to 14 days. Chronic antigen stimulation can lead to clonal expansion of MALT and progress to malignant transformation manifesting as lymphoma. The lymphoma originates in B cells in the marginal zone of MALT and expresses the CD20 surface antigen. Eradication of *H. pylori* infection is associated with a high rate of response and long-term remission for these tumors and is the treatment of choice given its efficacy and ease of use. Regression of these lymphomas occurs slowly, and serial endoscopy will be needed to document this patient's response to therapy.

For MALT lymphoma that is not localized to the stomach or, rarely, that is localized to the stomach but does not respond to eradication of *H. pylori* infection, anti-CD20–directed therapy with rituximab may be effective. However, the initial treatment for this patient is eradication of *H. pylori* infection.

Although surgery can be used to treat localized gastrointestinal lymphomas, it is generally performed in the setting of a complication, such as hemorrhage or perforation, because other therapies are less invasive and may be as effective as or more effective than surgery.

Obtaining a PET scan to complete staging before making treatment recommendations is not needed for this patient. Marginal zone lymphomas are less likely to be detected by PET than follicular and aggressive lymphomas; therefore, the test is less sensitive and is unlikely to change management in the absence of other abnormal findings on CT scanning or clinical examination.

Radiation therapy is quite effective in the treatment of gastric marginal zone lymphoma, with high local control rates and relatively low toxicity. However, radiation would generally be reserved for patients for whom *H. pylori* eradication therapy has failed, those with residual or recurrent disease, or those who are *H. pylori*-negative and thus not likely to respond to antibiotic therapy.

KEY POINT

- The initial treatment for gastric mucosa-associated lymphoid tissue lymphoma associated with *Helicobacter pylori* infection is proton pump inhibitor and antibiotic therapy.

Bibliography

Zucca E, Bertoni F. The spectrum of MALT lymphoma at different sites: biological and therapeutic relevance. Blood. 2016;127:2082-92. [PMID: 26989205] doi:10.1182/blood-2015-12-624304

Item 88   Answer: A

Educational Objective: Provide chemoprevention in a patient at high risk for breast cancer.

Exemestane is the most appropriate preventive measure. This postmenopausal woman has lobular carcinoma in situ and atypical hyperplasia. These atypical lesions are associated with a 30% to 35% lifetime risk of breast cancer, and patients with these findings on breast biopsy are candidates for chemoprophylaxis with antiestrogens. Antiestrogen options include tamoxifen in both premenopausal and postmenopausal women as well as raloxifene and aromatase inhibitors (such as exemestane or anastrozole) in postmenopausal women. Because this patient had a deep venous thrombosis while taking oral contraceptives in the past, both tamoxifen and raloxifene are contraindicated, and exemestane is the best option if she is willing to take chemoprophylaxis.

Exemestane prophylaxis decreased the risk of invasive breast cancer by 65% in the National Cancer Institute of Canada (NCIC) Clinical Trials Group MAP.3 trial. Compared with placebo, there were no significant differences between the two arms in terms of skeletal fractures, cardiovascular events, other cancers, or treatment-related deaths. There were minimal differences in quality-of-life symptoms, such as vasomotor symptoms or arthralgia. Unlike tamoxifen and raloxifene, exemestane does not increase the risk for venous thromboembolic disease or endometrial cancer. Anastrozole, another aromatase inhibitor, has also been shown to decrease the risk of breast cancer in patients with high-risk conditions and is an alternate option for this patient.

Although vitamin D deficiency has been associated with a higher risk of breast cancer, there are no studies supporting high-dose vitamin D as an effective method to decrease the risk of breast cancer.

A low-fat diet has been shown to decrease breast cancer recurrence in patients with a diagnosis of estrogen receptor–negative invasive breast cancer but has not been shown to be of benefit in decreasing the risk of breast cancer in patients with atypical breast lesions or other high-risk conditions.

Both raloxifene and tamoxifen are contraindicated due to this patient's history of a deep venous thrombosis.

KEY POINT

- Patients with lobular carcinoma in situ and atypical hyperplasia are candidates for chemoprophylaxis with antiestrogens.

Bibliography

Goss PE, Ingle JN, Alés-Martínez JE, Cheung AM, Chlebowski RT, Wactawski-Wende J, et al; NCIC CTG MAP.3 Study Investigators. Exemestane for breast-cancer prevention in postmenopausal women. N Engl J Med. 2011;364:2381-91. [PMID: 21639806] doi:10.1056/NEJMoa1103507

Item 89   Answer: A

Educational Objective: Stage colorectal cancer.

A contrast-enhanced CT scan is the most appropriate imaging modality for staging of patients with a new diagnosis of colorectal cancer. The preoperative staging evaluation for colorectal cancer should include a complete colonoscopy (if technically feasible) and contrast-enhanced CT scans of the chest, abdomen, and pelvis. Preoperative measurement of serum carcinoembryonic antigen (CEA) levels is also routinely done. In addition to imaging the abdomen and pelvis, the chest should be imaged with CT to rule out pulmonary

metastases and to establish a baseline for surveillance. CT imaging with contrast provides the most reliable means of detecting the presence of metastatic disease to the lungs, liver, intra-abdominal lymph nodes, and peritoneum, which are the most common sites of metastatic spread; CT is also useful in planning appropriate therapy. Patients with local or locoregional rectal cancer require further preoperative staging with endorectal ultrasonography or a pelvic MRI to assess the depth of tumor penetration (T stage), degree of lymph node involvement (N stage), and any metastasis (M stage). Staging using the TNM cancer staging system is the most accurate predictor of outcome in patients with colorectal cancer.

CT colonography would not add to the information obtained from a completed colonoscopy. It is an acceptable alternative to a screening colonoscopy for healthy individuals at low risk but is not appropriate for individuals at high risk with unexplained microcytic anemia because it will not provide the option for biopsy if an abnormal result is found.

Liver MRI is a sensitive tool to identify liver metastases and is especially useful in the background of fatty liver, a condition that decreases the sensitivity of contrast CT. In clinical practice, liver MRI is reserved for patients with suspicious but not diagnostic lesions on CT or with contraindications to CT contrast agents.

National guidelines specifically do not recommend PET/CT scans for either preoperative staging or for postoperative surveillance. PET/CT scans have a higher false-positive and false-negative rates than is often appreciated, and have not been shown to improve the accuracy of preoperative staging.

KEY POINT

- Staging of patients with colorectal cancer should include a contrast-enhanced CT scan of the chest, abdomen, and pelvis to determine the extent of the cancer and to establish a baseline for surveillance.

Bibliography

Meyerhardt JA, Mangu PB, Flynn PJ, Korde L, Loprinzi CL, Minsky BD, et al; American Society of Clinical Oncology. Follow-up care, surveillance protocol, and secondary prevention measures for survivors of colorectal cancer: American Society of Clinical Oncology clinical practice guideline endorsement. J Clin Oncol. 2013;31:4465-70. [PMID: 24220554] doi:10.1200/JCO.2013.50.7442

Item 90   Answer: A

Educational Objective: Treat ductal carcinoma in situ.

Anastrozole is the most effective adjuvant therapy for ductal carcinoma in situ (DCIS) in postmenopausal women younger than 60 years. In the National Surgical Adjuvant Breast and Bowel Project (NSABP) B-35 clinical trial, 5 years of anastrozole was found to be more effective than 5 years of tamoxifen at decreasing both ipsilateral and contralateral breast cancer in postmenopausal women with DCIS who were younger than 60 years when starting treatment. Almost 95% of the anastrozole group was free from local or contralateral recurrence compared to 88% of the tamoxifen group. Overall 10-year survival, approximately 90%, was comparable between the two groups. In women age 60 years or older, anastrozole and tamoxifen yielded equivalent results. All women in this trial were postmenopausal and underwent lumpectomy and breast radiation. Unlike in invasive breast cancer, there is no survival advantage to treatment with antiestrogens for patients with DCIS, and such treatment is discussed as an option for patients who wish to decrease their risk of local recurrence and contralateral breast cancers. Because this patient is younger than 60 years, anastrozole is the most effective adjuvant antiestrogen option to achieve this goal.

Raloxifene is a selective estrogen receptor modulator (SERM) that can be used for breast cancer prophylaxis in patients with atypical breast lesions or in patients with a strong family history of breast cancer, but it is not an effective option for hormonal therapy in patients who have DCIS or invasive cancers.

Chemotherapy is not indicated in the treatment of DCIS. Chemotherapy is used as adjuvant treatment to decrease the risk of distant metastases in many invasive breast cancers, but in DCIS the risk of distant metastases is only 1%. Tamoxifen alone is an option for DCIS and could be discussed as an alternative to anastrozole, particularly in patients who wish to avoid potential anastrozole side effects, such as arthralgia and decreased bone density.

The 21-gene recurrence score testing is used in invasive cancers to determine the benefit of adding adjuvant chemotherapy in patients with estrogen receptor–positive cancers who will be treated with antiestrogen treatment. It is not helpful at determining the benefit of antiestrogen therapy in DCIS. The use of the 21-gene recurrence score in DCIS to determine if radiation can be safely omitted has been studied, but it is not yet approved for this use.

KEY POINT

- Anastrozole adjuvant therapy for ductal carcinoma in situ in postmenopausal patients younger than age 60 years decreases the risk of recurrent ipsilateral and contralateral breast cancer but does not decrease overall survival.

Bibliography

Margolese RG, Cecchini RS, Julian TB, Ganz PA, Costantino JP, Vallow LA, et al. Anastrozole versus tamoxifen in postmenopausal women with ductal carcinoma in situ undergoing lumpectomy plus radiotherapy (NSABP B-35): a randomised, double-blind, phase 3 clinical trial. Lancet. 2016;387:849-56. [PMID: 26686957] doi:10.1016/S0140-6736(15)01168-X

Item 91   Answer: E

Educational Objective: Evaluate for activating mutations in newly diagnosed metastatic nonsquamous non–small cell lung cancer.

The most appropriate management is to test for epidermal growth factor receptor (EGFR), ALK, and ROS1 alterations. Mutations in EGFR, translocation of the ALK and EML-4 genes, or mutation of the ROS1 gene have been identified in a few non–squamous cell lung cancers, usually adenocarcinomas.

Patients with EGFR mutations have been found to derive significant benefit from treatment with erlotinib, whereas those with ALK translocations and ROS1 mutations derive similar benefit from crizotinib; these agents are recommended as initial therapy in these patients when mutation status is known before treatment is initiated. In patients who must start treatment before mutation test results are available, these agents can be used later in treatment. Current standard care is to test for these molecular alterations in any patient diagnosed with nonsquamous metastatic non–small cell lung cancer. Although testing can also be considered in patients with squamous histologic findings, the likelihood of finding an alteration is very low.

Erlotinib would not be appropriate for this patient in the absence of a confirmed EGFR mutation because there is no evidence it is effective in patients without the mutation.

Prophylactic cranial irradiation is a standard treatment for patients with metastatic small cell lung cancer after chemotherapy. It is not indicated at the time of diagnosis in patients with non–small cell lung cancer.

Because this patient's thoracic spine lesion is not causing pain, there is no role for palliative radiotherapy at this time.

Patients are often treated with chemotherapy while the results of mutation testing are pending, but it is critical to obtain testing as soon as possible after diagnosis. For this reason, it is most appropriate to perform mutation testing before initiation of chemotherapy.

KEY POINT

- For nonsquamous metastatic non–small cell lung cancer, testing for molecular alterations in the epidermal growth factor receptor (EGFR), ALK, and ROS1 genes informs treatment options; patients with EGFR mutations derive significant benefit from treatment with erlotinib, whereas those with ALK translocations and ROS1 mutations derive similar benefit from crizotinib.

Bibliography

Dholaria B, Hammond W, Shreders A, Lou Y. Emerging therapeutic agents for lung cancer. J Hematol Oncol. 2016 Dec 9;9(1):138. [PMID: 27938382]

Item 92   Answer: A

Educational Objective: Manage very-low-risk prostate cancer with active surveillance.

The most appropriate management is active surveillance. The American College of Physicians recommends that clinicians inform men between 50 and 69 years of age about the limited potential benefits and substantial harms of screening for prostate cancer. The decision to screen should be based on the patient's general health and life expectancy and patient preferences. This patient has very-low-risk prostate cancer based on his biopsy findings and prostate-specific antigen (PSA) level at diagnosis. Management of such patients has evolved during the past several years. Although treatment is a reasonable consideration, recent literature supports the use of active surveillance, which is a program of scheduled assessments that include digital rectal examination, PSA measurement, and prostate biopsy. The purpose of active surveillance is to identify early evidence of cancer progression in an effort to limit treatment to those most likely to benefit. It is appropriate only for men with low-risk or very-low-risk prostate cancer who have a life expectancy of at least 10 years. Although no randomized data are available to support this strategy, available data indicate that the 15-year metastasis-free survival in appropriately selected patients is up to 97%. Active surveillance is currently considered appropriate standard care in this patient population.

Bone scan is not indicated for this asymptomatic patient because he has a very low likelihood of occult metastatic disease. A bone scan would be indicated only if there were signs or symptoms suggestive of osseous metastatic disease.

Leuprolide would be indicated for treatment of metastatic disease, and it can also be combined with radiation for treatment of high-risk or very-high-risk prostate cancer. However, it has no role in the treatment of an asymptomatic patient with very-low-risk prostate cancer.

Observation, sometimes called "watchful waiting," is distinct from active surveillance. These patients are provided palliative care if and when symptomatic progression requires medical intervention for control of symptoms. Observation is appropriate for elderly men with significant medical comorbidities that limit life expectancy. Treatment is not appropriate for these men based on their relatively short predicted life expectancy.

KEY POINT

- Active surveillance is a reasonable option in men with low-risk or very-low-risk prostate cancer who have a life expectancy of at least 10 years; active surveillance consists of scheduled assessments that include digital rectal examination, prostate-specific antigen measurement, and prostate biopsy.

Bibliography

Klotz L, Vesprini D, Sethukavalan P, Jethava V, Zhang L, Jain S, et al. Long-term follow-up of a large active surveillance cohort of patients with prostate cancer. J Clin Oncol. 2015;33:272-7. [PMID: 25512465] doi:10.1200/JCO.2014.55.1192

Item 93   Answer: B

Educational Objective: Perform lung cancer screening after treatment for head and neck cancer.

The most appropriate diagnostic test to perform next is low-dose noncontrast CT scan of the chest. Following definitive treatment for head and neck cancer, patients require ongoing surveillance to look for evidence of recurrence as well as evidence of second primary head and neck cancer. Especially in patients with smoking-related cancers, the risk of a second primary cancer is substantial. Surveillance consists of history, physical examination, and laryngoscopy to examine the entire upper aerodigestive tract.

This patient meets the criteria for screening for lung cancer, independent of the previous head and neck cancer. The U.S. Preventive Services Task Force (USPSTF) recommends annual low-dose CT imaging of the thorax for all patients 55 to 80 years of age who have a 30-pack-year history of smoking and are continuing to smoke or who have quit within the past 15 years. The history of head and neck cancer further increases the risk for subsequent lung cancer in this patient and heightens the importance of such screening.

There is currently no established role for imaging studies of the head and neck or PET/CT scan in the absence of signs or symptoms indicative of metastatic disease. Imaging is indicated, however, for evaluation of concerning signs or symptoms suggestive of cancer recurrence or a new primary cancer.

The most clearly defined risk factor for thyroid cancer is radiation exposure of the thyroid during childhood. Radiation treatment of childhood cancers is the most likely source of exposure, but other sources include fallout from atomic weapons and nuclear power plant accidents. There are no recommendations for thyroid cancer screening after radiation exposure in adulthood. Such patients should be screened periodically for hypothyroidism with a serum thyroid-stimulating hormone level, but routine thyroid ultrasonography is not recommended.

KEY POINT

- Many patients with head and neck cancer have significant smoking histories and should be offered lung cancer screening if they meet high-risk criteria.

Bibliography

Humphrey LL, Deffebach M, Pappas M, et al. Screening for lung cancer with low-dose computed tomography: a systematic review to update the US Preventive Services Task Force recommendation. Ann Intern Med. 2013 Sep 17;159(6):411-20. [PMID: 23897166]

Item 94   Answer: C

Educational Objective: Evaluate lymphadenopathy.

In this patient with multiple enlarged lymph nodes that have persisted for several weeks and with negative results on fine-needle aspiration, a surgical lymph node biopsy should be performed. A surgical biopsy is preferable to less invasive biopsy techniques because it provides more tissue for a definitive diagnosis and allows study of nodal architecture, provided the nodes being evaluated are easily and safely accessible (for example, cervical, axillary, or inguinal).

Although a core biopsy of lymph nodes can be performed and may be diagnostic, it may not provide adequate tissue, particularly if the samples are small and there is necrosis, fibrosis, or only partial or patchy involvement of the node. In the case of lymphoma, which is likely in this patient, up to 35% of core biopsies of lymph nodes must be followed by an excisional lymph node biopsy to fully classify lymphoma. However, core biopsy may be an appropriate next step if the nodes are deep (for example, retroperitoneal) in an attempt to avoid a more invasive procedure.

A PET/CT scan in this patient may be abnormal but will not be diagnostic and may be positive for inflammatory or infectious conditions as well as lymphoma and other malignancies. Although staging with PET/CT may eventually be needed in this patient, that test would be more appropriate after a diagnosis of lymphoma has been made.

Patients with soft, small, freely movable lymph nodes that are limited to the cervical or inguinal area and who have no other significant history or physical examination findings can be followed with serial examinations over 6 to 8 weeks and require no additional investigation. However, from 30% to 50% of patients with supraclavicular lymphadenopathy have an associated malignancy. Right supraclavicular lymphadenopathy is associated with cancer in the thorax, including the mediastinum, lungs, or esophagus. Left supraclavicular lymphadenopathy is associated with abdominal malignancy and lymphoma. Because fine-needle aspiration cytology is an insensitive test, particularly in the diagnosis of lymphoma, further evaluation with lymph node excision is indicated.

KEY POINT

- Diagnosis and classification of lymphoma are generally established based on lymph node biopsy.

Bibliography

Frederiksen JK, Sharma M, Casulo C, Burack WR. Systematic review of the effectiveness of fine-needle aspiration and/or core needle biopsy for subclassifying lymphoma. Arch Pathol Lab Med. 2015;139:245-51. [PMID: 25611108] doi:10.5858/arpa.2013-0674-RA

Item 95   Answer: A

Educational Objective: Manage metastatic non–small cell lung cancer with palliative care.

The most appropriate management in addition to platinum-based chemotherapy is palliative care consultation. In patients with metastatic non–small cell lung cancer, early institution of palliative care has been shown to improve both quality of life and survival. Palliative care does not preclude aggressive cancer treatment with platinum-based combination chemotherapy and other interventions. Palliative care complements cancer treatment through its emphasis on controlling both cancer- and treatment-related symptoms that may interfere with effective treatment. It also makes it easier for patients and treating physicians to decide when treatment is no longer indicated, either because of insufficient efficacy or problematic toxicity. Current standard care is to offer palliative care services at the time of diagnosis with metastatic non–small cell lung cancer and, by extension, in patients diagnosed with any advanced incurable cancer.

PET/CT scan plays no role in this patient's management, as CT and bone scans have already been performed and have already documented the extent of metastatic disease.

Prophylactic cranial irradiation is indicated in selected patients with small cell lung cancer, but it is not appropriate in patients with non–small cell lung cancer.

Epidermal growth factor receptor (*EGFR*) mutation testing is not indicated because this patient has squamous cell carcinoma and has a smoking history. The incidence of *EGFR* mutation in such a patient is very low, and routine testing is not indicated.

KEY POINT

- In patients with metastatic non–small cell lung cancer, early institution of palliative care has been shown to improve both quality of life and survival; palliative care does not preclude aggressive cancer treatment.

Bibliography

Temel JS, Greer JA, Muzikansky A, et al. Early palliative care for patients with metastatic non-small-cell lung cancer. N Engl J Med. 2010 Aug 19;363(8):733-42. [PMID: 20818875]

Item 96   Answer: B

Educational Objective: Treat mismatch repair–deficient colorectal cancer.

An immune checkpoint inhibitor is the most reasonable treatment. This patient now has metastatic colorectal cancer with a mismatch repair–deficient tumor. Tumors may be mismatch repair deficient either because of a germline mutation (Lynch syndrome) or a somatic mutation or epigenetic silencing that is limited to the tumor. In either case, these mismatch repair–deficient tumors represent the very limited subset of metastatic colorectal cancers that have shown substantial benefit in a few small studies from treatment with immune checkpoint inhibitors, such as pembrolizumab or nivolumab. Unfortunately, these mismatch repair–deficient tumors represent only a small minority of patients with metastatic cancer. For most patients with metastatic colorectal disease (greater than 95%), immune checkpoint inhibitors have thus far been essentially ineffective.

Epidermal growth factor receptor inhibitors such as panitumumab or cetuximab are inappropriate for consideration in a patient with a mutation in *KRAS* or any other *RAS* gene because they are potentially active only in tumors with nonmutated *KRAS*, *NRAS*, and *BRAF* genes.

Several trials have examined the efficacy of simultaneously targeting both vascular endothelial growth factor and the endothelial growth factor receptor with dual antibody therapy. However, this synergic approach has not been shown to be effective, and the results suggest that dual antibody therapy for this patient is not the next most reasonable treatment option.

Although supportive comfort care only should be considered in patients who are either too sick for treatment or who have exhausted all reasonable treatment options, such a course of action would not be the first consideration in a fully functional patient with a meaningful treatment option.

KEY POINT

- An immune checkpoint inhibitor, such as pembrolizumab, shows benefit in patients with metastatic mismatch repair–deficient colorectal cancer.

Bibliography

Le DT, Uram JN, Wang H, Bartlett BR, Kemberling H, Eyring AD, et al. PD-1 Blockade in Tumors with Mismatch-Repair Deficiency. N Engl J Med. 2015;372:2509-20. [PMID: 26028255] doi:10.1056/NEJMoa1500596

Item 97   Answer: A

Educational Objective: **Prevent recurrent pneumonia in a patient with chronic lymphocytic leukemia.**

This patient with chronic lymphocytic leukemia (CLL) has had three hospitalizations for pneumonia in the past year, and assessing his immunoglobulin levels would be appropriate. Patients with CLL frequently are hypogammaglobulinemic and are prone to sinus and pulmonary infection. Intravenous immunoglobulin G replacement therapy has been shown to reduce the risk of infections in patients with CLL with documented hypogammaglobulinemia. Surveillance for viral infections and early initiation of antimicrobial agents for presumed bacterial infections are also essential.

Although this patient has lymphocytosis, lymphadenopathy, and splenomegaly, their presence alone is not an indication to treat his underlying CLL in the absence of symptoms or more significant cytopenias.

Although the patient has only 5% neutrophils and 1% bands, his total leukocyte count is 34,000/µL (34 × 10⁹/L), and thus he is not significantly neutropenic. Even if he were neutropenic, long-term granulocyte colony-stimulating factor (G-CSF) injections would not be appropriate.

Ibrutinib is an appropriate therapy for CLL that requires treatment because it is taken orally, is relatively easy for most patients to tolerate, and is associated with high response rates in both untreated and previously treated patients. However, there is no clear benefit to immediate initiation of ibrutinib therapy in asymptomatic patients.

KEY POINT

- Intravenous immunoglobulin G replacement therapy reduces the risk of infections in patients with chronic lymphocytic leukemia with documented hypogammaglobulinemia.

Bibliography

Sánchez-Ramón S, Dhalla F, Chapel H. Challenges in the role of gammaglobulin replacement therapy and vaccination strategies for hematological malignancy. Front Immunol. 2016;7:317. [PMID: 27597852] doi:10.3389/fimmu.2016.00317

Item 98   Answer: D

Educational Objective: **Evaluate recurrent colorectal cancer.**

The *RAS* mutation status of an archived primary tumor specimen should be tested next. This patient has colon cancer that has metastasized to the liver and lungs in a pattern that is not surgically curable. Chemotherapy is the treatment of choice, and several different agents will be considered. This patient may be a candidate for treatment with an epidermal growth factor receptor inhibitor, such as cetuximab or panitumumab. All patients with metastatic colorectal cancer should have tumor genotyping to identify mutations in the *KRAS* and *NRAS* genes because cetuximab and panitumumab are inactive in the 40% to 50% of tumors that harbor these mutations. It is therefore standard practice to obtain *RAS* mutational status of tumors of patients with metastatic disease. *RAS* mutations, when they occur, occur early in carcinogenesis, such that the *RAS* mutation status of the primary tumor and a subsequent recurrence are very highly concordant, and rebiopsy of the tumor for *RAS* status is not necessary. The absence of *KRAS* or *NRAS* mutations does not predict therapeutic success with cetuximab or panitumumab; up to 40% of tumors with wild type (nonmutated) genes will not respond to these agents. Multigene sequencing may open some experimental options, but it does not yield actionable information in terms of standard management options at this time. Thus, the expense is not warranted outside of a potential research setting.

The presentation and imaging of this patient, who was at high risk for recurrence, are virtually diagnostic of metastatic colon cancer, and an invasive procedure, such as needle biopsy, for pathologic confirmation is neither required nor appropriate.

A PET/CT scan would not provide any additional information to the imaging that is already available and would not change management.

KEY POINT

- The *RAS* mutational status of tumors should be tested in patients with metastatic disease to determine if they are candidates for treatment with an epidermal growth factor receptor inhibitor, such as cetuximab or panitumumab.

Bibliography

Allegra CJ, Rumble RB, Hamilton SR, Mangu PB, Roach N, Hantel A, et al. Extended RAS gene mutation testing in metastatic colorectal carcinoma to predict response to anti-epidermal growth factor receptor monoclonal antibody therapy: American Society of Clinical Oncology provisional clinical opinion update 2015. J Clin Oncol. 2016;34:179-85. [PMID: 26438111] doi:10.1200/JCO.2015.63.9674

Item 99   Answer: C

Educational Objective: **Treat non–small cell lung cancer that responds to first-line chemotherapy with maintenance chemotherapy.**

The most appropriate treatment is pemetrexed maintenance chemotherapy. In the absence of a driver mutation, the current standard for management of patients with metastatic non–small cell lung cancer and good performance status is platinum-based chemotherapy. Many combinations can be used, including carboplatin and pemetrexed, which was used for this patient. Treatment is given for four to six cycles depending on response. There is no evidence to support continuation of treatment after six cycles. However, maintenance chemotherapy, such as with single-agent pemetrexed, has been shown to improve progression-free survival and, in some studies, overall survival. Therefore, maintenance chemotherapy is an appropriate option for patients with metastatic non–small cell lung cancer who respond to first-line platinum-based chemotherapy. Either the nonplatinum agent used for first-line treatment is continued as a single agent ("continuation maintenance") or an alternative agent, most commonly docetaxel, is used ("switch maintenance").

Continuation of platinum-based chemotherapy with a different partner agent is not indicated for this patient. There is no evidence supporting the use of carboplatin beyond six cycles in patients with metastatic non–small cell lung cancer. In addition, this patient has been diagnosed with adenocarcinoma, and currently available evidence indicates that gemcitabine is not effective in patients with adenocarcinoma.

Because this patient did not have an epidermal growth factor receptor (*EGFR*) mutation, there is no role for erlotinib treatment. Erlotinib is effective only in patients with an identified activating *EGFR* mutation.

For patients with metastatic disease, radiation is reserved for palliation of cancer-related symptoms, most commonly pain. It has no role in treatment of the cancer.

KEY POINT

- Maintenance chemotherapy is an appropriate option for patients with metastatic non–small cell lung cancer who respond to first-line platinum-based chemotherapy.

Bibliography

Ciuleanu T, Brodowicz T, Zielinski C, et al. Maintenance pemetrexed plus best supportive care versus placebo plus best supportive care for non-small-cell lung cancer: a randomised, double-blind, phase 3 study. Lancet. 2009 Oct 24;374(9699):1432-40. [PMID: 19767093]

Item 100   Answer: C

Educational Objective: Treat early-stage laryngeal cancer.

The most appropriate treatment in this patient with early-stage laryngeal cancer is radiation therapy. In early-stage laryngeal cancer, it is important to consider predicted efficacy and anticipated voice quality and other potential functional impairments when deciding on a treatment plan. For patients with early-stage disease, cure rates are high with surgery and with radiation. For patients treated with surgery, the use of adjuvant radiation or combined chemotherapy and radiation is recommended based on findings at surgery. However, open hemilaryngectomy results in suboptimal functional outcomes and is associated with complications, including bleeding, infection, laryngocutaneous fistula, and aspiration. Radiation is highly effective with low morbidity, and functional outcomes are generally superior in patients with laryngeal cancer who are treated with radiation compared with those treated with surgery. Radiation therapy often causes xerostomia, thickening of saliva, mucositis, dysphagia, odynophagia, and malnutrition.

Use of combined chemotherapy and radiation is appropriate for patients with locally advanced laryngeal cancer who need total laryngectomy for effective treatment. The most commonly used agent is high-dose cisplatin. Cetuximab, a monoclonal antibody directed against the epidermal growth factor receptor, is also an accepted care option in this setting. However, these therapies are not indicated in patients with early-stage laryngeal cancer, who are effectively treated with radiation alone.

KEY POINT

- Early-stage laryngeal cancer is most appropriately treated with radiation alone because it is highly effective in that area, has low morbidity, and is associated with superior voice quality compared with patients who are treated with surgery.

Bibliography

Chera BS, Amdur RJ, Morris CG, Kirwan JM, Mendenhall WM. T1N0 to T2N0 squamous cell carcinoma of the glottic larynx treated with definitive radiotherapy. Int J Radiat Oncol Biol Phys. 2010;78:461-6. [PMID: 20153124] doi:10.1016/j.ijrobp.2009.08.066

Item 101   Answer: E

Educational Objective: Treat stage I rectal cancer.

The most appropriate treatment is surgery. Based on the information available, this person has a T2N0, stage I midrectal cancer. Patients with rectal tumors that are not full thickness and do not have lymph node involvement (stage I) on pretreatment imaging usually undergo surgery, with a total mesorectal excision being the preferred procedure. The mesorectum is a fatty sheath covering the rectum that contains the regional lymph nodes. A total mesorectal excision entails a sharp dissection of the pelvis outside of the mesorectum to allow removal of the mesorectum fully intact en bloc with the rectum. Because this patient's tumor is 8 cm from the anal verge, this is a midrectal tumor. Resection of such a tumor would be anticipated to be sphincter sparing and so would not be anticipated to require a permanent colostomy. However, considerable expertise is required to avoid complications with this procedure, which should be performed only by a subspecialized surgeon.

If postoperative findings upstage the tumor to stage II or III, then consideration of further interventions, such as radiation or chemotherapy, may be warranted. However, data do not support a role for adding either chemotherapy or radiation therapy to the management of surgically confirmed stage I rectal cancer.

KEY POINT

- Rectal cancers without full thickness penetration of the bowel wall or involved lymph nodes are stage I and are treated with surgical resection.

Bibliography

Allegra CJ, Yothers G, O'Connell MJ, Beart RW, Wozniak TF, Pitot HC, et al. Neoadjuvant 5-FU or capecitabine plus radiation with or without oxaliplatin in rectal cancer patients: a phase III randomized clinical trial. J Natl Cancer Inst. 2015;107. [PMID: 26374429] doi:10.1093/jnci/djv248

Item 102   Answer: C

Educational Objective: Prevent chemotherapy-induced neutropenia.

This patient has fever and neutropenia caused by her chemotherapy and should start granulocyte colony-stimulating factor (G-CSF) with her next cycle of chemotherapy. Febrile neutropenia is defined as a single fever (101 °F [38.3 °C]) or sustained elevated temperature (38 °C [100.4 °F]) in a patient with a current or anticipated absolute neutrophil count less than 500 cells/µL (0.5×10^9/L). Most infections are believed to arise from the patient's endogenous flora. Neutropenia typically occurs 5 to 15 days after administration of chemotherapy. G-CSF and granulocyte-macrophage colony-stimulating factor can be given prophylactically to patients receiving chemotherapeutic regimens that carry a high risk of neutropenia and as secondary prophylaxis in patients such as this one, who have had a previous episode.

In this patient, initiating G-CSF or pegylated G-CSF on day 2 of her next cycle of chemotherapy would reduce the risk of another bout of febrile neutropenia and help maintain the dose intensity of her chemotherapy.

Reducing this patient's dose of chemotherapy for the next cycle would not be an appropriate strategy to avoid neutropenia because she is a young patient being treated with curative intent, and reducing her chemotherapy dosages might compromise her outcome. The prophylactic use of G-CSF is a better strategy.

There is little benefit to starting G-CSF once a patient already has fever and neutropenia. Although there may be a slightly more rapid return of neutrophils, the benefit is minimal, and there is no demonstrated reduction in mortality.

Fluoroquinolone prophylaxis is typically reserved for high-risk patients with ongoing neutropenia. High-risk patients typically include those undergoing allogeneic hematopoietic cell transplantation or receiving induction chemotherapy for acute leukemia. Neither of these applies to this patient.

KEY POINT

- Granulocyte colony-stimulating factor is effective for prophylaxis and secondary prophylaxis of neutropenia in patients undergoing chemotherapy but has little benefit in patients who are currently neutropenic.

Bibliography

Smith TJ, Bohlke K, Lyman GH, et al; American Society of Clinical Oncology. Recommendations for the use of WBC growth factors: American Society of Clinical Oncology Clinical practice guideline update. J Clin Oncol. 2015 Oct 1;33(28):3199-212. doi: 10.1200/JCO.2015.62.3488. [PMID: 26169616]

Item 103   Answer: B

Educational Objective: Treat a gastrointestinal stromal tumor with imatinib.

The most appropriate management for this patient is oral imatinib for 3 years. Gastrointestinal stromal tumors (GISTs) most commonly occur in the stomach, although they can arise anywhere in the digestive tract. Although rare, they are the most common sarcoma of the digestive tract. Location outside of the stomach, larger size, and higher mitotic index are all factors that increase the risk of recurrence after resection and indicate use of adjuvant therapy. Almost all GISTs have an activating mutation in the c-KIT proto-oncogene, leading to constitutive activation of the KIT receptor tyrosine kinase. Therefore, she should be treated with the small-molecule receptor tyrosine kinase inhibitor imatinib, which blocks c-KIT tyrosine kinase phosphorylation. In such high-risk patients, recurrence-free survival and overall survival are superior in patients who receive 3 years of imatinib therapy compared with 1 year of therapy.

Rituximab is a genetically engineered chimeric monoclonal antibody against CD20, a B-cell specific surface antigen. CD20 regulates cell cycle initiation. Rituximab binds to the antigen on the cell surface, activating complement-dependent B-cell cytotoxicity, and binds to human Fc receptors, mediating cell killing through an antibody-dependent cellular toxicity. Rituximab is used in the treatment of rheumatoid arthritis, ANCA-related vasculitis, chronic lymphocytic leukemia, and non-Hodgkin lymphoma. As predicted by its mechanism of action, it is not effective in the treatment of GIST.

Because GISTs are relatively resistant to radiation therapy, such treatment is not used after a complete resection.

Small gastric GISTs with low mitotic indices may often be managed with surgery alone, but because this patient has a GIST with several factors that increase the risk of recurrence, observation without further therapy is not sufficient.

KEY POINT

- High-risk gastrointestinal stromal tumors should be treated with surgery and 3 years of adjuvant imatinib.

Bibliography

Joensuu H, Eriksson M, Sundby Hall K, Hartmann JT, Pink D, Schütte J, et al. One vs three years of adjuvant imatinib for operable gastrointestinal stromal tumor: a randomized trial. JAMA. 2012;307:1265-72. [PMID: 22453568] doi:10.1001/jama.2012.347

Item 104   Answer: B

Educational Objective: Manage superior vena cava syndrome.

This patient has symptoms, signs, and CT scan findings consistent with superior vena cava (SVC) syndrome due to a mediastinal malignancy, with symptoms developing over 2 weeks, and should receive a mediastinoscopy. It is important to establish a tissue diagnosis before treatment. There are no peripheral sites to biopsy in this case: the only abnormal result found on imaging and examination is the mediastinal mass. Although some patients may be unable to have surgery if they are in severe respiratory distress, are hemodynamically unstable, or have evidence of cerebral edema, most patients who present with SVC syndrome can tolerate a surgical biopsy. Mediastinoscopy with biopsy

CONT.

has a diagnostic yield of over 90% and is more likely than core biopsies to obtain specimens adequate for determining nodal architecture and histologic subtype if a lymphoma is present. SVC syndrome is caused by thrombosis or other nonmalignant obstructions in about 35% of cases. Of malignant causes, approximately 75% are due to lung cancers, with non–small cell lung cancers most common. Lymphoma and metastatic cancer each cause about 10% of cases; thymoma, germ cell cancer, and mesothelioma are each present in 1% to 3% of cases.

Dexamethasone is often used to treat SVC syndrome and, particularly in lymphomas, may decrease symptoms. However, dexamethasone may obscure histologic findings in lymphomas, and a biopsy should be done before starting the patient on glucocorticoids.

Percutaneous intravascular stents can be placed in patients with respiratory distress before tissue biopsy, but this patient is not having respiratory distress and does not require stent placement.

Radiation requires an initial tissue diagnosis and is used as initial treatment in some but not all malignancies that cause SVC syndrome. If this patient has a lymphoma, as is clinically most likely, she would be treated with initial chemotherapy.

KEY POINT

- Most patients with superior vena cava syndrome do not require emergency intervention, and a tissue biopsy should be obtained.

Bibliography
Wilson LD, Detterbeck FC, Yahalom J. Clinical practice. Superior vena cava syndrome with malignant causes. N Engl J Med. 2007;356:1862-9. Erratum in: N Engl J Med. 2008 Mar 6;358(10):1083. [PMID: 17476012]

Item 105   Answer: C

Educational Objective: Treat locally advanced head and neck cancer.

The most appropriate treatment is cisplatin plus radiation. Treatment of head and neck cancer in the adjuvant setting depends heavily on the results of pathologic analysis of the resection specimen. This should include assessment of human papillomavirus (HPV) status based on tumor staining for p16, a viral protein. HPV has been found to be responsible for most oropharynx cancers (tonsil and base of tongue). Most patients diagnosed with HPV-associated head and neck cancer are younger than expected and do not have traditional risk factors, such as the patient in this case. Positivity for HPV has a significant impact on prognosis but does not yet affect treatment decision making. Options for treatment include no adjuvant therapy, radiation alone, and combined chemotherapy and radiation. No adjuvant therapy is required for early-stage cancers with no high-risk pathologic features, such as poorly differentiated histology and lymphovascular invasion. For early-stage cancers with high-risk features and for some

locally advanced cancers (specifically any node-positive cancer), radiation alone is appropriate. Combined chemotherapy and radiation has been shown to improve survival in patients with locally advanced cancer after surgery when there are positive surgical margins or evidence of nodal metastases with extracapsular extension. Extracapsular extension refers to squamous cell carcinoma that breaks through the outer capsule of the lymph node and extends into surrounding tissues. Notably, the number of lymph nodes involved has not been clearly shown to be a predictor of benefit with combined chemotherapy and radiation adjuvant therapy. This patient underwent surgery and had evidence of extracapsular extension; therefore, combined cisplatin and radiation is the most appropriate adjuvant treatment.

Chemotherapy alone, either with single-agent cisplatin or cisplatin-based combination chemotherapy, is not indicated. Adjuvant chemotherapy has not been shown to improve survival or other treatment outcomes in this setting.

Vaccination of children before sexual activity is important in the primary prevention of HPV infection and the reduction of the incidence of oropharyngeal, cervical, and anal cancers associated with this virus. Immunization plays no role in patients who are already infected with HPV.

Radiation alone is not indicated owing to the presence of extracapsular extension.

KEY POINT

- Combined chemotherapy and radiation improves survival in patients with locally advanced head and neck cancer after surgery when there are positive surgical margins or evidence of nodal metastases with extracapsular extension.

Bibliography
Adelstein D, Gillison ML, Pfister DG, Spencer S, Adkins D, Brizel DM, et al. NCCN guidelines insights: head and neck cancers, version 2.2017. J Natl Compr Canc Netw. 2017;15:761-770. [PMID: 28596256] doi:10.6004/jnccn.2017.0101

Item 106   Answer: B

Educational Objective: Treat stage II non–small cell lung cancer with adjuvant chemotherapy after resection.

The most appropriate treatment is adjuvant chemotherapy. Most (80%) lung cancers are non–small cell lung cancers (NSCLCs), with the most common type being adenocarcinoma of the lung. Current treatment options for NSCLCs include surgical resection, radiation therapy, chemotherapy, and targeted therapies. Several studies have found a small but significant survival benefit associated with adjuvant chemotherapy in patients with stage II and stage III NSCLC. Although both cisplatin- and carboplatin-based chemotherapy regimens have been studied, only cisplatin-based chemotherapy has been shown to improve survival. At least four different cisplatin-based combination regimens can be used for adjuvant chemotherapy treatment; however, patients must be selected carefully because toxicity can be substantial. Based on this survival benefit, cisplatin-based chemotherapy is recommended after surgery for stage II and stage III NSCLC in patients such as this one without contraindications to chemotherapy.

Combined chemotherapy and radiation has not been shown to improve outcomes in patients with NSCLC after surgery with negative margins. Combined chemotherapy and radiation is used, however, as a primary therapy for patients with stage III lung cancer with clinically evident mediastinal lymphadenopathy noted at the time of initial evaluation; this is because this group of patients does not typically fare well with surgery.

Radiation as a single modality has no role in the adjuvant treatment of resected NSCLC in the absence of positive surgical margins. In the presence of positive margins, it is reasonable to recommend radiation.

Observation is not recommended as a routine management strategy because of the survival benefit associated with chemotherapy treatment. Observation would be appropriate only for a patient who could not be treated with chemotherapy owing to medical contraindications or personal preference.

KEY POINT

- Adjuvant cisplatin-based chemotherapy for stage II and stage III non–small cell lung cancer provides a survival advantage.

Bibliography

Pignon JP, Tribodet H, Scagliotti GV; LACE Collaborative Group. Lung adjuvant cisplatin evaluation: a pooled analysis by the LACE Collaborative Group. J Clin Oncol. 2008 Jul 20;26(21):3552-9. [PMID: 18506026]

Item 107   Answer: D

Educational Objective: Manage cancer of unknown primary site in a patient with poor performance status.

This patient should receive supportive management and hospice care. He has moderately differentiated adenocarcinoma of unknown primary site with extensive metastatic disease and severe debilitation, jaundice, and evidence of substantial nutritional deficiency as indicated by cachexia, bitemporal wasting, and hypoalbuminemia. This is a patient who is too debilitated and deconditioned to have a realistic chance of benefit from chemotherapy, and the most appropriate management is to focus on symptom control and comfort. Hospice care would be the most effective means of accomplishing these goals.

In a more medically fit patient with adenocarcinoma in a predominantly abdominal pattern, treatment with a gastrointestinal chemotherapy regimen, such as 5-fluorouracil (5-FU), leucovorin, and oxaliplatin (FOLFOX); 5-FU, leucovorin, and irinotecan (FOLFIRI); or 5-FU, leucovorin, irinotecan, and oxaliplatin (FOLFIRINOX) would be a reasonable

consideration; however, this patient is too debilitated to tolerate these treatments.

A platinum-based germ cell regimen would be appropriate for a younger patient with a midline poorly differentiated carcinoma, but this patient does not meet these criteria and, again, is too sick to tolerate this treatment.

Hepatic arterial embolization is an appropriate consideration for patients with well-differentiated neuroendocrine tumors or primary liver cancer who are well enough to tolerate such treatments and whose disease is largely confined to the liver.

KEY POINT

- Patients with several comorbidities and poor performance status are unlikely to benefit from aggressive chemotherapy, and such treatment is likely to cause serious or life-threatening toxicity.

Bibliography

Fizazi K, Greco FA, Pavlidis N, Daugaard G, Oien K, Pentheroudakis G; ESMO Guidelines Committee. Cancers of unknown primary site: ESMO Clinical Practice Guidelines for diagnosis, treatment and follow-up. Ann Oncol. 2015;26 Suppl 5:v133-8. [PMID: 26314775] doi:10.1093/annonc/mdv305

Item 108   Answer: C

Educational Objective: Diagnose renal cell carcinoma in a patient with erythrocytosis.

The most appropriate diagnostic test to perform next is CT scan of the abdomen. Although symptomatic erythrocytosis is most commonly associated with myeloproliferative neoplasms, such as polycythemia vera, it is important to assess for all possible causes. This patient has symptomatic erythrocytosis in the setting of a markedly elevated erythropoietin level and in the absence of organomegaly. This combination of findings is most consistent with autonomous production of erythropoietin, most commonly by an underlying tumor. Tumors known to be associated with this paraneoplastic syndrome include kidney cancer and, less frequently, hepatocellular carcinoma, cerebellar hemangioblastoma, pheochromocytoma, and uterine myomata. Clues to tumor-related erythrocytosis may include microscopic hematuria (kidney cancer); abnormal liver chemistry test results, hepatitis B, hemochromatosis, or cirrhosis (hepatocellular); headache, abnormal neurological findings (hemangioblastoma); hypertension, abnormal electrolyte levels, or hyperglycemia (pheochromocytoma); and menorrhagia (uterine myomata). In the absence of suggestive symptoms or findings, a CT scan of the abdomen is indicated as the first study for further evaluation of this patient.

Bone marrow biopsy and serum *JAK-2* mutation testing can be done to evaluate for possible underlying polycythemia vera. However, polycythemia vera is most commonly seen in the setting of a low or an undetectable erythropoietin level, not with a markedly elevated level as seen in this patient. In addition, polycythemia vera is commonly associated with an elevated leukocyte and platelet count, as well as hepatosplenomegaly, but these are not present in this patient. These findings make the diagnosis of polycythemia vera less likely; therefore, testing to evaluate for that diagnosis is not indicated as initial management.

Chest radiography has no role in this patient's evaluation because lung cancer is not associated with paraneoplastic erythrocytosis. In addition, chest radiography cannot evaluate for any of the cancers that are associated with erythrocytosis.

KEY POINT

- Erythrocytosis is a common paraneoplastic syndrome associated with kidney cancer.

Bibliography

Morais C, Johnson DW, Vesey DA, Gobe GC. Functional significance of erythropoietin in renal cell carcinoma. BMC Cancer. 2013 Jan 10;13:14. [PMID: 23305401]

Item 109   Answer: D

Educational Objective: Treat oligometastatic liver metastases of colorectal cancer.

The most appropriate management is resection of all lesions. The role of postoperative surveillance in patients with colorectal cancer is to identify surgically curable recurrence, such as oligometastatic liver disease or lung metastases. The liver is the primary metastatic site for patients with colorectal cancer. About one third of patients with metastatic disease will have it confined to the liver and will be amenable to surgical resection and cure, with or without adjuvant chemotherapy. The criteria for surgical resection of hepatic metastases have expanded from the "three lesions or less" rule. Most patients with good performance status can be considered for surgical resection unless they have one of three conditions: tumor involvement of the common artery or portal vein or common bile duct; more than 70% liver involvement, more than six involved segments, or involvement of all three hepatic veins; and a predicted inadequate hepatic reserve after resection. This patient has recurrent colorectal cancer in a single organ in an oligometastatic pattern. As such, he is a candidate for surgery with curative intent.

Hepatic arterial embolization is not routinely used to treat colorectal cancer because colorectal tumors tend not to be very vascular. Further, it is a palliative, noncurative intervention. It is more appropriately considered in the management of unresectable neuroendocrine tumors or primary liver cancers.

A needle biopsy should not be done because it will not change management. The clinical presentation in this patient is compelling enough to diagnose recurrent colorectal cancer; a negative needle biopsy specimen would be assumed to be a false negative and would not alter management. Surgical resection would be the appropriate intervention regardless of the results of a biopsy.

Because this cancer is potentially curable, palliative chemotherapy should not be considered.

KEY POINT

- Patients with recurrent colorectal cancer in a single organ in an oligometastatic pattern are candidates for surgery with curative intent.

Bibliography

Smith JJ, D'Angelica MI. Surgical management of hepatic metastases of colorectal cancer. Hematol Oncol Clin North Am. 2015;29:61-84. [PMID: 25475573] doi:10.1016/j.hoc.2014.09.003

Item 110   Answer: A

Educational Objective: Treat carcinoma of unknown primary site in a woman with isolated axillary lymph node metastases.

The most appropriate management is to treat an axillary presentation of adenocarcinoma in a woman as a likely primary breast cancer. Patients with cancer of unknown primary involving a single lymph node or single lymph node region may have potentially treatable disease. Women with isolated axillary lymphadenopathy that is found to be an adenocarcinoma or a poorly differentiated carcinoma should be assumed to have locoregional breast cancer until proved otherwise. Breast MRI is indicated in this setting and reveals a primary breast mass in 50% to 70% of patients. In addition, immunohistochemical staining for estrogen receptor, progesterone receptor, HER2 expression, and other breast cancer–specific markers should be performed on the biopsy specimen to help establish the diagnosis of breast tumor and guide therapy.

If the breast MRI scan is normal, the patient should be managed as for primary breast cancer and should undergo axillary lymph node dissection. Although in the past mastectomy was typically recommended in this setting, if no primary cancer is detected on the mammogram or breast MRI scan, axillary dissection with subsequent breast and axillary radiation is an accepted alternative to mastectomy. In patients with triple-negative breast cancer with axillary node involvement, adjuvant chemotherapy is indicated and can be given either before or after axillary dissection.

The management and prognosis are similar whether or not a primary breast cancer is identified, and, in the absence of distant metastases, patients should be treated with curative intent. Women who are found to have other sites of metastatic adenocarcinoma in addition to the axillary lymph node should be treated for metastatic breast cancer.

Letrozole is a hormonal therapy used for hormone receptor–positive breast cancers. This patient's cancer is estrogen and progesterone receptor–negative, and she would not receive any benefit from adjuvant hormonal therapy.

Radiation to the breast and axilla will be recommended after completing surgery and adjuvant chemotherapy but is not given as initial management before these other modalities.

Given the potential curability of this cancer, observation alone would also be inadequate.

> **KEY POINT**
>
> - Women with isolated axillary lymph-node adenocarcinoma metastases should be presumptively considered to have locoregional breast cancer and should be treated as such.

Bibliography

Fizazi K, Greco FA, Pavlidis N, Daugaard G, Oien K, Pentheroudakis G; ESMO Guidelines Committee. Cancers of unknown primary site: ESMO Clinical Practice Guidelines for diagnosis, treatment and follow-up. Ann Oncol. 2015;26 Suppl 5:v133-8. [PMID: 26314775] doi:10.1093/annonc/mdv305

Item 111   Answer: D

Educational Objective: Prevent tumor lysis syndrome in a patient with Burkitt lymphoma.

The most appropriate treatment is the administration of rasburicase along with intravenous hydration with normal saline and furosemide. Malignancies associated with rapid cell turnover can release large quantities of electrolytes and procoagulants into the circulation, causing the potentially life-threatening complication of tumor lysis syndrome. Spontaneous tumor lysis syndrome occurs commonly in patients with leukemia and Burkitt lymphoma and after treatment of bulky large B-cell lymphoma or advanced chronic lymphocytic leukemia. Rapid cell breakdown results in hyperkalemia, hyperphosphatemia, hyperuricemia, hypocalcemia, and disseminated intravascular coagulation. Hyperuricemia can lead to uric acid nephropathy and acute kidney injury. In this patient, proceeding with rasburicase, intravenous hydration, and furosemide with plans for prompt initiation of systemic therapy is appropriate. Rasburicase can rapidly and effectively lower serum urate levels and reduce the risk of acute uric acid nephropathy seen with tumor lysis syndrome. Because of its rapid onset of action and ability to lower urate levels quickly, which may be renoprotective, rasburicase should be administered before initiation of chemotherapy in patients with underlying kidney disease or those with signs of kidney disease, including an elevated serum creatinine level and a low urine output. Intravenous hydration with diuretics to maintain a high urine output is also key to reducing the risk of kidney failure and managing hyperkalemia and hyperphosphatemia, as well as hyperuricemia.

Large-volume intravenous hydration with normal saline plus administration of allopurinol to limit hyperuricemia is usually effective to prevent tumor lysis syndrome. However, this patient has hyperuricemia and an elevated serum creatinine level, making rasburicase preferred to allopurinol.

Whereas glucocorticoids and radiation therapy may be effective at shrinking this patient's tumors, such therapy will not prevent and will likely exacerbate tumor lysis syndrome.

> **KEY POINT**
>
> - Burkitt lymphoma often presents with early signs of tumor lysis, and it is important to institute tumor lysis syndrome prophylaxis before initiation of chemotherapy.

Bibliography

Casulo C, Friedberg J. Treating Burkitt lymphoma in adults. Curr Hematol Malig Rep. 2015;10:266-71. [PMID: 26013028] doi:10.1007/s11899-015-0263-4

Item 112   Answer: C

Educational Objective: Treat breast cancer using ovarian suppression along with aromatase-inhibitor therapy.

The most appropriate treatment is leuprolide and an aromatase inhibitor. Two prospective randomized clinical trials have shown the superiority of ovarian suppression with leuprolide plus an aromatase inhibitor, such as exemestane, over ovarian suppression plus tamoxifen or tamoxifen alone in premenopausal women with higher-risk hormone receptor–positive early breast cancer.

Analyzing the trials together, disease-free survival at 5 years was 91.1% in the ovarian-suppression-plus-exemestane group and 88.3% in the ovarian-suppression-plus-tamoxifen group. Overall survival was the same in both groups. Compared with tamoxifen alone, ovarian suppression with tamoxifen improved disease-free survival, which was further improved by ovarian suppression plus exemestane. The benefit was particularly dramatic in women younger than 35 years who had a 15.7% absolute improvement in 5-year disease-free survival with the use of ovarian suppression and exemestane compared to tamoxifen alone. Adverse effects were seen more frequently in the patients on ovarian suppression, and by 4 years, 21% of patients had stopped ovarian suppression due to side effects. In patients who do not tolerate initial treatment with ovarian suppression and exemestane, ovarian suppression with tamoxifen can be used, transitioning to an aromatase inhibitor after 2 to 3 years if tolerated.

An aromatase inhibitor is ineffective in premenopausal women unless concomitant ovarian suppression is given.

The benefit of ovarian suppression alone is similar to tamoxifen alone and inferior to the option of ovarian suppression and an aromatase inhibitor.

In patients who require initial chemotherapy and remain premenopausal, treatment with tamoxifen alone has a higher risk of breast cancer recurrence than ovarian suppression plus an aromatase inhibitor.

> **KEY POINT**
>
> - Ovarian suppression along with antiestrogen therapy is recommended to decrease breast cancer recurrence in women with high-risk, early-stage, hormone receptor–positive breast cancer who remain premenopausal after chemotherapy.

Bibliography

Pagani O, Regan MM, Walley BA, Fleming GF, Colleoni M, Láng I, et al; TEXT and SOFT Investigators. Adjuvant exemestane with ovarian suppression in premenopausal breast cancer. N Engl J Med. 2014;371:107-18. [PMID: 24881463] doi:10.1056/NEJMoa1404037

Item 113   Answer: E

Educational Objective: Manage a residual mass after treatment of diffuse large B-cell lymphoma.

For this patient with a residual mass after treatment for diffuse large B-cell lymphoma, the appropriate management is observation with serial CT scanning to ensure that the mass is stable. This patient's current CT and PET scan results demonstrate an excellent response to therapy. Her disease was characterized by bulky retroperitoneal lymphadenopathy, and it is probable that the residual mass found on CT scan represents scar tissue rather than viable tumor. Bulky lymphoma masses, when treated with effective systemic therapy, often do not show complete resolution by CT scan. The PET scan results also suggest the absence of active disease, although PET scan is not 100% sensitive or specific. In this circumstance, observation by serial CT (with or without further PET scanning) is most appropriate.

An autologous stem cell transplant could be an appropriate option for a patient with relapsed or residual disease. Even if the PET scan showed higher residual uptake, given the potential for false-positive CT and PET scan results, proceeding to further therapy without tissue documentation of recurrence would not be appropriate.

Although biopsy could be considered to document the presence or absence of viable lymphoma (and should be done to definitively document disease before initiation of any salvage treatment), this procedure could be deferred in a patient with a low suspicion for disease who has a favorable CT scan and metabolic response by PET, unless there are reasons to expect residual or progressive disease.

Consolidative radiation therapy has been used for patients with large cell lymphoma and initial bulky disease and residual mass. This treatment can decrease the risk of local recurrence; however, routine use has not been proven to improve survival or cure, and many patients without active disease would be irradiated.

KEY POINT

- In a patient with a residual mass after treatment of bulky diffuse large B-cell lymphoma, observation with serial CT scanning is appropriate if diagnostic testing shows a low likelihood of active disease.

Bibliography

Thanarajasingam G, Bennani-Baiti N, Thompson CA. PET-CT in staging, response evaluation, and surveillance of lymphoma. Curr Treat Options Oncol. 2016;17:24. [PMID: 27032646] doi:10.1007/s11864-016-0399-z

Item 114   Answer: B

Educational Objective: Treat advanced ovarian cancer with intravenous and intraperitoneal chemotherapy.

The most appropriate initial treatment for this patient with advanced ovarian cancer is intravenous (IV) and intraperitoneal (IP) cisplatin and paclitaxel chemotherapy. This treatment is associated with a 16-month improvement in median overall survival in women with stage III ovarian cancer and no residual mass greater than 1 cm after surgical debulking compared with intravenous chemotherapy alone. Patients receiving IP/IV chemotherapy have a higher incidence of toxicities, including leukopenia, thrombocytopenia, fever, infection, fatigue, pain, and gastrointestinal events. Less than half of patients starting IP/IV therapy can complete all six cycles of therapy. However, the National Cancer Institute encourages the use of IP/IV chemotherapy for optimally debulked stage III ovarian cancer. Obstacles to the widespread adoption of IP/IV chemotherapy include not only the higher toxicities but also placement of an IP catheter and training of nursing staff in IP chemotherapy administration. The original IP/IV regimen required hospitalization for the first 3 days of each cycle. Modified regimens that allow all treatment to be given on an outpatient basis are now accepted options.

High-dose chemotherapy with hematopoietic stem cell transplantation is not recommended for the treatment of ovarian cancer, neither as initial treatment nor after recurrence.

Patients with left colon or rectosigmoid resections had a higher risk of discontinuing IP therapy, so this approach is no longer recommended in patients who undergo bowel resection. The types of catheters used have improved, with fewer catheter-related problems.

Olaparib is approved for use to treat relapsed ovarian cancer in women with *BRCA1* or *BRCA2* germline mutations. This oral poly(ADP-ribose) polymerase (PARP) inhibitor is FDA approved as monotherapy for patients with germline *BRCA*-mutated advanced ovarian cancer previously treated with three or more lines of chemotherapy. Patients with germline *BRCA1*- or *BRCA2*-associated cancers show responses in ovarian, breast, pancreatic, and prostate cancers, with a 31% response rate and median duration of response of 7 months in platinum-resistant ovarian cancers. Olaparib is not used as initial therapy in ovarian cancer.

KEY POINT

- Intravenous and intraperitoneal cisplatin and paclitaxel chemotherapy is a treatment option for patients with advanced ovarian cancer.

Bibliography

Wright AA, Cronin A, Milne DE, et al. Use and effectiveness of intraperitoneal chemotherapy for treatment of ovarian cancer. J Clin Oncol. 2015 Sep 10;33(26):2841-7. [PMID: 26240233]

Item 115   Answer: C

Educational Objective: Treat a patient with a metastatic well-differentiated gastrointestinal neuroendocrine tumor.

The most appropriate management for this patient is to not intervene now and repeat the CT scan in 3 months. Neuroendocrine tumors can arise from the endocrine cells of the pancreas or neuroendocrine cells of the aerodigestive tract. These two entities look and behave similarly; however, several anticancer agents that show activity against pancreatic neuroendocrine tumors show little or no activity against aerodigestive tumors. This patient is asymptomatic with an incidental finding of a well-differentiated, low-grade, small-bowel gastrointestinal neuroendocrine tumor (previously known as carcinoid) with multiple small metastases to the liver. The liver is overwhelmingly the most common site of metastasis, and diagnosis is often established through an incidental finding of hepatomegaly or abnormal findings on an imaging study. Such tumors are often asymptomatic and indolent, and asymptomatic patients may do well, with minimal growth and no symptoms for years, even with metastatic disease. As such, there is no urgency to intervene. Follow-up examination and imaging at approximately 3 months is appropriate. Although perhaps 25% of metastatic gastrointestinal neuroendocrine tumors will elaborate serotonin, a hormone causing diarrhea or facial flushing (carcinoid syndrome), most patients have a hormonally nonfunctional tumor and thus do not require treatment for these symptoms. In patients whose disease appears stable on the 3-month CT scan, further monitoring with serial imaging at 3- to 6-month intervals is appropriate.

Hepatic arterial embolization may be helpful in shrinking liver metastases or reducing hormonal output from functional tumors and may be considered in a patient with progressive or symptomatic disease.

Obstruction of the bowel from a well-differentiated neuroendocrine primary tumor is very uncommon, so prophylactic surgery to remove the primary bowel tumor in an asymptomatic patient with metastases is not indicated.

Chemotherapy for gastrointestinal neuroendocrine tumors is of limited utility in asymptomatic patients with small volume disease that has not been demonstrated to be progressive. In these patients, the toxicities of treatment outweigh the benefit.

KEY POINT

- Well-differentiated, low-grade, metastatic gastrointestinal neuroendocrine tumors are often indolent and asymptomatic and do not require immediate treatment.

Bibliography

Singh S, Asa SL, Dey C, Kennecke H, Laidley D, Law C, et al. Diagnosis and management of gastrointestinal neuroendocrine tumors: an evidence-based Canadian consensus. Cancer Treat Rev. 2016;47:32-45. [PMID: 27236421] doi:10.1016/j.ctrv.2016.05.003

Item 116   Answer: D

Educational Objective: Treat hormone receptor-positive breast cancer in a premenopausal patient with primary breast radiation and tamoxifen.

In addition to primary breast radiation, this patient should receive adjuvant tamoxifen. She has a 2.5-cm, node-negative, hormone receptor-positive, *HER2*-negative breast cancer. Gene-expression assays, such as the 21-gene recurrence score, are helpful in determining the benefit of adding adjuvant chemotherapy to tamoxifen in patients with node-negative, hormone receptor-positive, *HER2*-negative breast cancer. The 21-gene recurrence score has been shown to be not only prognostic for the risk of distant recurrence but also predictive for the magnitude of benefit of adding chemotherapy to tamoxifen.

A prospective trial of patients with hormone receptor-positive, *HER2*-negative, node-negative breast cancers with 21-gene recurrence scores of 0 to 10 was published in November 2015. The 5-year rate of freedom from recurrence of breast cancer at a distant or local site was 98.7% with endocrine therapy alone. This is standard care for patients with early breast cancer with these characteristics.

Adjuvant chemotherapy, given either alone or followed by tamoxifen, does not improve the disease-free or overall survival in patients with hormone receptor-positive, node-negative breast cancers with low-risk recurrence scores. The SOFT (Suppression of Ovarian Function Trial) study showed that the combination of ovarian suppression and an aromatase inhibitor is superior to tamoxifen in patients with higher-risk early breast cancer who require initial chemotherapy and remain premenopausal, but it is not superior to tamoxifen alone in women with low-risk breast cancers who do not need adjuvant chemotherapy.

KEY POINT

- Primary breast radiation and tamoxifen are indicated for premenopausal patients with node-negative, hormone receptor-positive, *HER2*-negative breast cancer with low-risk recurrence scores.

Bibliography

Tevaarwerk AJ, Wisinski KB, O'Regan RM. Endocrine therapy in premenopausal hormone receptor-positive breast cancer. J Oncol Pract. 2016 Nov;12(11):1148-1156. [PMID: 27858538]

Item 117   Answer: E

Educational Objective: Manage prostate cancer in a patient with significant comorbidities.

The most appropriate management in this patient with early-stage prostate cancer and significant medical comorbidities is observation. His medical history is consistent with a predicted life expectancy of less than 5 years, his voiding symptoms are better after treatment with an α-blocker, and he has no other symptoms attributable to his cancer. Based on the typically indolent course of a low-grade localized prostate cancer, this patient will most likely die as a result of one of his other medical conditions rather than his prostate cancer. He is also at significant risk for complications associated with treatment. These issues should all be discussed with the patient so he can understand the competing issues involved and thereby permit him to be an active participant in decision making.

Observation is distinct from active surveillance. Observation consists of periodic follow-up to assess symptoms related to cancer progression that require palliation. Active surveillance, however, is a plan to defer definitive prostate cancer therapy until there is evidence of cancer progression based on evidence from systematic monitoring, including changes in prostate-specific antigen level and findings on digital rectal examination, biopsy results, or both. Because this patient's early-stage cancer is not appropriate for treatment, he is not a candidate for active surveillance.

Androgen deprivation therapy is not a recommended treatment for early-stage prostate cancer and will expose this patient to unnecessary side effects, including decreased libido and erectile dysfunction, osteoporosis, fatigue, gynecomastia, and hot flushes.

Bone scan is very unlikely to reveal bone metastases in asymptomatic men who have low-risk prostate cancer and, therefore, is not indicated.

Radiation is not appropriate for this patient because of his short predicted life expectancy, the indolent course of early-stage prostate cancer, and prostate radiation side effects, including bladder, bowel, and rectum injury along with erectile dysfunction.

KEY POINT

- For men with early-stage prostate cancer who have limited life expectancy or significant medical comorbidities, observation is the most appropriate management.

Bibliography

Daskivich TJ, Fan KH, Koyama T, et al. Effect of age, tumor risk, and comorbidity on competing risks for survival in a U.S. population-based cohort of men with prostate cancer. Ann Intern Med. 2013 May 21;158(10):709-17. [PMID: 23689764]

Item 118   Answer: D

Educational Objective: Avoid unnecessary imaging in a patient with stage IIB invasive breast cancer.

No imaging studies are necessary for this patient with stage IIB invasive breast cancer. Patients with clinical stages I and II invasive breast cancers are at low risk for metastases at the time of diagnosis of their initial breast cancer. There is a lack of evidence suggesting that routine imaging studies improve the detection of metastatic disease or survival. Clinical staging based on history, physical examination,

and serum liver chemistry tests and alkaline phosphatase measurements is the standard for confirming that patients have early-stage breast cancer. Staging imaging studies are recommended only if signs or symptoms suggest metastatic disease.

Bone scan is indicated for patients with localized bone pain or elevated serum alkaline phosphatase levels.

Chest CT is recommended for patients who have pulmonary symptoms or abnormal results on lung examination. Abdominal and possibly pelvic CT is indicated in patients with abnormal results on serum liver chemistry tests or with abnormal alkaline phosphatase levels, abdominal symptoms, or abnormal findings on physical examination of the abdomen or pelvis.

PET scan is not indicated in the staging of clinical stage I, II, or operable stage III breast cancer. In patients with large stage III cancers or inflammatory breast cancer, staging imaging studies are indicated and detect occult distant metastases in 10% to 21% of patients.

Despite a campaign to educate physicians about the lack of benefit of staging imaging studies in clinical stages I to II breast cancer, these tests continue to be done in a large percentage of patients with early breast cancer. A study from Ontario showed that after publication of the American Clinical Society's "Top Five" 2012 guidelines recommending against routine imaging studies in stages I and II breast cancer, 84% of patients with operable early-stage cancer had at least one imaging staging study. Radiologically evident metastases were found in only 2 of 200 patients, both of whom had clinical stage III breast cancer.

KEY POINT

- Clinical staging based on history, physical examination, and serum liver chemistry tests and alkaline phosphatase measurements is the standard to confirm early-stage breast cancer; staging imaging studies are recommended only if signs or symptoms suggest metastatic disease.

Bibliography

Schnipper LE, Smith TJ, Raghavan D, Blayney DW, Ganz PA, Mulvey TM, et al. American Society of Clinical Oncology identifies five key opportunities to improve care and reduce costs: the top five list for oncology. J Clin Oncol. 2012;30:1715-24. [PMID: 22493340] doi:10.1200/JCO.2012.42.8375

Item 119   Answer: A

Educational Objective: Treat hairy cell leukemia.

This patient has hairy cell leukemia, a low-grade B-cell disorder characterized by cytopenia and splenomegaly without lymphadenopathy. Hairy cells (classic appearance of thread-like projections emanating from the cell surface) are typically seen in the peripheral blood smear, and findings on flow cytometry demonstrate positivity for surface markers CD20, CD11c, CD25, and CD103. Cladribine is an appropriate initial therapy for hairy cell leukemia.

Cladribine, as well as another purine nucleoside analogue, pentostatin, is associated with complete response rates exceeding 80% to 90%. A single 5- or 7-day course of cladribine is often all that is required. Many patients have durable remissions, although a significant minority do relapse and require retreatment with the same or alternate agents.

Interferon-alfa therapy is active in the treatment of hairy cell leukemia but is rarely used anymore given its toxicity and inferior response rate compared to other agents.

Hairy cell leukemia is typically CD20 positive and should respond to rituximab. However, clinical trials of rituximab have shown mixed results. Many experts reserve rituximab for patients failing two cycles of a purine nucleoside analogue. Rituximab is not given as initial therapy.

Hypersplenism in hairy cell leukemia may play a larger role in the mechanism of cytopenias compared to other lymphoproliferative disorders. Splenectomy can be an effective treatment for relieving symptoms and ameliorating cytopenias associated with hairy cell leukemia. Before effective systemic therapies were available, splenectomy was the initial treatment of choice. However, splenectomy does not treat the underlying marrow infiltration and is no longer considered appropriate initial therapy.

Some patients with hairy cell leukemia are asymptomatic and do not require immediate therapy. However, this patient has fatigue and anemia, so observation would not be appropriate.

KEY POINT

- Initial therapy for hairy cell leukemia is a purine nucleoside analogue, either cladribine or pentostatin.

Bibliography

Getta BM, Park JH, Tallman MS. Hairy cell leukemia: past, present and future. Best Pract Res Clin Haematol. 2015;28:269-72. [PMID: 26614906] doi:10.1016/j.beha.2015.10.015

Item 120   Answer: A

Educational Objective: Diagnose transformed follicular lymphoma.

This patient has a 7-year history of follicular lymphoma with a recent onset of systemic symptoms and a rapidly enlarging right inguinal lymph node. Biopsy of the right inguinal node would be appropriate to evaluate for histologic progression of disease. Transformation to diffuse large B-cell lymphoma occurs in approximately 30% of patients with follicular lymphoma. Transformation may be suggested by a change in the clinical pattern of disease, such as the development of new systemic symptoms or rapid progression of a localized area of disease. In addition, a rise in serum lactate dehydrogenase level or markedly higher areas of standardized uptake values on PET scanning should raise suspicion of transformation. In such cases, a new lymph node biopsy is required to establish the occurrence of transformation. In this patient, rapid progression in just one area of disease, the onset of systemic symptoms, and a high serum lactate dehydrogenase level raise suspicion for transformation. If transformation to another, more aggressive lymphoma is demonstrated, a more aggressive course of treatment would be appropriate. Thus, a new biopsy in this setting is important to optimize management.

Idelalisib, a PI3K kinase inhibitor, is an oral agent that has shown significant activity for the treatment of relapsed follicular lymphoma. It has a reasonably high rate of partial response. It would be appropriate in this patient if transformation is excluded.

Radiation for palliation to a single symptomatic site can be considered for relapsed follicular lymphoma. However, this patient has systemic symptoms, and active systemic options are available; therefore, single-site palliative radiation would not be preferred at this time.

Treating with additional chemotherapy would be a reasonable option for this patient, given her excellent and prolonged initial response, if she has documented relapse of follicular lymphoma and requires retreatment. However, transformation to a large B-cell lymphoma should first be excluded because it may require a different treatment strategy.

KEY POINT

- Transformation of follicular lymphoma to an aggressive non-Hodgkin lymphoma may be suggested by a change in the clinical pattern of disease, such as the development of new systemic symptoms or rapid progression of a localized area of disease.

Bibliography

Casulo C, Burack WR, Friedberg JW. Transformed follicular non-Hodgkin lymphoma. Blood. 2015;125:40-7. [PMID: 25499449] doi:10.1182/blood-2014-04-516815

Item 121   Answer: A

Educational Objective: Evaluate isolated inguinal lymphadenopathy.

The most appropriate diagnostic test to perform is an anoscopy. In the United States, approximately 35,000 patients receive a diagnosis of cancer of unknown primary (CUP) annually. The clinical evaluation should not involve an exhaustive search for a primary site because detection of an asymptomatic and occult primary tumor does not improve outcome. In a patient with CUP, it is important to look for treatable subgroups. Patients with CUP who have lymphadenopathy in a single lymph node or single lymph node region belong to a potentially more treatable subgroup of patients with CUP. Most patients with carcinoma, especially squamous cell carcinoma, involving inguinal lymph nodes have a primary site in the genital or anorectal area. In women this necessitates a careful examination of the vulva, vagina, and cervix. Men require a careful examination of the penis. Men and women should have a careful examination of the perineal skin, a digital rectal examination, and an anoscopy. This patient's examination is complete except for digital rectal examination and anoscopy. The anal region drains directly to the inguinal lymph nodes.

Cancers of the anus that metastasize to the inguinal nodes are local-regionally advanced but not distantly metastatic and are potentially curable with a combination of chemotherapy and radiation therapy.

A bone scan would not be useful in identifying a treatable primary source and would not be indicated in a patient with an enlarged inguinal lymph node in the absence of specific bone pain.

Colonoscopy and upper endoscopy would be indicated in a patient presenting with gastrointestinal symptoms, unexplained anemia, or blood in the stool.

Although PET scans may sometimes suggest the location of a primary tumor, these findings are rarely definitive and do not improve long-term outcome.

Measurement of serum tumor marker levels, such as carcinoembryonic antigen, CA-19-9, CA-15-3, and CA-125, is rarely helpful and virtually never diagnostic.

KEY POINT

- Squamous cell carcinoma or poorly differentiated carcinoma presenting as isolated inguinal lymphadenopathy should prompt a careful examination of the vulva, vagina, and cervix in women, penis in men, and perineal skin and anus in both men and women.

Bibliography

Fizazi K, Greco FA, Pavlidis N, Daugaard G, Oien K, Pentheroudakis G; ESMO Guidelines Committee. Cancers of unknown primary site: ESMO Clinical Practice Guidelines for diagnosis, treatment and follow-up. Ann Oncol. 2015;26 Suppl 5:v133-8. [PMID: 26314775] doi:10.1093/annonc/mdv305

Item 122   Answer: D

Educational Objective: Treat stage II colon cancer without high-risk features.

No further treatment is needed. This patient has stage II colorectal cancer (invades full thickness of the bowel [T3]), and lymph nodes are not involved [N0]). Patients with stage II colon cancer do not have a clear survival advantage with administration of adjuvant chemotherapy; consequently, surgery alone is the acceptable standard practice for most patients. Exceptions are patients with stage II colon cancer with characteristics associated with a high risk for recurrence (T4 primary tumor [invasion into adjacent structures or through the peritoneum], lymphovascular invasion, inadequate lymph node sampling [fewer than 12 lymph nodes examined], poorly differentiated histology, elevated postoperative carcinoembryonic antigen (CEA), or clinical perforation or obstruction). In these patients, the prognosis is similar to that of patients with stage III disease, and adjuvant chemotherapy may be appropriate. Exposing this patient to the toxicity of chemotherapy is not warranted, as data do not support a survival benefit in such patients. For patients with stage II disease and a high risk for recurrence, treatment with 5-fluororuracil/leucovorin or capecitabine may be appropriate. Patients with stage II disease with a substantial number of high-risk features may at times be considered for oxaliplatin-containing chemotherapy, such as parenteral 5-fluorouracil, leucovorin, and oxaliplatin (FOLFOX).

Patients with stage III disease (lymph node metastases) are routinely treated with oxaliplatin-containing regimens, such as FOLFOX, after resection. The combination of capecitabine plus intravenous oxaliplatin is also an acceptable regimen for adjuvant treatment of patients with stage III colon cancer.

Because local recurrence of colon cancer rarely develops and because it can be difficult to isolate the small bowel from the radiation field, radiation therapy, either alone or in combination with chemotherapy, does not have a role in the routine management of patients with stage III colon cancer. In addition, radiation to the small bowel may cause substantial toxicity.

KEY POINT

- Patients with stage II colon cancer without high-risk features are unlikely to benefit from adjuvant treatment.

Bibliography

Dotan E, Cohen SJ. Challenges in the management of stage II colon cancer. Semin Oncol. 2011;38:511-20. [PMID: 21810510] doi:10.1053/j.seminoncol.2011.05.005

Item 123   Answer: C

Educational Objective: Treat melanoma with a solitary brain metastasis.

Surgical resection of the brain lesion in this patient with previous melanoma would be the most appropriate treatment. Assuming the lesion is surgically accessible, resection would provide a tissue diagnosis confirming the suspicion of metastatic melanoma, provide the best long-term local control, and offer the best potential for cure. Postoperative radiosurgery to the tumor bed may be considered to reduce the risk for recurrence. Melanoma may be associated with solitary or oligometastatic disease, and metastasectomy can be curative in a significant minority of these patients. Metastasectomy with or without systemic medical therapy is associated with increased overall survival compared to systemic medical therapy alone in patients with stage IV melanoma. Based on a cohort analysis of data from a randomized clinical trial, surgery was associated with a median overall survival of 15.8 months compared to 6.9 months with systemic therapy alone. The 4-year overall survival also favored the surgery group, 20.8% versus 7% in the group receiving systemic therapy alone.

Immunotherapy with nivolumab, pembrolizumab, or ipilimumab plus nivolumab is used in the treatment of metastatic melanoma but would not be recommended as first-line therapy if there is a resectable isolated metastasis, as in this patient.

Gamma knife or other forms of radiosurgery can provide high rates of local control while minimizing radiation exposure to the rest of the brain. With a large mass, however, surgical resection would provide a better probability of long-term control.

Treatment with BRAF/MEK inhibitor combination therapy, such as dabrafenib plus trametinib or vemurafenib plus cobimetinib, is effective for *BRAF*-mutated melanoma and can target disease in the brain, but these agents would not be preferred as initial therapy here because they are less effective than metastasectomy in increasing survival and offering a chance of cure.

Whole brain radiation therapy is reserved for patients with multiple metastases that are not amenable to focal therapies (surgery or radiosurgery). Although whole brain radiation therapy does decrease the risk of newer metastases, it is associated with an increased risk of late neurologic dysfunction.

KEY POINT

- Melanoma may be associated with solitary or oligo-metastatic disease, and metastasectomy will prolong survival and can be curative in these patients.

Bibliography

Deutsch GB, Kirchoff DD, Faries MB. Metastasectomy for stage IV melanoma. Surg Oncol Clin N Am. 2015;24:279-98. [PMID: 25769712] doi:10.1016/j.soc.2014.12.006

Item 124   **Answer:**   **C**

Educational Objective: Treat locally advanced anal cancer.

Pelvic radiation therapy with concurrent chemotherapy is the most appropriate treatment. Anal carcinoma is a rare but increasing cause of cancer and accounts for approximately 2% of gastrointestinal cancers. Most anal cancers are squamous cell carcinomas and are associated with human papillomavirus (HPV) infection, particularly HPV 16 and HPV 18. Risk factors for anal cancer include HPV infection; sexually transmitted infections; multiple sex partners; men having sex with men; receptive anal intercourse; history of vaginal, cervical, or vulvar cancer; immunosuppression due to hematologic malignancy; solid organ transplantation; or HIV infection. Most patients present with a perianal lesion or mass associated with rectal bleeding or anal discomfort. This patient has locally invasive, node-positive squamous cell cancer of the anus. Curative-intent treatment with the combination of pelvic radiation therapy and concurrent systemic chemotherapy is indicated. This would be appropriate for patients with stages I, II, and III anal cancer. Mitomycin plus fluorouracil has been the standard chemotherapy regimen in patients with anal cancer for the past 50 years, although capecitabine, an oral fluorouracil prodrug, is now often used instead of parenteral fluorouracil.

Randomized studies of anal cancer treatment have shown radiation plus chemotherapy to be superior to radiation alone and 5-fluorouracil plus mitomycin to be superior to 5-fluorouracil alone.

Surgery for anal cancer is reserved as a salvage treatment for either local recurrence or incomplete response to chemotherapy plus radiation therapy, and is potentially curative. However, because definitive surgery must remove the anal sphincter, a placement of a permanent colostomy would be required.

HPV vaccine is approved for and has been shown to prevent anal HPV infection and anal intraepithelial neoplasia, precursors of anal cancer. However, HPV immunization is not an effective therapy for anal cancer once it has developed.

KEY POINT

- Anal cancer is often curable with combined chemotherapy and radiation, avoiding surgery.

Bibliography

James RD, Glynne-Jones R, Meadows HM, Cunningham D, Myint AS, Saunders MP, et al. Mitomycin or cisplatin chemoradiation with or without maintenance chemotherapy for treatment of squamous-cell carcinoma of the anus (ACT II): a randomised, phase 3, open-label, 2×2 factorial trial. Lancet Oncol. 2013;14:516-24. [PMID: 23578724] doi:10.1016/S1470-2045(13)70086-X

Item 125   **Answer:**   **B**

Educational Objective: Treat early-stage breast cancer with extended aromatase-inhibitor therapy.

The most appropriate management for this patient with early-stage breast cancer is to continue anastrozole for 5 years. In the North America Breast Cancer Group MA.17R trial, 1918 postmenopausal women with hormone receptor–positive early breast cancer who had completed 5 years of an aromatase inhibitor were randomly assigned to 5 years of letrozole or placebo. Most of the women had also received 5 years of tamoxifen before starting aromatase inhibitor therapy. The 5-year disease-free survival rate was 95% with letrozole versus 91% with placebo. Overall survival was the same in both groups. Patients on letrozole had a higher incidence of bone pain, bone fractures, and new-onset osteoporosis. This patient has tolerated anastrozole therapy well, has preserved bone density, and remains at higher risk (tumor size greater than 2 cm and pathologically involved lymph nodes). Extending aromatase inhibitor therapy to 10 years is reasonable for this patient.

Tamoxifen can be used sequentially with an aromatase inhibitor during the first 5 years of hormonal therapy. Studies have demonstrated equivalent results between sequential therapy (2 years of either tamoxifen or an aromatase inhibitor followed by 3 years of the other agent) compared with 5 years of an aromatase inhibitor. However, no data show benefit of tamoxifen, either as a single agent or in combination with an aromatase inhibitor, after completing 5 years of an aromatase inhibitor.

KEY POINT

- Extending aromatase-inhibitor therapy beyond 5 years to 10 years in postmenopausal women with hormone receptor–positive early breast cancer is associated with an increase in the 5-year disease-free survival rate but not overall survival.

Bibliography

Goss PE, Ingle JN, Pritchard KI, Robert NJ, Muss H, Gralow J, et al. Extending aromatase-inhibitor adjuvant therapy to 10 years. N Engl J Med. 2016;375:209-19. [PMID: 27264120] doi:10.1056/NEJMoa1604700

Item 126   Answer: B

Educational Objective: Manage metastatic lung cancer in a patient with poor performance status.

The most appropriate management is palliative care consultation. This patient has advanced metastatic non–small cell lung cancer and very poor performance status, and he had several months of symptoms before hospitalization. Although systemic chemotherapy and other treatments can help many patients with advanced non–small cell lung cancer, data clearly indicate that not all patients benefit. In particular, patients with poor performance status have not been shown to benefit from systemic treatment of their cancer. In those patients, the most appropriate intervention is palliative care consultation. Evidence suggests that patients with metastatic non–small cell lung cancer who have palliative care consultation at the time of diagnosis have decreased depression and prolonged life by 2.7 months. In addition, goals of care should be discussed, as well as the low likelihood of efficacy associated with systemic treatment.

Ablation of liver metastases plays no role in the management of patients with non–small cell lung cancer and poor performance status, particularly in the setting of extensive extrahepatic cancer, such as in this patient.

Platinum-based chemotherapy is associated with significant potential toxicity in patients with poor performance status and is not recommended.

Given the presence of obvious extensive metastatic disease, radiation treatment would be recommended only for palliation. However, this patient is experiencing systemic effects from his cancer and does not have any specific lesion needing local palliation.

KEY POINT

- Patients with non–small cell lung cancer and poor performance status do not benefit from systemic treatment of their cancer; in such patients, the most appropriate intervention is palliative care consultation.

Bibliography

Bade BC, Silvestri GA. Palliative care in lung cancer: a review. Semin Respir Crit Care Med. 2016 Oct;37(5):750-759. [PMID: 27732996]

Item 127   Answer: B

Educational Objective: Treat neoplastic epidural spinal cord compression.

This patient should receive immediate decompressive surgery. Once spinal cord compression is diagnosed, treatment must be started urgently to prevent irreversible loss of neurologic function. Glucocorticoids should be given immediately and promptly followed by surgery, external beam radiation, or stereotactic body radiation. A study of 101 patients with epidural spinal cord compression showed that patients who received surgery followed by radiotherapy had better outcomes and lower morbidity and mortality than those who received radiotherapy alone. Candidates for surgery include those with a life expectancy of at least 3 months and the absence of comorbidities that would otherwise be a contraindication to surgery.

Radiation therapy would never be done electively in a patient with epidural cord compression because delays in treatment lead to further neurologic deterioration.

Palliative care and supportive care alone might be appropriate in a patient with a very poor prognosis who does not want any further active antineoplastic therapy. Patients in this situation must be aware of the high likelihood of neurologic deterioration, including loss of ambulation and loss of control of bowel and bladder function. In most patients with metastatic cancer, treatment to avoid these complications is recommended.

Urgent radiation would be appropriate in patients who are not surgical candidates because of comorbidities, who have an expected survival of less than 3 months, or who refuse surgery. This patient has a life expectancy of more than 3 months and has no medical contraindications to surgery.

KEY POINT

- Initial administration of dexamethasone followed by decompressive surgery for epidural spinal cord compression is recommended in patients who are acceptable surgical candidates and who have an expected survival of at least 3 months.

Bibliography

Patchell RA, Tibbs PA, Regine WF, et al. Direct decompressive surgical resection in the treatment of spinal cord compression caused by metastatic cancer: a randomised trial. Lancet. 2005 Aug 20-26;366(9486):643-8. [PMID: 16112300]

Item 128   Answer: B

Educational Objective: Manage a *BRCA2* mutation carrier with prophylactic bilateral salpingo-oophorectomy.

The most appropriate recommendation for this patient is bilateral salpingo-oophorectomy by age 40 to 45 years. This patient has tested positive for a pathogenic *BRCA2* mutation. Although she has no family history of ovarian cancer, she has a 12% lifetime risk for ovarian cancer. Prophylactic bilateral salpingo-oophorectomy (BSO) is strongly recommended for both *BRCA1* and *BRCA2* mutation carriers. Risk-reducing BSO markedly reduces the risk for ovarian cancer and, if done while premenopausal, decreases the risk for breast cancer by 50%. For *BRCA1* mutation carriers, the risk for ovarian cancer increases substantially after age 35 years, and thus prophylactic BSO is recommended between the ages of 35 and 40 years and after completion of childbearing. *BRCA1* carriers who delay BSO until age 40 years will have a 4% risk of being diagnosed with an ovarian cancer. For *BRCA2* carriers, however, the risk of ovarian cancer before age 50 is only 1%. Therefore, it is reasonable to delay risk-reducing BSO until age 40 to

45 years in *BRCA2* mutation carriers, particularly if they have already undergone prophylactic bilateral mastectomy. BSO can reduce the risk of ovarian, fallopian tube, or primary peritoneal cancers by 80% and decrease all-cause mortality to age 70 years by 77%.

Because this patient desires further childbearing and is only 38 years old, she can safely delay BSO until age 40 to 45 years and until childbearing is complete.

Screening with annual or semiannual pelvic ultrasonography and CA-125 is not effective and has been removed as a screening recommendation from *BRCA1* and *BRCA2* management guidelines.

Oral contraceptive use decreases the risk for ovarian cancer by as much as 50% with prolonged use and can be used in *BRCA1* and *BRCA2* carriers but is not an adequate substitute for prophylactic BSO.

KEY POINT

- Prophylactic bilateral salpingo-oophorectomy is recommended for both *BRCA1* and *BRCA2* mutation carriers, which markedly reduces the risk for ovarian cancer and, if done while premenopausal, decreases the risk for breast cancer by 50%.

Bibliography

Finch AP, Lubinski J, Møller P, Singer CF, Karlan B, Senter L, et al. Impact of oophorectomy on cancer incidence and mortality in women with a BRCA1 or BRCA2 mutation. J Clin Oncol. 2014;32:1547-53. [PMID: 24567435] doi:10.1200/JCO.2013.53.2820

Item 129   Answer: D

Educational Objective: Diagnose chronic lymphocytic leukemia.

This patient's elevated lymphocyte count and the identification of smudge cells on the peripheral blood smear, together with the presence of lymphadenopathy on physical examination, point to a possible diagnosis of chronic lymphocytic leukemia (CLL). B-cell CLL is the most common form of adult leukemia, accounting for 10% of hematologic malignancies. Patients are usually asymptomatic at presentation, with CLL identified by a lymphocytosis on a routine complete blood count. Flow cytometry is the most appropriate test to make an initial diagnosis of CLL. It can be easily performed on peripheral blood and will show B-cell antigens (CD19, CD20, and CD23), coexpression of CD5 (usually a T-cell marker), and low levels of a monoclonal surface immunoglobulin. In most cases, CLL can be suspected based on the complete blood count and review of a peripheral blood smear. However, other conditions may present with lymphocytosis, which flow cytometry can help distinguish from typical CLL. Other conditions include reactive lymphocytosis, T-cell leukemias, and other B-cell lymphoproliferative disorders involving the blood, such as mantle cell and marginal zone lymphomas and hairy cell leukemia.

A bone marrow aspiration and biopsy can be used to diagnose CLL and will provide prognostic information based on the extent of marrow involvement. However, flow cytometry has replaced bone marrow examination, which is not routinely needed as part of diagnosing or staging the disease, although it may still be useful in evaluating atypical cases or the mechanisms of cytopenia in patients with CLL.

A CT scan may show lymphadenopathy or nonpalpable splenomegaly in patients with CLL; however, it does not provide additional information that is helpful in the management of disease in asymptomatic patients.

Prognosis for patients with CLL is determined by gene mutation status (immune globulin variable heavy-chain mutation) and fluorescence in situ hybridization or array-based karyotyping. In patients with CLL, a deletion of chromosome 17p is concerning because it is associated with a short median survival (less than 3 years). These cytogenetic and molecular genetic studies may have implications in choice of therapies. However, these studies would not typically be ordered until a definitive diagnosis of CLL is obtained.

KEY POINT

- Flow cytometry on peripheral blood is the most appropriate test to make an initial diagnosis of chronic lymphocytic leukemia.

Bibliography

Strati P, Shanafelt TD. Monoclonal B-cell lymphocytosis and early-stage chronic lymphocytic leukemia: diagnosis, natural history, and risk stratification. Blood. 2015;126:454-62. [PMID: 26065657] doi:10.1182/blood-2015-02-585059

Item 130   Answer: A

Educational Objective: Treat metastatic renal cell carcinoma.

The most appropriate management is left radical nephrectomy. Renal cell carcinomas arise in the renal cortex and are the most common type of tumors affecting the kidney. Patients with renal cell carcinoma are often asymptomatic until they have advanced disease, but possible symptoms include hematuria, an abdominal mass, abdominal pain, and unexplained weight loss. However, the classic triad of flank pain, hematuria, and a palpable abdominal mass occurs in only approximately 9% of patients. This patient most likely has metastatic kidney cancer based on identification of a large kidney mass associated with a suspicious pulmonary nodule and anemia. However, there is no histologic diagnosis of cancer at this point. Debulking nephrectomy has been shown to improve survival in patients diagnosed with metastatic kidney cancer, particularly in those with limited metastatic disease. Patients with lung-only metastasis and good performance status benefit most. In this patient, therefore, nephrectomy would serve two purposes. It would confirm the diagnosis and also serve as treatment for her metastatic kidney cancer. Following nephrectomy it would be appropriate to consider metastasectomy for removal of the isolated pulmonary lesion.

Nivolumab, a monoclonal antibody directed against programmed death receptor 1, is currently FDA approved for treatment of advanced clear cell carcinoma of the kidney. However, nivolumab is not recommended as first-line treatment and should not be started before establishing a histologic diagnosis of clear cell carcinoma. Clear cell carcinoma has not been confirmed in this patient, so the use of nivolumab would be premature.

PET/CT scan plays no role in the evaluation of a patient suspected of having kidney cancer. The presence or absence of fluorodeoxyglucose avidity would not influence management.

External beam radiation does not play a role in the treatment of metastatic kidney cancer except for palliative treatment of metastatic sites, such as painful osseous metastatic lesions. In this patient with a large kidney mass and one site of metastatic disease, surgery is indicated. Radiation has not been shown to improve outcomes in this setting and is not recommended.

KEY POINT

- Debulking nephrectomy improves survival in patients diagnosed with metastatic kidney cancer, particularly in those with limited metastatic disease.

Bibliography

Flanigan RC, Salmon SE, Blumenstein BA, et al. Nephrectomy followed by interferon alfa-2b compared with interferon alfa-2b alone for metastatic renal-cell cancer. N Engl J Med. 2001 Dec 6;345(23):1655-9. [PMID: 11759643]

Item 131   Answer: D

Educational Objective: Manage advanced-stage follicular lymphoma in an asymptomatic patient.

For this 75-year-old man with advanced-stage follicular lymphoma who is asymptomatic and does not have bulky disease, observation is an appropriate management strategy. There is no proof that earlier therapy for stage III to IV (nodes on both sides of the diaphragm [III]; noncontiguous extranodal involvement [IV]) follicular lymphoma provides benefit over deferring therapy until needed, provided the patient is comfortable with a strategy of surveillance. Patients with nonbulky follicular lymphoma who are not symptomatic may survive many years without the need for therapy.

Spontaneous tumor lysis syndrome occurs commonly in patients with leukemia and Burkitt lymphoma and after treatment of bulky large B-cell lymphoma or advanced chronic lymphocytic leukemia. Tumor lysis syndrome results in hyperkalemia, hyperphosphatemia, hyperuricemia, hypocalcemia, and disseminated intravascular coagulation. Hyperuricemia can lead to urate nephropathy and acute kidney injury. Prevention of tumor lysis syndrome is accomplished with large-volume intravenous hydration with normal saline plus administration of allopurinol to limit hyperuricemia.

Because this patient will not likely be receiving chemotherapy, there is no need for allopurinol to prevent tumor lysis syndrome. Even if he were to be treated, tumor lysis is not common in low-grade lymphomas in the absence of bulky disease or preexisting renal disease or hyperuricemia.

Although follicular lymphomas are sensitive to radiation, and radiation therapy may be used for palliation of symptomatic bulky sites of disease or for cure in patients with localized (stage I to II) follicular lymphoma, this patient clearly has disseminated disease with diffuse lymphadenopathy, and systemic therapy would be appropriate if needed.

Follicular lymphoma associated with symptomatic systemic disease requires multiagent therapy that traditionally includes rituximab plus cyclophosphamide, doxorubicin, vincristine, and prednisone (R-CHOP); rituximab plus cyclophosphamide, vincristine, and prednisone (R-CVP); or rituximab and bendamustine. This patient is asymptomatic and does not yet require systematic therapy.

KEY POINT

- Patients with nonbulky follicular lymphoma who are not symptomatic may survive many years without the need for therapy.

Bibliography

Blood. 2016 Apr 28;127(17):2055-63. doi: 10.1182/blood-2015-11-624288. Epub 2016 Mar 17. Follicular lymphoma: evolving therapeutic strategies. Kahl BS, Yang DT.

Item 132   Answer: D

Educational Objective: Screen for breast cancer in a patient with previous chest wall radiation.

Annual mammography or breast MRI starting now is the most appropriate screening strategy in this patient. She has a history of radiation to the chest wall to treat Hodgkin lymphoma at age 19 years and is at high risk for breast cancer. Among this group, the cumulative breast cancer incidence by age 40 to 45 years ranges from 13% to 20% and is similar to that in BRCA gene mutation carriers. The risk varies with the dose of radiation used, and the strength of the screening recommendation is highest for women who received the highest dose of radiation (20 Gy or higher). For women with low- to moderate-dose chest radiation (less than 20 Gy), the decision to screen should be an individual one, taking into account additional risk factors and patients' values. The increased risk for breast cancer begins within 8 years after treatment. The International Late Effects of Childhood Cancer Guideline Harmonization Group recommends that for women who received chest wall radiation before the age of 30 years, screening should begin at age 25 years or 8 years after completion of radiation therapy, whichever is last. The Guideline Harmonization Group notes that the ideal screening modality is unknown because of a lack of sufficient evidence, but breast MRI, mammography, or a combination of mammography and breast MRI are all reasonable choices. National Comprehensive Cancer Network guidelines recommend annual mammography and MRI starting after age 25 for patients receiving radiation between ages 10 and 30, beginning 8 to 10 years after irradiation.

This patient completed radiation at the age of 19 years. According to the Guideline Harmonization Group, her breast cancer screening should start at age 27 years (8 years after radiation or age 25 years, whichever is last), not 30 years.

Patients at average risk for breast cancer should start screening every 2 years by age 50 years, with the option to start mammographic screening between ages 40 and 50 years being an individualized decision. This patient, however, is at high, not average, risk.

KEY POINT

- The International Late Effects of Childhood Cancer Guideline Harmonization Group recommends that for women who received chest wall radiation before the age of 30 years, breast screening should begin at age 25 years or 8 years after completion of radiation therapy, whichever is last.

Bibliography

Mulder RL, Kremer LC, Hudson MM, et al; International Late Effects of Childhood Cancer Guideline Harmonization Group. Recommendations for breast cancer surveillance for female survivors of childhood, adolescent, and young adult cancer given chest radiation: a report from the International Late Effects of Childhood Cancer Guideline Harmonization Group. Lancet Oncol. 2013 Dec;14(13):e621-9. doi:10.1016/S1470-2045(13)70303-6. [PMID: 24275135]

Item 133   Answer: B

Educational Objective: Manage fertility in a patient with early-stage breast cancer.

Fertility specialist consultation before chemotherapy is appropriate for this patient with early-stage breast cancer. Current guidelines recommend addressing the possibility of chemotherapy-related infertility with all patients treated with chemotherapy during their reproductive years and referring them as early as possible in the treatment process to reproductive specialists. The risk of infertility after chemotherapy for breast cancer is related to patient age, treatment type and doses, and pretreatment fertility. Even if women resume menses after chemotherapy, they may have infertility and are at risk for premature menopause. In women, embryo cryopreservation is a proven fertility preservation method. Current methods allow egg harvesting to occur at any point in the menstrual cycle. Patients who carry deleterious *BRCA1* or *BRCA2* mutations have the option of preimplantation genetic selection and implanting only embryos that do not have the deleterious mutation. Studies to date show no increase in the risk for disease recurrence with fertility preservation methods.

Fertility consultation after chemotherapy is less likely to be beneficial given the exposure of ovarian follicles to the chemotherapy agent. The ovarian response to ovarian stimulation and the quality of the oocytes decrease after even one round of chemotherapy.

There is insufficient evidence regarding the use of a gonadotropin-releasing hormone agonist such as goserelin during chemotherapy to preserve ovarian function, and it should not replace established methods of fertility preservation.

There is no reason to recommend against future childbearing in patients with early-stage breast cancer. Pregnancy after breast cancer diagnosis is associated with no difference in disease-free survival and a slightly reduced risk of death.

KEY POINT

- Fertility specialist consultation is recommended for all patients before chemotherapy during their reproductive years.

Bibliography

Loren AW, Mangu PB, Beck LN, Brennan L, Magdalinski AJ, Partridge AH, et al; American Society of Clinical Oncology. Fertility preservation for patients with cancer: American Society of Clinical Oncology clinical practice guideline update. J Clin Oncol. 2013;31:2500-10. [PMID: 23715580] doi:10.1200/JCO.2013.49.2678

Item 134   Answer: B

Educational Objective: Treat localized gastroesophageal cancer.

The most reasonable treatment strategy is neoadjuvant chemotherapy plus radiation therapy. Although only 30% to 40% of patients with gastroesophageal cancer have potentially resectable disease at presentation, patients with local and locoregional disease are typically treated surgically. Unfortunately, recurrence rates are high, and cure rates with surgical resection alone remain low. Studies have shown that administration of neoadjuvant chemotherapy improves outcome to a modest but statistically significant degree. Neoadjuvant chemotherapy plus radiation therapy is given before a planned curative-intent surgery to patients who are believed to have fully resectable disease to eradicate any micrometastatic disease that might be present outside of the surgical field and thus increase the chance for cure. There is often confusion between neoadjuvant chemotherapy and conversion chemotherapy. The key distinction between neoadjuvant chemotherapy and conversion chemotherapy is that in conversion chemotherapy, the patient's tumor is not believed to be currently resectable but could possibly become resectable if adequate tumor regression can be accomplished with chemotherapy. Thus, both neoadjuvant and conversion chemotherapy are given with a plan for surgery to follow; however, neoadjuvant therapy is administered to patients with micrometastatic disease thought to be resectable, whereas conversion therapy is given to shrink visible tumors in patients with unresectable disease in whom disease might become resectable with adequate tumor regression.

Adjuvant therapy is given after curative-intent surgery to eradicate any residual micrometastatic disease and increase the chance for cure. Because of the low cure rates for locoregional therapy for esophageal cancer, chemotherapy has been added to many treatment regimens, and many patients are currently treated with combination chemoradiation following surgery for resectable disease. However, the optimal treatment regimen and the overall effectiveness of different treatment approaches have not yet been established. However, there is no evidential support for adjuvant radiation therapy (surgery followed by radiation therapy) for patients with localized gastroesophageal cancer.

Palliative therapy is given to patients with incurable cancer to prolong survival or control symptoms. Palliative care should be considered for patients with poor performance status due to chronic medical comorbidities, for those who have not been able to tolerate initial treatment attempts, or for those who have exhausted standard treatment options.

KEY POINT

- Neoadjuvant therapy is given before a planned curative-intent surgery to patients with fully resectable disease to eradicate micrometastatic and increase the chance for cure.

Bibliography

van Hagen P, Hulshof MC, van Lanschot JJ, Steyerberg EW, van Berge Henegouwen MI, Wijnhoven BP, et al; CROSS Group. Preoperative chemoradiotherapy for esophageal or junctional cancer. N Engl J Med. 2012;366:2074-84. [PMID: 22646630] doi:10.1056/NEJMoa1112088

Item 135   Answer: B

Educational Objective: Treat superficial bladder cancer.

The most appropriate treatment is intravesicular bacillus Calmette-Guérin (BCG) for six treatments followed by periodic cystoscopy. Bladder cancer is the most commonly diagnosed cancer of the urinary tract. In the United States, almost all bladder cancer is transitional cell carcinoma. Risk factors include advanced age, white ethnicity, various occupational exposures, and cigarette smoking. Smoking is the most important risk factor and encompasses current and former smokers and persons exposed to secondhand smoke. Persons at occupational risk include metal workers, painters, miners, textile workers, and leather workers. The most common presenting symptom of bladder cancer is gross hematuria. Most patients diagnosed with bladder cancer will be found to have non-muscle invasive disease, which can be purely exophytic or can involve limited bladder wall invasion. For patients with non-muscle invasive cancer, transurethral resection of the bladder tumor (TURBT) is the standard initial management. For those with high-grade or recurrent low-grade cancer, standard care is to follow TURBT with six rounds of intravesical chemotherapy, most commonly BCG or mitomycin given directly into the bladder. This procedure is done both for treatment of the identified lesion and to help prevent additional bladder tumors from developing. The risk of either recurrent cancer or a new bladder cancer arising elsewhere is significant. Therefore, after BCG or mitomycin treatment, it is essential

to perform cystoscopy 3 months after treatment and subsequently at 3- to 6-month intervals to look for new cancers. Patients with noninvasive bladder cancer have an excellent prognosis, and cancer-related deaths rarely occur. Patients who develop recurrent disease with favorable tumor characteristics may be retreated with intravesicular therapy but, if higher-risk tumors are found, may require cystectomy.

Cisplatin-based chemotherapy has no role in the treatment of non-muscle invasive cancer. It is used most often as a neoadjuvant treatment before surgery in patients with muscle-invasive cancer. The role of adjuvant chemotherapy in muscle-invasive cancer is much less clear.

Partial cystectomy is not needed for the treatment of early-stage, non-muscle invasive bladder cancer. However, it has a role in selected patients with muscle-invasive cancer.

KEY POINT

- Initial treatment for high-grade or recurrent low-grade bladder cancer is transurethral resection of the bladder tumor followed by intravesical chemotherapy and periodic cystoscopy.

Bibliography

Hall MC, Chang SS, Dalbagni G, et al. Guideline for the management of nonmuscle invasive bladder cancer (stages Ta, T1, and Tis): 2007 update. J Urol. 2007 Dec;178(6):2314-30. [PMID: 17993339]

Item 136   Answer: D

Educational Objective: Properly apply the results of clinical oncology trials to individual patients.

The patient would most likely achieve efficacy results inferior to those in the published trial. Patients who participate in clinical trials typically have a good to excellent performance status, performing most of their normal activities of living. Patients who are sedentary, with limited exercise tolerance and limited caloric intake, are substantially less likely to benefit from treatment than patients who are more medically fit. Patients with a poor performance status, such as this one, would also be more likely to experience greater toxicity with aggressive treatment than would a more medically fit patient. Consequently, the results of clinical trials, which typically comprise medically fit patients with a good performance status, cannot be directly extrapolated to patients with poor health and poor performance status, such as this one.

KEY POINT

- Results of clinical trials in patients with cancer, usually encompassing medically fit patients with good performance status, cannot be extrapolated to patients with poor health and performance status.

Bibliography

Tinetti ME. The gap between clinical trials and the real world: extrapolating treatment effects from younger to older adults. JAMA Intern Med. 2014;174:397-8. [PMID: 24424303] doi:10.1001/jamainternmed.2013.13283

Item 137   Answer: B

Educational Objective: Treat advanced breast cancer using palbociclib with antiestrogen therapy.

Letrozole plus palbociclib is the most appropriate treatment for this patient with advanced breast cancer that recurs after completing previous adjuvant aromatase inhibitor therapy. Palbociclib is an oral cyclin-dependent kinase 4 and 6 (CDK4 and CDK6) inhibitor that is synergistic with endocrine therapies in vitro. In vitro studies suggest that breast cancer that has become resistant to hormonal therapy remains dependent on cyclin D1-CDK4 for proliferation. Two studies have shown benefit to the combination of antiestrogen therapy with palbociclib for hormone receptor–positive, *HER2*-negative advanced breast cancer, with an increased response rate and an approximate doubling of progression-free survival compared to hormonal therapy alone. Therapy with palbociclib was associated with increased adverse effects, including fatigue, nausea, and neutropenia.

Based on these studies, palbociclib has been approved for use with either letrozole as first-line therapy or fulvestrant for women with hormone receptor–positive, *HER2*-negative advanced breast cancer. As first-line therapy, an aromatase inhibitor with palbociclib is typically preferred.

The aromatase inhibitor exemestane alone is unlikely to be effective in a patient who has relapsed a few years after receiving treatment with another aromatase inhibitor and is an inferior choice to combination hormonal therapy and palbociclib.

Raloxifene can be used as chemoprophylaxis to lower the risk of breast cancer in patients with increased risk due to atypical breast lesions or strong family history but is not an active agent for treatment of breast cancer.

Tamoxifen is not typically recommended as first-line therapy for advanced hormone receptor–positive, *HER2*-negative breast cancer. As a second-line agent after previous aromatase inhibitor treatment, it has an overall response rate of only 10%.

KEY POINT

- Patients with widely metastatic hormone receptor–positive, *HER2*-negative breast cancer can benefit from combination antiestrogen therapy with palbociclib.

Bibliography

Turner NC, Ro J, André F, et al; PALOMA3 Study Group. Palbociclib in hormone-receptor-positive advanced breast cancer. N Engl J Med. 2015 Jul 16;373(3):209-19. [PMID: 26030518]

Item 138   Answer: A

Educational Objective: Treat stage III colon cancer.

The most appropriate treatment is the FOLFOX regimen of 5-fluorouracil (5-FU), leucovorin, and oxaliplatin. This patient has stage IIIC colon cancer. Stage III is defined by metastases to the local-regional lymph nodes, and stage IIIC is defined by metastases to four or more nodes. Stage III colon cancer is potentially curable, although the risk of treatment failure increases with the number of nodes, and four or more positive nodes is a worrisome prognostic indicator. Currently all patients with stage III cancer are recommended to receive adjuvant chemotherapy after definitive surgery, as large randomized trials have shown that this modestly improves the likelihood of cure. For over a decade, the combination of oxaliplatin plus a fluoropyrimidine, such as 5-FU or its oral prodrug, capecitabine, have been the accepted standard management for stage III colon cancer. The drug 5-FU is usually given with the reduced folate leucovorin, which is inactive alone but causes 5-FU to bind more tightly to its target enzyme.

Oxaliplatin with oral capecitabine (CAPOX) is also an acceptable regimen for adjuvant treatment of stage III colon cancer. Use of oral capecitabine requires a highly reliable, motivated patient who is able to adhere to a complex oral medication schedule.

Local recurrence in colon cancer, unlike rectal cancer, is rare, so radiation therapy is not a routine part of the management of colon cancer. Further, it can be difficult to isolate the small bowel from the radiation field, which results in unnecessary toxicity. Therefore, radiation therapy does not have a role in the routine management of patients with stage III colon cancer, either alone or combined with chemotherapy.

KEY POINT

- The FOLFOX regimen of 5-fluorouracil, leucovorin, and oxaliplatin or oxaliplatin with oral capecitabine (CAPOX) is the most appropriate adjuvant therapy for stage III colon cancer.

Bibliography

André T, de Gramont A, Vernerey D, Chibaudel B, Bonnetain F, Tijeras-Raballand A, et al. Adjuvant fluorouracil, leucovorin, and oxaliplatin in stage II to III colon cancer: updated 10-year survival and outcomes according to BRAF mutation and mismatch repair status of the MOSAIC study. J Clin Oncol. 2015;33:4176-87. [PMID: 26527776] doi:10.1200/JCO.2015.63.4238

Item 139   Answer: C

Educational Objective: Evaluate anemia in a patient with chronic lymphocytic leukemia.

Obtaining a direct antiglobulin (Coombs) test would be the appropriate initial diagnostic step to help guide management in this patient with chronic lymphocytic leukemia (CLL) with anemia. Concomitant autoimmune disease, including immune thrombocytopenia and hemolytic anemia, is common among patients with CLL. Anemia in patients with CLL can have many mechanisms, including myelophthisis (replacement of normal marrow elements by fibrosis or tumor) from the CLL itself, hypersplenism, chemotherapy, pure red cell aplasia, and autoimmune hemolytic anemia. The patient's reticulocytosis is strongly suggestive of a hemolytic anemia. Identifying the mechanism of anemia can help guide therapy. If the patient has a positive direct antiglobulin test result suggestive of a secondary immunohemolytic anemia, glucocorticoids would be the appropriate first treatment for this patient.

Parvovirus has a tropism for erythrocyte precursors and is a known cause of aplastic crisis in patients with underlying hematologic disorders, iron deficiency, and immunosuppression. Patients with CLL and others with immunosuppression can have prolonged infections resulting in persistent anemia. However, reticulocytopenia (as opposed to the reticulocytosis as seen in this patient) would be characteristic for this complication.

A bone marrow aspiration and biopsy can help determine the mechanism of anemia in patients with CLL to assess for the extent of marrow replacement, for evaluation of hypoplasia from chemotherapy, to look for secondary myelodysplasia or pure red cell aplasia, or suggest evidence of erythroid hyperplasia, which could be seen in hypersplenism or an immunohemolytic disease. However, if the result of a direct antiglobulin test is positive and reticulocytosis is present, bone marrow aspiration and biopsy would not be needed.

Ibrutinib, an oral Bruton kinase inhibitor, is effective in CLL and mantle cell lymphoma. Although ibrutinib can cause some marrow suppression, this is not typical and would not be associated with reticulocytosis.

Hypersplenism (with or without immunohemolysis) may have a role in this patient's anemia, and eventually splenectomy may be an appropriate treatment. However, establishing the mechanism of the anemia and initiating systemic treatment would be preferable and a less invasive option.

KEY POINT

- Autoimmune hemolytic anemia is common in patients with chronic lymphocytic leukemia; a direct antiglobulin (Coombs) test can confirm the diagnosis and guide treatment.

Bibliography

Molica S, Polliack A. Autoimmune hemolytic anemia (AIHA) associated with chronic lymphocytic leukemia in the current era of targeted therapy. Leuk Res. 2016;50:31-36. [PMID: 27657651] doi:10.1016/j.leukres.2016.09.002

Item 140   Answer: B

Educational Objective: Screen for *PD-L1* expression in metastatic non-small cell lung cancer

Up until recently, the accepted front-line treatment for patients with metastatic non-small cell lung cancer was platinum-based chemotherapy in all patients except those found to have a driver mutation, in whom small molecule inhibitors, such as erlotinib, are indicated. However, pembrolizumab has recently been approved by the FDA for the initial treatment of metastatic non-small cell lung cancer positive for expression of programmed cell death ligand 1 (*PDL1*). Pembrolizumab is a monoclonal antibody directed against *PDL1*, and it blocks binding of this ligand to the programmed death receptor 1 receptor, preventing the cancer from silencing cellular immunity. This agent was found to improve overall survival compared to platinum-based chemotherapy in a phase III trial that enrolled 305 patients with advanced non-small cell lung cancer who had at least 50% tumor cell positivity for *PD-L1*. In this study, overall survival was 10.3 months with pembrolizumab compared to 6 months with platinum-based chemotherapy. Based on this data, it has now become standard practice to test all patients newly diagnosed with metastatic non-small cell lung cancer for *PD-L1* expression.

Liver biopsy can help confirm the presence of metastatic disease but is not indicated in patients with imaging findings consistent with metastatic disease whose diagnosis has been confirmed by biopsy of the primary lesion.

PET/CT scan has no role in the evaluation or management of patients with known metastatic disease and would not be indicated for this patient.

Pulmonary function tests also play no role in the management of patients with metastatic disease. They are typically indicated in patients who are being considered for surgery for early-stage disease.

KEY POINT

- It has now become standard practice to test all patients newly diagnosed with metastatic non-small cell lung cancer for programmed cell death ligand 1 expression.

Bibliography

Reck M, Rodríguez-Abreu D, Robinson AG, Hui R, Csoszi T, Fülöp A, et al; KEYNOTE-024 Investigators. Pembrolizumab versus chemotherapy for PD-L1-positive non-small-cell lung cancer. N Engl J Med. 2016;375:1823-1833. [PMID: 27718847]

Item 141   Answer: B

Educational Objective: Treat midline poorly differentiated carcinoma of unknown primary site.

The most appropriate treatment is a germ cell chemotherapy regimen of cisplatin and etoposide. Cancer of unknown primary (CUP) is a diagnosis of exclusion established in patients with a solid metastatic tumor after a detailed medical history and physical examination have been done and imaging studies or other diagnostic studies have not identified a primary tumor site. Diagnostic efforts should focus on identifying whether a patient is among the approximately 20% of patients with CUP who fall into identifiable subgroups with a more favorable prognosis and who can benefit from a specific treatment strategy. A biopsy obtained from the site that can be sampled in the safest, least invasive manner is done, and specimens are often evaluated by immunohistochemical stains consistent with the tumor's pattern of presentation to attempt to establish a diagnosis of a more treatable subtype of CUP. The patient is a young man with a poorly differentiated CUP site that is predominantly midline in presentation. In the absence of an identified primary tumor, these patients should be treated presumptively for metastatic germ cell tumor. The absence of abnormal findings on testicular examination or ultrasonography or the absence of germ-cell specific markers, such as α-fetoprotein and β-human chorionic gonadotropin, does not exclude this diagnosis or this course of action. Even if these evaluation results are negative, an unrecognized germ cell tumor may still exist, and these patients should be treated for this possibility with a platinum-based chemotherapy regimen.

A chemotherapy regimen focused on digestive tract malignancies, such as fluorouracil and irinotecan, would be appropriate palliation for a pattern of CUP consistent with a gastrointestinal primary tumor, such as disease predominantly below the diaphragm with liver or peritoneal involvement. However, this patient has bulky lymphadenopathy below and above the diaphragm, making a digestive malignancy unlikely.

The extent of retroperitoneal lymphadenopathy and mediastinal lymphadenopathy makes initial treatment with either radiation therapy or surgery inappropriate.

KEY POINT

- Young men with poorly differentiated carcinoma that is characterized by centrally located bulky retroperitoneal or mediastinal lymphadenopathy may have an unrecognized germ cell tumor and are best treated with a platinum-based chemotherapy regimen.

Bibliography
Fizazi K, Greco FA, Pavlidis N, Daugaard G, Oien K, Pentheroudakis G; ESMO Guidelines Committee. Cancers of unknown primary site: ESMO Clinical Practice Guidelines for diagnosis, treatment and follow-up. Ann Oncol. 2015;26 Suppl 5:v133-8. [PMID: 26314775] doi:10.1093/annonc/mdv305

Item 142   Answer: C

Educational Objective: Define an inclusionary predictive tumor marker.

The finding of a *BRAF* V600E mutation is best described in this situation as an inclusionary predictive marker. Predictive markers help identify specific aspects of the tumor that can guide clinicians in determining which therapies are or are not appropriate for particular patients. For example, specific *BRAF*-targeted treatment, such as vemurafenib and dabrafenib, is indicated only in the subset of patients in whom the *BRAF* V600E mutation is found, and patients with this mutation are predicted to respond favorably to these agents. Conversely, the absence of the *BRAF* V600E mutation in patients with metastatic melanoma excludes consideration of such therapy and strongly predicts an absence of benefit from such a treatment.

An exclusionary predictive marker excludes patients from treatment that otherwise might have been used. Examples of exclusionary predictive markers are the *KRAS* or

NRAS mutations in patients with colorectal cancer, the presence of which would exclude the activity of an anti-epidermal growth factor receptor (EGFR)-targeted therapy. Patients with these gene mutations have disease that is not only found to be highly resistant to these agents, but they can also experience accelerated tumor growth with the use of such treatments.

Prognostic markers would quantitate a patient's risk of recurrence but would not indicate whether the outcome was more or less likely to be influenced by a certain treatment or intervention. Whereas predictive markers provide actionable information that is useful in guiding therapy, prognostic markers do not provide actionable information and therefore typically do not guide therapy and provide little to no value in clinical management.

KEY POINT

- Inclusionary predictive tumor markers identify which therapies are more likely to be effective.

Bibliography
Nair M, Sandhu SS, Sharma AK. Prognostic and predictive biomarkers in cancer. Curr Cancer Drug Targets. 2014;14(5):477-504. [PMID: 24807144]

Item 143   Answer: D

Educational Objective: Recommend genetic counseling to an asymptomatic patient with a family history of *BRCA*-related cancers.

The most appropriate management for this patient is referral to a genetic counselor. This patient has a family history suggestive of an inherited breast and ovarian cancer susceptibility gene and is interested in genetic testing. Both her mother and maternal aunt had cancers suggestive of a *BRCA1* or *BRCA2* mutation. Women with triple-negative breast cancers diagnosed before age 60 years are recommended to have *BRCA1* and *BRCA2* genetic testing, as are women with ovarian cancer diagnosed at any age. Referral to a genetic counselor or other suitably trained health care provider is the best option for genetic risk assessment. The U.S. Preventive Services Task Force has published guidelines for risk assessment and recommends referral to a genetic counselor for asymptomatic women who have not been diagnosed with a *BRCA*-related cancer but have a family history of *BRCA*-related cancers. These guidelines include screening tools designed to identify a family history that may be associated with an increased risk for *BRCA1* or *BRCA2* mutations. Family history factors suggesting an increased likelihood of *BRCA* mutations include breast cancer diagnosis before age 50 years, bilateral breast cancer, family history of breast and ovarian cancer, presence of breast cancer in one or more male family members, multiple cases of breast cancer in the family, one or more family member with two primary types of *BRCA*-related cancer, and Ashkenazi Jewish ethnicity. Genetic counseling should always occur before any genetic test is performed. The essential components of counseling include informing the patient of the test purpose, implications of diagnosis, alternative testing options (including foregoing testing), and any possible risks and benefits. The National Society of Genetic Counselors Web site (http://nsgc.org) can be used to locate a genetic counselor.

Direct-to-consumer tests may not include the appropriate type of genetic testing. In addition, genetic testing should be done after pretest genetic counseling, which is not always available in patients being tested by direct-to-consumer commercial genetic tests.

Although *BRCA1* and *BRCA2* testing for the three mutations most common in the Ashkenazi Jewish population (called multisite testing) is recommended for Ashkenazi Jewish women with breast cancer diagnosed at any age, comprehensive *BRCA1* and *BRCA2* testing is recommended if additional criteria for *BRCA1/2* testing are met.

KEY POINT

- Asymptomatic patients with a family history of *BRCA*-related cancers should receive genetic counseling for genetic risk assessment.

Bibliography

Moyer VA; U.S. Preventive Services Task Force. Risk assessment, genetic counseling, and genetic testing for BRCA-related cancer in women: U.S. Preventive Services Task Force recommendation statement. Ann Intern Med. 2014;160:271-81. [PMID: 24366376]

Item 144   Answer: A

Educational Objective: Evaluate suspected testicular cancer.

The most appropriate management is to measure β-human chorionic gonadotropin and α-fetoprotein levels. In the setting of unilateral testicular swelling or a palpable testicular mass in a young man, cancer is a diagnosis of exclusion. This patient has unilateral testicular swelling. Physical examination and ultrasonography both point to the presence of a testicular mass. Although extrinsic processes can cause testicular swelling, ultrasonography is very accurate in differentiation of intrinsic from extrinsic testicular pathology. In a patient found to have a testicular mass, the diagnosis of cancer must be confirmed histologically. Germ cell tumors are the most common type of testicular cancer. These tumors can be pure seminomas or nonseminomas. However, before histologic confirmation, α-fetoprotein and β-human chorionic gonadotropin levels should be measured to most accurately determine stage and prognosis. The serum α-fetoprotein level is never elevated in patients with pure seminomas, and β-human chorionic gonadotropin is elevated in only approximately 20% of patients with pure seminomas. Nonseminomatous germ cell tumors can contain elements of seminoma, but those elements are mixed with tumors with nonseminomatous histologies, which include yolk sac tumor, choriocarcinoma, and embryonal carcinoma. This distinction is important for determining the correct treatment. However, these measurements do not determine diagnosis and are not a substitute for histologic evaluation. Because levels will fall after orchiectomy, measurement before surgery is

recommended. Failure of the levels to fall suggests inadequate therapy, and elevation of the levels after treatment suggests recurrent disease.

Needle biopsy is contraindicated in the evaluation of testicular masses owing to the risk of biopsy tract seeding.

Chest radiography and CT of the abdomen and pelvis are done after a diagnosis is established. CT of the chest is indicated if the chest radiograph is abnormal or lung metastases are strongly suspected. PET-CT has little role in the evaluation of men with confirmed testicular cancer in part because of a high rate of false-positive results. It would not be indicated before establishing a diagnosis.

Radical inguinal orchiectomy is essential for establishing a diagnosis of testicular cancer in the most expeditious and safest way possible. However, it should be performed after tumor markers are measured.

KEY POINT

- Before histologic confirmation of testicular cancer, α-fetoprotein and β-human chorionic gonadotropin levels should be measured to most accurately determine stage and prognosis.

Bibliography

Mir MC, Pavan N, Gonzalgo ML. Current clinical applications of testicular cancer biomarkers. Urol Clin North Am. 2016 Feb;43(1):119-25. doi:10.1016/j.ucl.2015.08.011. [PMID: 26614034]

Item 145   Answer: A

Educational Objective: Treat symptomatic brain metastases.

This patient has evidence of brain metastases in the setting of metastatic hormone receptor-negative, *HER2*-positive breast cancer and should receive dexamethasone. She has headache and ataxia but no signs or symptoms of severe intracranial edema or impending herniation. Glucocorticoids are indicated as initial treatment in all patients with symptomatic brain metastases; they improve neurologic symptoms in 75% of patients, usually reducing intracranial pressure and improving neurologic symptoms within hours. Dexamethasone given either intravenously or orally is typically used because of its minimal mineralocorticoid effect and long half-life. Doses should be tapered to the lowest effective dose after stereotactic radiation and then tapered over several weeks. For patients on glucocorticoids for longer than 6 weeks, prophylaxis against pneumocystis pneumonia is recommended. Patients should be monitored for symptoms of gastritis or peptic ulcer, but there is no evidence that prophylaxis with H_2-blockers or proton-pump inhibitors is effective at preventing these complications. Patients should also be monitored for steroid myopathy.

Only about 25% of patients with brain metastases have seizures, and prophylactic antiepileptic therapy is not recommended in patients who have not had seizures. When antiepileptic drug therapy is used, newer agents, such as levetiracetam, are preferred to older agents, given the more favorable safety profiles and less potential for drug-drug interactions.

Mannitol and mechanical hyperventilation would be used in patients with severe edema at risk for herniation but are not indicated in this patient. Similarly, neurosurgical decompression would be recommended in patients with severe edema or impending herniation unable to wait for a response to dexamethasone or unresponsive to other treatments.

Whole brain radiation is less desirable in patients with good prognostic tumors and a limited number of brain metastases; stereotactic radiation would be recommended instead, but only after initial glucocorticoid treatment to improve peritumoral edema.

KEY POINT

- Patients with symptomatic brain metastases should be initially treated with glucocorticoids.

Bibliography

Lin X, DeAngelis LM. Treatment of brain metastases. J Clin Oncol. 2015;33:3475-84. [PMID: 26282648] doi:10.1200/JCO.2015.60.9503

Item 146   Answer: C

Educational Objective: Manage posttreatment surveillance for a patient with cervical cancer.

The most appropriate posttreatment surveillance for this patient with cervical cancer is a history, physical examination, and gynecologic examination every 3 months to monitor for local recurrence. Guidelines for posttreatment surveillance of patients with cervical cancer recommend a thorough history and examination every 3 to 6 months for the first 2 years, then every 6 to 12 months for years 2 through 5. Higher-risk patients, such as those treated with chemotherapy or radiation, should be evaluated every 3 months for 2 years, then every 6 months for years 2 through 5; those with lower-risk disease treated with surgery alone should be evaluated every 6 months for 2 years, then annually through year 5. The main goals of surveillance are to detect central pelvic (not involving the pelvic sidewall) recurrences that might be amenable to curative therapy and to address treatment-related symptoms. Treatment-related symptoms include bladder and bowel dysfunction; dyspareunia; difficulty achieving sexual arousal and orgasm; hot flushes; lymphedema of the lower extremities; fatigue; and mood disturbances related to fear of recurrence, altered body image, and loss of fertility. Patients also should be educated at these visits about symptoms that might indicate recurrence, including vaginal bleeding or new abdominal or pelvic pain. Most recurrences are symptomatic and are detected within 2 years of primary treatment, with nearly all detected by 5 years. Additional laboratory or imaging studies should be directed by signs or symptoms suggesting possible recurrence rather than done as routine studies in asymptomatic patients. Although annual cervical or vaginal cytology, or both, is recommended, it is unlikely that an asymptomatic recurrence will be found by cytology alone. In addition, pelvic radiation may alter tissue histology and make cytology interpretation difficult.

There is no evidence that routine imaging studies with either ultrasonography or CT results in better patient outcomes than clinical monitoring, or that the response to palliative therapy is improved by such surveillance techniques. Routine laboratory studies are also not recommended.

KEY POINT

- Posttreatment surveillance of patients with cervical cancer is limited to a thorough history and examination every 3 to 6 months for the first 2 years, then every 6 to 12 months for years 2 through 5; frequency of visits can be tailored to the patient's risk.

Bibliography

Elit L, Fyles AW, Devries MC, Oliver TK, Fung-Kee-Fung M; Gyneocology Cancer Disease Site Group. Follow-up for women after treatment of cervical cancer: a systematic review. Gynecol Oncol. 2009 Sep;114(3):528-35. [PMID: 19560188]

Item 147   Answer: B

Educational Objective: Treat stage III lung cancer with combined chemotherapy and radiation.

The most appropriate treatment is combined chemotherapy and radiation. Treatment for stage III non–small cell lung cancer, which is defined in most cases by the presence of mediastinal lymphadenopathy, can vary significantly based on the extent of the primary tumor and the extent of associated lymphadenopathy. Patients with extensive primary tumors, such as this patient whose tumor invades the mediastinum, are not candidates for surgery. Patients with bulky, multistation (widespread mediastinal or hilar lymph node involvement) lymphadenopathy in the mediastinum do not fare well after surgery. These patients should be treated with combined chemotherapy and radiation, which has been shown to improve outcomes compared with either chemotherapy alone or radiation alone.

In highly selected patients with stage III disease, surgery may be considered an appropriate therapeutic option. For patients with T3N1 disease, surgery can be done as initial therapy, although the procedure should include mediastinal lymph node dissection. In patients with negative mediastinal lymph nodes, adjuvant chemotherapy should be given. In patients with positive mediastinal lymph nodes, sequential chemotherapy and radiation is recommended. However, this patient has bulky mediastinal disease and is clearly not a candidate for surgery.

Pembrolizumab is a monoclonal antibody directed against programmed death receptor 1 (PD-1) that is indicated for treatment of recurrent metastatic non–small cell lung cancer. It has no role in the treatment of locally advanced non–small cell lung cancer and would not be indicated for this patient.

Radiation alone is inferior to combined chemotherapy and radiation and is not typically recommended. It would be recommended only for patients who were not candidates for combined chemotherapy and radiation based on comorbid conditions. However, this patient does not have any comorbid conditions that would preclude chemotherapy.

As noted previously, this patient has bulky mediastinal disease and is clearly not a candidate for surgery; therefore, surgical resection is not appropriate.

KEY POINT

- Patients with non–small cell lung cancer who have extensive primary tumors or bulky, multistation lymphadenopathy in the mediastinum are not candidates for surgery and instead should be treated with combined chemotherapy and radiation.

Bibliography

Tam K, Daly M, Kelly K. Treatment of locally advanced non-small cell lung cancer. Hematol Oncol Clin North Am. 2017 Feb;31(1):45-57. doi:10.1016/j.hoc.2016.08.009. [PMID: 27912833]

Item 148   Answer: B

Educational Objective: Evaluate metastatic gastroesophageal junction adenocarcinoma for *HER2* amplification.

This patient's tumor tissue should be assessed for human epidermal growth factor receptor 2 (*HER2*) amplification. He has metastatic adenocarcinoma of the distal esophagus. Approximately 25% of gastroesophageal cancers demonstrate *HER2* amplification; such tumors achieve a superior response to chemotherapy when the anti-*HER2* monoclonal antibody trastuzumab is added to standard chemotherapy. For this reason, determination of *HER2* amplification status is necessary when initiating chemotherapy for patients with a gastroesophageal tumor.

BRAF mutation status is of paramount importance in patients with melanoma, 40% of whom will have *BRAF*-mutated tumors that are highly likely to respond to tyrosine kinase inhibitors targeting *BRAF*. However, such mutations are exceedingly rare in upper gastrointestinal malignancies, and *BRAF*-targeting agents have thus far failed to show activity in *BRAF*-mutated gastrointestinal malignancies.

RAS mutation status is relevant to the use of anti-epidermal growth factor receptor (*EGFR*) monoclonal antibodies in colorectal cancer. These agents have not been shown to be active in upper gastrointestinal malignancies and are not part of the treatment paradigm.

Neither a PET/CT scan nor a barium swallow will add useful information for this patient because the available CT imaging is sufficient for establishing a treatment plan. Any further information regarding extent of disease that might be found on a PET/CT would not be expected to change management. A barium swallow is unlikely to provide clinically useful information about the extent of his tumor or additional information about his swallowing capacity.

KEY POINT

- Upper gastrointestinal tumors should be assessed for human epidermal growth factor receptor 2 (*HER2*) amplification to guide chemotherapy.

Bibliography

Jomrich G, Schoppmann SF. Targeting HER 2 and angiogenesis in gastric cancer. Expert Rev Anticancer Ther. 2016;16:111-22. [PMID: 26567753] doi:10.1586/14737140.2016.1121110

Item 149   Answer: B

Educational Objective: Treat castrate-sensitive metastatic prostate cancer with androgen deprivation therapy and docetaxel.

The most appropriate management is leuprolide plus docetaxel. Standard therapy for metastatic prostate cancer or evidence of disseminated disease based on an elevated serum prostate-specific antigen (PSA) is androgen deprivation therapy (ADT). ADT consists of inhibiting androgen synthesis by using a gonadotropin-releasing hormone (GnRH) agonist (such as leuprolide) or blocking the androgen receptor with an antiandrogen agent (such as flutamide or bicalutamide). Bilateral orchiectomy is a reasonable alternative to GnRH agonist therapy, particularly in the very elderly. ADT is typically combined with docetaxel chemotherapy in patients with extensive metastatic disease. This patient has castrate-sensitive metastatic prostate cancer. He presented with clinical metastatic disease and had a significant response to treatment with leuprolide, based on both a reduction in his PSA level and improvement in pain related to his metastatic lesion to the lumbar spine. Two randomized trials have confirmed a survival benefit associated with combined ADT and docetaxel chemotherapy for men with castrate-sensitive metastatic prostate cancer. Based on the observed improvement in survival, use of docetaxel in this setting is now accepted standard care and should be recommended unless a contraindication to chemotherapy exists. Myelosuppression is the most common side effect of docetaxel. Hepatic dysfunction or compromised bone marrow function are contraindications to its use. This patient's medical history does not indicate any contraindication to treatment with docetaxel.

Continuation of leuprolide alone would not be recommended in a patient who is a candidate for docetaxel chemotherapy based on the demonstrated improvement in survival in men treated with six cycles of docetaxel.

Although radiation to the lumbar spine would be indicated for pain control or for treatment of neurologic compromise due to nerve compression by metastatic disease, this patient has no evidence of neurologic compromise, and his pain improved with leuprolide treatment. Therefore, radiation is not indicated at this time.

KEY POINT

- In men with clinical metastatic prostate cancer that is castrate sensitive, docetaxel along with continuation of androgen deprivation therapy has been shown to improve survival and is accepted as standard care.

Bibliography

James ND, Sydes MR, Clarke NW, et al; STAMPEDE Investigators. Addition of docetaxel, zoledronic acid, or both to first-line long-term hormone therapy in prostate cancer (STAMPEDE): survival results from an adaptive, multiarm, multistage, platform randomized controlled trial. Lancet. 2016 Mar 19;387(10024):1163-77. [PMID: 26719232]

Index

A

NAME AND ADDRESS (Please complete.)

_____
Last Name   First Name   Middle Initial

_____
Address

_____
Address cont.

_____
City   State   ZIP Code

_____
Country

_____
Email address

B

Order Number

(Use the 10-digit Order Number on your
MKSAP materials packing slip.)

C

ACP ID Number

(Refer to packing slip in your MKSAP materials
for your 8-digit ACP ID Number.)

ACP® American College of Physicians
Leading Internal Medicine, Improving Lives

Medical Knowledge Self-Assessment Program® 18

TO EARN *CME Credits and/or MOC Points* YOU MUST:

1. Answer all questions.
2. Score a minimum of 50% correct.

==

TO EARN *FREE* INSTANTANEOUS *CME Credits and/or MOC Points* ONLINE:

1. Answer all of your questions.
2. Go to **mksap.acponline.org** and enter your ACP Online username and password to access an online answer sheet.
3. Enter your answers.
4. You can also enter your answers directly at **mksap.acponline.org** without first using this answer sheet.

To Submit Your Answer Sheet by Mail or FAX for a $20 Administrative Fee per Answer Sheet:

1. Answer all of your questions and calculate your score.
2. Complete boxes A-H.
3. Complete payment information.
4. Send the answer sheet and payment information to ACP, using the FAX number/address listed below.

D

Required Submission Information if Applying for MOC

Birth Month and Day | | | | | |
                       M M   D D

ABIM Candidate Number | | | | | | |

COMPLETE FORM BELOW ONLY IF YOU SUBMIT BY MAIL OR FAX

Last Name   First Name   MI

Payment Information. Must remit in US funds, drawn on a US bank.
The processing fee for each paper answer sheet is $20.

☐ Check, made payable to ACP, enclosed

Charge to   ☐ **VISA**   ☐ **MasterCard**   ☐ **AMERICAN EXPRESS**   ☐ **DISCOVER**

Card Number _____

Expiration Date _____/_____   Security code (3 or 4 digit #s) _____
                    MM   YY

Signature _____

Fax to: 215-351-2799

Mail to:
Member and Customer Service
American College of Physicians
190 N. Independence Mall West
Philadelphia, PA 19106-1572

1 Ⓐ Ⓑ Ⓒ Ⓓ Ⓔ
2 Ⓐ Ⓑ Ⓒ Ⓓ Ⓔ
3 Ⓐ Ⓑ Ⓒ Ⓓ Ⓔ
4 Ⓐ Ⓑ Ⓒ Ⓓ Ⓔ
5 Ⓐ Ⓑ Ⓒ Ⓓ Ⓔ

6 Ⓐ Ⓑ Ⓒ Ⓓ Ⓔ
7 Ⓐ Ⓑ Ⓒ Ⓓ Ⓔ
8 Ⓐ Ⓑ Ⓒ Ⓓ Ⓔ
9 Ⓐ Ⓑ Ⓒ Ⓓ Ⓔ
10 Ⓐ Ⓑ Ⓒ Ⓓ Ⓔ

11 Ⓐ Ⓑ Ⓒ Ⓓ Ⓔ
12 Ⓐ Ⓑ Ⓒ Ⓓ Ⓔ
13 Ⓐ Ⓑ Ⓒ Ⓓ Ⓔ
14 Ⓐ Ⓑ Ⓒ Ⓓ Ⓔ
15 Ⓐ Ⓑ Ⓒ Ⓓ Ⓔ

16 Ⓐ Ⓑ Ⓒ Ⓓ Ⓔ
17 Ⓐ Ⓑ Ⓒ Ⓓ Ⓔ
18 Ⓐ Ⓑ Ⓒ Ⓓ Ⓔ
19 Ⓐ Ⓑ Ⓒ Ⓓ Ⓔ
20 Ⓐ Ⓑ Ⓒ Ⓓ Ⓔ

21 Ⓐ Ⓑ Ⓒ Ⓓ Ⓔ
22 Ⓐ Ⓑ Ⓒ Ⓓ Ⓔ
23 Ⓐ Ⓑ Ⓒ Ⓓ Ⓔ
24 Ⓐ Ⓑ Ⓒ Ⓓ Ⓔ
25 Ⓐ Ⓑ Ⓒ Ⓓ Ⓔ

26 Ⓐ Ⓑ Ⓒ Ⓓ Ⓔ
27 Ⓐ Ⓑ Ⓒ Ⓓ Ⓔ
28 Ⓐ Ⓑ Ⓒ Ⓓ Ⓔ
29 Ⓐ Ⓑ Ⓒ Ⓓ Ⓔ
30 Ⓐ Ⓑ Ⓒ Ⓓ Ⓔ

31 Ⓐ Ⓑ Ⓒ Ⓓ Ⓔ
32 Ⓐ Ⓑ Ⓒ Ⓓ Ⓔ
33 Ⓐ Ⓑ Ⓒ Ⓓ Ⓔ
34 Ⓐ Ⓑ Ⓒ Ⓓ Ⓔ
35 Ⓐ Ⓑ Ⓒ Ⓓ Ⓔ

36 Ⓐ Ⓑ Ⓒ Ⓓ Ⓔ
37 Ⓐ Ⓑ Ⓒ Ⓓ Ⓔ
38 Ⓐ Ⓑ Ⓒ Ⓓ Ⓔ
39 Ⓐ Ⓑ Ⓒ Ⓓ Ⓔ
40 Ⓐ Ⓑ Ⓒ Ⓓ Ⓔ

41 Ⓐ Ⓑ Ⓒ Ⓓ Ⓔ
42 Ⓐ Ⓑ Ⓒ Ⓓ Ⓔ
43 Ⓐ Ⓑ Ⓒ Ⓓ Ⓔ
44 Ⓐ Ⓑ Ⓒ Ⓓ Ⓔ
45 Ⓐ Ⓑ Ⓒ Ⓓ Ⓔ

46 Ⓐ Ⓑ Ⓒ Ⓓ Ⓔ
47 Ⓐ Ⓑ Ⓒ Ⓓ Ⓔ
48 Ⓐ Ⓑ Ⓒ Ⓓ Ⓔ
49 Ⓐ Ⓑ Ⓒ Ⓓ Ⓔ
50 Ⓐ Ⓑ Ⓒ Ⓓ Ⓔ

51 Ⓐ Ⓑ Ⓒ Ⓓ Ⓔ
52 Ⓐ Ⓑ Ⓒ Ⓓ Ⓔ
53 Ⓐ Ⓑ Ⓒ Ⓓ Ⓔ
54 Ⓐ Ⓑ Ⓒ Ⓓ Ⓔ
55 Ⓐ Ⓑ Ⓒ Ⓓ Ⓔ

56 Ⓐ Ⓑ Ⓒ Ⓓ Ⓔ
57 Ⓐ Ⓑ Ⓒ Ⓓ Ⓔ
58 Ⓐ Ⓑ Ⓒ Ⓓ Ⓔ
59 Ⓐ Ⓑ Ⓒ Ⓓ Ⓔ
60 Ⓐ Ⓑ Ⓒ Ⓓ Ⓔ

61 Ⓐ Ⓑ Ⓒ Ⓓ Ⓔ
62 Ⓐ Ⓑ Ⓒ Ⓓ Ⓔ
63 Ⓐ Ⓑ Ⓒ Ⓓ Ⓔ
64 Ⓐ Ⓑ Ⓒ Ⓓ Ⓔ
65 Ⓐ Ⓑ Ⓒ Ⓓ Ⓔ

66 Ⓐ Ⓑ Ⓒ Ⓓ Ⓔ
67 Ⓐ Ⓑ Ⓒ Ⓓ Ⓔ
68 Ⓐ Ⓑ Ⓒ Ⓓ Ⓔ
69 Ⓐ Ⓑ Ⓒ Ⓓ Ⓔ
70 Ⓐ Ⓑ Ⓒ Ⓓ Ⓔ

71 Ⓐ Ⓑ Ⓒ Ⓓ Ⓔ
72 Ⓐ Ⓑ Ⓒ Ⓓ Ⓔ
73 Ⓐ Ⓑ Ⓒ Ⓓ Ⓔ
74 Ⓐ Ⓑ Ⓒ Ⓓ Ⓔ
75 Ⓐ Ⓑ Ⓒ Ⓓ Ⓔ

76 Ⓐ Ⓑ Ⓒ Ⓓ Ⓔ
77 Ⓐ Ⓑ Ⓒ Ⓓ Ⓔ
78 Ⓐ Ⓑ Ⓒ Ⓓ Ⓔ
79 Ⓐ Ⓑ Ⓒ Ⓓ Ⓔ
80 Ⓐ Ⓑ Ⓒ Ⓓ Ⓔ

81 Ⓐ Ⓑ Ⓒ Ⓓ Ⓔ
82 Ⓐ Ⓑ Ⓒ Ⓓ Ⓔ
83 Ⓐ Ⓑ Ⓒ Ⓓ Ⓔ
84 Ⓐ Ⓑ Ⓒ Ⓓ Ⓔ
85 Ⓐ Ⓑ Ⓒ Ⓓ Ⓔ

86 Ⓐ Ⓑ Ⓒ Ⓓ Ⓔ
87 Ⓐ Ⓑ Ⓒ Ⓓ Ⓔ
88 Ⓐ Ⓑ Ⓒ Ⓓ Ⓔ
89 Ⓐ Ⓑ Ⓒ Ⓓ Ⓔ
90 Ⓐ Ⓑ Ⓒ Ⓓ Ⓔ

91 Ⓐ Ⓑ Ⓒ Ⓓ Ⓔ
92 Ⓐ Ⓑ Ⓒ Ⓓ Ⓔ
93 Ⓐ Ⓑ Ⓒ Ⓓ Ⓔ
94 Ⓐ Ⓑ Ⓒ Ⓓ Ⓔ
95 Ⓐ Ⓑ Ⓒ Ⓓ Ⓔ

96 Ⓐ Ⓑ Ⓒ Ⓓ Ⓔ
97 Ⓐ Ⓑ Ⓒ Ⓓ Ⓔ
98 Ⓐ Ⓑ Ⓒ Ⓓ Ⓔ
99 Ⓐ Ⓑ Ⓒ Ⓓ Ⓔ
100 Ⓐ Ⓑ Ⓒ Ⓓ Ⓔ

101 Ⓐ Ⓑ Ⓒ Ⓓ Ⓔ
102 Ⓐ Ⓑ Ⓒ Ⓓ Ⓔ
103 Ⓐ Ⓑ Ⓒ Ⓓ Ⓔ
104 Ⓐ Ⓑ Ⓒ Ⓓ Ⓔ
105 Ⓐ Ⓑ Ⓒ Ⓓ Ⓔ

106 Ⓐ Ⓑ Ⓒ Ⓓ Ⓔ
107 Ⓐ Ⓑ Ⓒ Ⓓ Ⓔ
108 Ⓐ Ⓑ Ⓒ Ⓓ Ⓔ
109 Ⓐ Ⓑ Ⓒ Ⓓ Ⓔ
110 Ⓐ Ⓑ Ⓒ Ⓓ Ⓔ

111 Ⓐ Ⓑ Ⓒ Ⓓ Ⓔ
112 Ⓐ Ⓑ Ⓒ Ⓓ Ⓔ
113 Ⓐ Ⓑ Ⓒ Ⓓ Ⓔ
114 Ⓐ Ⓑ Ⓒ Ⓓ Ⓔ
115 Ⓐ Ⓑ Ⓒ Ⓓ Ⓔ

116 Ⓐ Ⓑ Ⓒ Ⓓ Ⓔ
117 Ⓐ Ⓑ Ⓒ Ⓓ Ⓔ
118 Ⓐ Ⓑ Ⓒ Ⓓ Ⓔ
119 Ⓐ Ⓑ Ⓒ Ⓓ Ⓔ
120 Ⓐ Ⓑ Ⓒ Ⓓ Ⓔ

121 Ⓐ Ⓑ Ⓒ Ⓓ Ⓔ
122 Ⓐ Ⓑ Ⓒ Ⓓ Ⓔ
123 Ⓐ Ⓑ Ⓒ Ⓓ Ⓔ
124 Ⓐ Ⓑ Ⓒ Ⓓ Ⓔ
125 Ⓐ Ⓑ Ⓒ Ⓓ Ⓔ

126 Ⓐ Ⓑ Ⓒ Ⓓ Ⓔ
127 Ⓐ Ⓑ Ⓒ Ⓓ Ⓔ
128 Ⓐ Ⓑ Ⓒ Ⓓ Ⓔ
129 Ⓐ Ⓑ Ⓒ Ⓓ Ⓔ
130 Ⓐ Ⓑ Ⓒ Ⓓ Ⓔ

131 Ⓐ Ⓑ Ⓒ Ⓓ Ⓔ
132 Ⓐ Ⓑ Ⓒ Ⓓ Ⓔ
133 Ⓐ Ⓑ Ⓒ Ⓓ Ⓔ
134 Ⓐ Ⓑ Ⓒ Ⓓ Ⓔ
135 Ⓐ Ⓑ Ⓒ Ⓓ Ⓔ

136 Ⓐ Ⓑ Ⓒ Ⓓ Ⓔ
137 Ⓐ Ⓑ Ⓒ Ⓓ Ⓔ
138 Ⓐ Ⓑ Ⓒ Ⓓ Ⓔ
139 Ⓐ Ⓑ Ⓒ Ⓓ Ⓔ
140 Ⓐ Ⓑ Ⓒ Ⓓ Ⓔ

141 Ⓐ Ⓑ Ⓒ Ⓓ Ⓔ
142 Ⓐ Ⓑ Ⓒ Ⓓ Ⓔ
143 Ⓐ Ⓑ Ⓒ Ⓓ Ⓔ
144 Ⓐ Ⓑ Ⓒ Ⓓ Ⓔ
145 Ⓐ Ⓑ Ⓒ Ⓓ Ⓔ

146 Ⓐ Ⓑ Ⓒ Ⓓ Ⓔ
147 Ⓐ Ⓑ Ⓒ Ⓓ Ⓔ
148 Ⓐ Ⓑ Ⓒ Ⓓ Ⓔ
149 Ⓐ Ⓑ Ⓒ Ⓓ Ⓔ
150 Ⓐ Ⓑ Ⓒ Ⓓ Ⓔ

151 Ⓐ Ⓑ Ⓒ Ⓓ Ⓔ
152 Ⓐ Ⓑ Ⓒ Ⓓ Ⓔ
153 Ⓐ Ⓑ Ⓒ Ⓓ Ⓔ
154 Ⓐ Ⓑ Ⓒ Ⓓ Ⓔ
155 Ⓐ Ⓑ Ⓒ Ⓓ Ⓔ

156 Ⓐ Ⓑ Ⓒ Ⓓ Ⓔ
157 Ⓐ Ⓑ Ⓒ Ⓓ Ⓔ
158 Ⓐ Ⓑ Ⓒ Ⓓ Ⓔ
159 Ⓐ Ⓑ Ⓒ Ⓓ Ⓔ
160 Ⓐ Ⓑ Ⓒ Ⓓ Ⓔ

161 Ⓐ Ⓑ Ⓒ Ⓓ Ⓔ
162 Ⓐ Ⓑ Ⓒ Ⓓ Ⓔ
163 Ⓐ Ⓑ Ⓒ Ⓓ Ⓔ
164 Ⓐ Ⓑ Ⓒ Ⓓ Ⓔ
165 Ⓐ Ⓑ Ⓒ Ⓓ Ⓔ

166 Ⓐ Ⓑ Ⓒ Ⓓ Ⓔ
167 Ⓐ Ⓑ Ⓒ Ⓓ Ⓔ
168 Ⓐ Ⓑ Ⓒ Ⓓ Ⓔ
169 Ⓐ Ⓑ Ⓒ Ⓓ Ⓔ
170 Ⓐ Ⓑ Ⓒ Ⓓ Ⓔ

171 Ⓐ Ⓑ Ⓒ Ⓓ Ⓔ
172 Ⓐ Ⓑ Ⓒ Ⓓ Ⓔ
173 Ⓐ Ⓑ Ⓒ Ⓓ Ⓔ
174 Ⓐ Ⓑ Ⓒ Ⓓ Ⓔ
175 Ⓐ Ⓑ Ⓒ Ⓓ Ⓔ

176 Ⓐ Ⓑ Ⓒ Ⓓ Ⓔ
177 Ⓐ Ⓑ Ⓒ Ⓓ Ⓔ
178 Ⓐ Ⓑ Ⓒ Ⓓ Ⓔ
179 Ⓐ Ⓑ Ⓒ Ⓓ Ⓔ
180 Ⓐ Ⓑ Ⓒ Ⓓ Ⓔ

MK7010